CHRONIC FATIGUE SYNDROME

A Treatment Guide

CHRONIC FATIGUE SYNDROME

SYNDROME

A Treatment Guide

ERICA F. VERRILLO

LAUREN M. GELLMAN

St. Martin's Griffin ✖ New York

We dedicate this book . . .

to the millions of people
around the world who have suffered
the ravages of CFIDS in silence

to those who have raised their voices
for those who couldn't

to those who have labored to find
the cause and the cure

and to those who have
held our hands

Preface

Throughout this book we have examined the practical problems surrounding chronic fatigue and immune dysfunction syndrome (CFIDS). Rather than delve into debates concerning theoretical and political issues, we have focused on the clinical aspects of CFIDS. We have taken great pains to present material in an objective, unbiased fashion regardless of our personal preferences.

Compiling information about an illness as complex as CFIDS can be daunting. Despite the difficulties surrounding such a project, the task has been more than worthwhile. In assembling a book that attempts to answer primary treatment questions, we have not only responded to a basic need in the CFIDS community, but have satisfied our own quest for knowledge as well. It is this knowledge, combined with the firm belief that experience is the best teacher, that has enabled us to overcome some of the limitations of the illness we both have. For us this book not only represents the sum total of over 15 years of knowledge and experience, it is the book we wish we could have had when we first became ill.

We gratefully acknowledge the input of Dr. Charles Lapp, Dr. David Bell, and Dr. Thomas Steinbach who reviewed this book for medical accuracy. Finally, any errors remaining are our own.

Erica F. Verrillo
Lauren M. Gellman
October 1997

Contents

I
AN OVERVIEW

II
THE MULTIFACETED SYMPTOMS OF CFIDS

III
TREATMENT OPTIONS

IV
COPING AND MANAGEMENT STRATEGIES

APPENDICES

A Note to Our Readers . . .

Throughout this book we have used the name chronic fatigue and immune dysfunction syndrome (CFIDS) to refer to the illness known to the lay public as chronic fatigue syndrome (CFS). We have chosen CFIDS because it is the name currently endorsed by the National CFIDS Association and is accepted by most informed clinicians and researchers in this country. However, despite the addition of "immune dysfunction," CFIDS does not adequately describe this illness any more than CFS does. The inclusion of the word "fatigue" as part of the name of an illness has led to misconceptions and sometimes dismissal of what should be regarded as a serious and debilitating illness. No other medical condition is named after a single symptom, much less a symptom associated with a number of other illnesses. (Fatigue is characteristic of Parkinson's disease, cancer, multiple sclerosis, and numerous other chronic conditions.) CFIDS should not set a precedent.

A number of suggestions have been offered as alternatives, including ME (myalgic encephalomyelitis, the name currently used in the United Kingdom and Canada), low natural killer cell syndrome (LINKS, as it is known in Japan), post-viral syndrome, Nightingale's disease, and chronic immune dysfunction syndrome (CIDS). Dr. Katrina Berne, author of *Running on Empty,* has compiled a list of 40 names from those of a more descriptive nature, such as autonomic nervous system dysfunction syndrome, to names that honor pioneering clinicians, such as Cheney-Peterson disease or Ramsay's disease.

There is currently widespread interest in changing the name of this illness to one that is less misleading. We encourage our readers to make their voices heard on this issue so that this illness can receive the appropriate recognition and attention that it deserves.

Introduction:
The Treatment Dilemma

Healing is a matter of time,
but it is also sometimes a matter of opportunity.
— HIPPOCRATES —

CFIDS is one of those diseases for which receiving a diagnosis can bring as much frustration as relief. All too often a person who has spent years searching for a diagnosis expects that identification of the illness will bring with it, if not a cure, at the very least an effective treatment plan. Unfortunately, most of us who have had the illness identified for us have also been told that CFIDS has "no known cause or cure," a phrase that invariably creates enough hopelessness to offset any relief the diagnosis may have offered.

The lack of known cause or cure, while discouraging, certainly does not imply that an illness cannot be treated, or that those who suffer from it will not recover. Throughout the ages, physicians have successfully treated diseases on the basis of their knowledge of symptoms and human physiologic responses rather than on test results. And because human physiology has not changed much over the past 40,000 years, for the most part remedies have remained remarkably consistent. For example, the Chinese medical system, which relies heavily on nutrition and the use of herbs, was codified more than 5000 years ago. Herbal remedies, pharmaceutical derivatives, massage and manual manipulation techniques, nutritional therapy, and stress reduction methods (meditation, yoga) are treatments that have withstood the test of time, and still form the mainstay of medical systems throughout the world.

The premise of this book is that the absence of a cure does not in any way imply that there is no treatment for CFIDS. To make the grounds for

1

this position clear, consider the popular concept that an illness "attacks." Cure, in this conceptual framework, consists of killing the attacker. In CFIDS, the attacker is unknown, unidentified, and perhaps not even a single factor; thus counterattack is impossible. The victim is left with only two choices: lie back and let nature take its course (which in CFIDS can be agonizing) or look for alternative points of view. The alternative we suggest is to view CFIDS as a form of systemic *damage* that must be gradually, methodically, and thoughtfully repaired. Or, to use an analogy, if CFIDS is like falling into a hole, as some patients have observed, recovery is like climbing out of the hole, step by step, rung by rung.

The purpose of treatment is to provide rungs. Each treatment that relieves a symptom can serve to haul a person with CFIDS one step farther out of the hole. And with every treatment that successfully accomplishes its purpose, the body becomes stronger and more footholds are available. People who have had CFIDS for a long time are well aware that this approach can lead to significant improvement, enough so that return to work or recommencement of a social life is possible. For example, statements like "With B_{12} shots and Kutapressin I had enough stamina to go on vacation with my family" are heard frequently enough to warrant attention. If each person measures a treatment by what it can restore to his or her life, that standard provides a basis and framework for recovery.

With that image in mind, we have compiled a list of treatments, therapies, and techniques that have been successfully used by people with CFIDS. None of these treatments is guaranteed. That is to say, what works wonders for one person may not work for another. Nor are they cures. None has been claimed to completely eradicate the disease. But some may relieve the worst symptoms or decrease the severity of the illness. For people who are unable to leave their beds, have lost their jobs, or would like to resume at least the semblance of a normal life, a 10%, 20%, or 30% improvement is not to be dismissed. The key to determining which of these treatments will be effective is knowledge. Understanding your illness—your symptoms, your responses, your ups and downs—is the greatest favor you can do for yourself and your doctor. Dr. Patricia Salvato, a CFIDS specialist practicing in Houston, Texas, expresses this idea quite well: "Well-informed patients simply make for better partners in healthcare, and, when knowledge is shared, everybody benefits; there is an unbelievable amount of healing in just the sharing of new knowledge" (*Mass CFIDS Update,* Summer 1996).

This book is divided into four main parts. Part I is an overview of CFIDS to help orient the reader. CFIDS, along with some of its most notable characteristics, is presented as it feels to the patient. Possible causes of

CFIDS are presented in brief (without entering into polemics), followed by diagnosis, tests, and finally prognosis.

Part II deals exclusively with symptoms. This is a guide to understanding the body's reaction to CFIDS and is a key resource for devising appropriate treatment plans. Each entry describes a CFIDS symptom from the perspective of the patient. Following the description is an explanation (or as close as we can get; many explanations are only tentative) of why the symptom occurs in CFIDS. At the end of each symptom are treatment tips, recommendations for further reading, and resources for additional information. The reading recommendations are nearly all patient-oriented, nontechnical books, rather than medical articles. For those interested in research, a bibliography is provided at the end of this book. The "see" section at the end of each symptom provides cross-references to relevant parts of the book.

Part III consists of a treatment dictionary, divided into three chapters: pharmaceuticals and prescription drugs, nutritional supplements and botanicals, and alternative and complementary medical and supportive therapies. The short introduction explains that, although people with CFIDS can, and do, respond quite differently to treatments, there are, nevertheless, certain guidelines each person should be aware of.

Part IV discusses some useful coping techniques and what are commonly referred to as "lifestyle adjustments." Although this discussion comes last, we do not mean to imply that learning to cope with CFIDS is in any way less important than treating the illness. Coping and management strategies can sometimes determine the rate of recovery a person will make so their importance can hardly be overstated. The three areas discussed are stress, the home environment, and diet. Stress is one of the primary obstacles for people with CFIDS and some useful management tips are provided. Toxins in the home, the most important environment for people with disabling illnesses, and how to keep your living area safe will be of special interest to those with multiple chemical sensitivities (MCS), an illness in its own right and certainly a significant problem for a subset of patients with CFIDS. Making generalizations about diet is difficult indeed when patients with CFIDS can have such varied food sensitivities. Nevertheless, the topic is important because diet can make an enormous difference in how a person with CFIDS feels.

The final chapter of this book concerns children with CFIDS. Although children experience the same symptoms as adults with CFIDS, their needs are different. This chapter provides some special tips for parents of children with CFIDS, as well as resources that respond to the specific needs of children.

The information found in this book was gathered from a variety of sources: medical articles, books about CFIDS, newspaper and journal articles, research reviews, personal accounts, interviews, and survey results. Although we relied on published sources for specific information concerning the mechanisms and treatment options available to people with CFIDS, unpublished sources such as letters, telephone conversations, interviews, questionnaires, and Internet discussion groups were invaluable in assessing the effectiveness of specific treatments and therapies. The rich and varied experience of the CFIDS community itself forms the ballast of the book, for this is, above all, a book that reflects our own efforts to find treatment for this baffling disease.

I

AN OVERVIEW

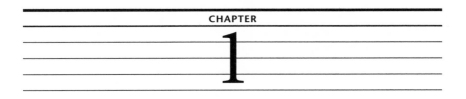

The Many Faces of CFIDS

Four Patients' Stories

Sarah . . . Sarah first became ill in August 1987, when she was 32 years old. At that time she was completing a teacher training program and rearing two young children. The first symptom she noticed was an inability to fall asleep, and stay asleep, at night. She also had severe headaches, which she attributed to the aftermath of the flu. She did not become alarmed, however, until she tried to pick up her infant son and her legs gave way. As a former swimmer, she was highly attuned to her body and realized that the loss of strength in her legs was unusual. She started experiencing pain and stiffness in her joints as well. She was surprised that exercise made her feel much worse, exacerbating the insomnia and pain. Hardest of all for a student, she was finding it difficult to concentrate and to retain information. As she told her doctor, she felt like her "batteries had run out." She was falling asleep at 4 o'clock in the afternoon, although she had had energy to spare just a few weeks earlier. Her doctor chalked up her symptoms to stress and suggested that she "take it easy." Sarah's problems did not resolve with rest, however. When she appeared a few weeks later with a sore throat, low-grade fever, and swollen glands, the doctor suspected a virus. Blood tests revealed a low white blood cell count, indicative of a viral infection. By the end of the semester she was so exhausted she decided to take a leave of absence. She felt much better, but her symptoms persisted. Her doctor ordered endocrine system tests and recommended that she see both a neurologist and a gastroenterologist. None of their tests revealed any abnormalities. At that point her doctor thought she might have CFIDS and recommended she "stay home and rest." After a year and a half, Sarah returned to school, still feeling "run down," but able to function if she took naps and did not overexert herself.

Samantha... Samantha's history goes back to 1964, when she contracted a severe case of mononucleosis as a freshman in college. Her recovery was so slow she did not feel like she ever got over the illness. In the following years she periodically felt extremely tired and "just not able to get up and get going." By the early 1970s she exhibited obvious allergies for the first time to pollens, molds, and animal dander. She also began to have some mild muscle and joint pain. By the mid-1970s she began to have chronic gastrointestinal problems. "It seemed that one day I could eat anything I wanted; the next day was just a disaster. Whenever I ate, it hurt. When I didn't eat, it hurt. I experienced severe weight loss." She was sent to one gastroenterologist after another. They diagnosed irritable bowel syndrome.

Samantha continued to work but was hospitalized from time to time. She tried a number of treatments but nothing seemed to help. "I had severe reactions to the drugs they were giving me. I began to shake; sometimes I could not write out a check. Every time I went to the doctor with a physical complaint, whether it was my doctor or a specialist, I was referred to a psychologist. I felt like no one was listening to me, no one was treating my physical problems, and I might as well give up."

By the end of 1992 Samantha could barely make it to work, much less stay the entire day. "I would sit down at my desk, take one look at a page of work, start to try and work on it, and become so exhausted that I would go into another office, which had carpeting on the floor, and sleep. When I woke up I would be so exhausted I could barely summon enough energy to drive home. I was way behind on my paperwork. By the last month of that year I could barely attend meetings. That summer I rested, but the symptoms did not improve." At this point, Samantha was desperate to discover what was wrong with her.

The first real clue came through a newspaper article about the local CFIDS support group. Upon reading the case histories of two of the people in the group, she felt she was reading her own story. Through the group, she learned there was a national organization and that there were experts. She chose to go to a renowned specialist, who diagnosed a classic case of CFIDS. For Samantha, a woman who had been ill with an unnamed illness for most of her life, the diagnosis was an indescribable relief. "He gave me a diagnosis and validated the illness for me, as well as suggesting treatments that to this day I continue. Most important over time has been the feeling of having been given back the sense of who I am. He gave me back my belief in myself, restored my confidence, and left me with the feeling that this incredible saga of the past 20 years had not been in vain. Now I know that throughout all those things that have happened—throughout all the years of confusion, frustration, and pain—the core of who I am has always been there."

In the 3 years since her diagnosis, Samantha has improved but not recovered. She can drive, take care of herself, and is supervising the building of a new house—a vast improvement over the days when she could not even leave her bed or comb her hair.

Jeanette ... Jeanette, a 65-year-old woman with four grown children and eight grandchildren, had always been healthy. In 1992 she took a trip to mainland China, after which several people became sick with a respiratory illness. Shortly after she returned home, she had her carpets cleaned. The next day she had a slight headache, which progressed to a severe flu-like illness with headache, chills, drenching sweats, and high-grade fever. Because she seemed to have no respiratory involvement, her doctor believed it was not the flu. He treated her for malaria, although she did not test positive for it. Then he treated her for Lyme disease, also in the absence of positive test results. Finally, she was sent to a well-known clinic for diagnosis. That team of doctors decided that she had an unknown viral illness and told her it would gradually improve over time. She was bedridden for several months, during which time she experienced significant deterioration. Finally, she was referred to a clinic in New Jersey that specialized in the treatment of chronic fatigue syndrome. The physician at the clinic prescribed various medicines, most of which made her feel worse. She tried vitamins, minerals, enzymes, nutritious foods. The only help she found was a transient boost from Ritalin (methylphenidate), which enabled her to get up for 2 hours in the morning and an hour later in the day. Most things made her feel sicker and more tired. Eventually, Ritalin seemed to stop helping too.

Of the symptoms she now has, Jeanette describes the most debilitating as the need to lie down "at least 22 hours a day. I even have to lie down to eat because it takes all my energy to stand up for the 5 or 10 minutes it takes to prepare my meal. In the mornings I can be up for an hour—if I'm careful. Of course, if I overdo, I pay for it for several days or perhaps weeks."

Nick ... Nick, a 29-year-old landscaper with his own business, first became seriously ill in 1992 after contracting the flu. After several months, he felt a little better and resumed working part time. However, he never felt completely recovered. About a year later, he was diagnosed with CFIDS. Over the course of the following year, he tried many different therapies and treatments, both conventional and alternative, and saw significant improvement. In 1995, 3 years after having contracted the illness, he visited a nationally known CFIDS specialist and was told he was "in recovery." This was welcome news for Nick. He continued weight lifting to recover his strength and followed a low sugar, high protein diet, which seemed to make a difference. Currently, Nick is troubled by cognitive problems, joint pain, and fatigue. While he has made significant improvement since his early years with CFIDS, he is not recovering at the rate he would like and is quite discouraged by the periodic setbacks.

At first glance these four people have very different stories to tell. A young man never recovers from a bout with the flu. A 30-year-old woman feels dragged out for years with an unknown virus but is able to function. A teenager becomes ill with "mono" in the early 1960s and not only never recovers completely but feels progressively worse over the next 30 years. A grandmother becomes so ill after a trip abroad that suddenly her life comes to a halt.

The above accounts, although dissimilar in many respects, are familiar to CFIDS specialists around the globe—a flu-like ailment that doesn't resolve and, in fact, seems to produce myriad other debilitating symptoms; a series of misdiagnoses from skeptical doctors; a period of confinement to bed or home, which in Jeanette's case has lasted for years; and medications that only seem to make matters worse.

CFIDS is, without doubt, one of the most complex, multifaceted, baffling illnesses the medical world has encountered. It has thus far defied anyone to identify its cause, find a cure, or even formulate a good case definition. It is hard to describe and even harder to diagnose because its symptoms can range from allergies to vertigo and can occur in every imaginable combination. Most confusing, however, is the range in severity of CFIDS, from mere inconvenience to an utterly disabling disease. People with severe CFIDS, like Jeanette, can be completely bedridden, unable to perform basic tasks without assistance, whereas those with milder illness, like Sarah, may be able to work full time but feel nagged by a persistent feeling that their energy has waned, or their "get-up-and-go" just got up and went.

The enormous variation in severity and symptoms of CFIDS, combined with a paucity of information regarding the transmissibility, extent, and nature of the illness, has helped contribute to the many misconceptions about CFIDS. These misconceptions, half-truths, and outright errors have not only led to a certain complacency on the part of the medical establishment but have made it difficult for people who have the illness to recognize it in themselves, much less seek out appropriate treatments. Despite their lack of knowledge, however, it is possible, just on the basis of the clinical experience of the many doctors who have observed and treated patients with CFIDS, to make some generalizations about the salient characteristics of the illness. An understanding of these often eases the task of identifying possible CFIDS in patients with various "nonspecific" symptoms.

Distinctive Features

One of the most notable characteristics of CFIDS is that it often arises suddenly. Many, if not most, patients with CFIDS can give the precise date they first started experiencing symptoms. Often these patients describe the onset as "flu-like," with many symptoms typical of a viral infection. The sudden onset of the illness is what allows a good diagnostician to distinguish CFIDS from many of the ailments and conditions CFIDS can resemble, such as allergies, endocrine abnormalities, multiple sclerosis, and mood disorders, none of which develops from one moment to the next.

To complicate matters for the diagnostician, and for the patient seeking a diagnosis, CFIDS does not always come on suddenly after a flu-like illness. It can also develop with deceptive slowness, its symptoms emerging one by one until the patient's life is irrevocably changed. In these cases it may be difficult for the person experiencing the symptoms to recognize that anything is amiss until months or even years have passed, especially if that person maintains a busy, active life. In these cases there is a strong tendency to attribute the growing signs of illness to stress, overwork, or aging. Samantha, a former licensed professional counselor and school psychologist, presents a good example of how CFIDS can manifest itself slowly and insidiously. It is now thought that close to half of CFIDS cases can develop in just this manner. Needless to say, these are the hardest for a doctor to diagnose. The patient may go from doctor to doctor for years before a tentative diagnosis is reached.

Another important characteristic is that CFIDS symptoms generally wax and wane. This may help distinguish CFIDS from many of the other diseases and conditions that may share similar symptoms with CFIDS. Typically, someone who contracts CFIDS suddenly will experience a period of pronounced illness for several months, followed by shorter periods of remission and relapse. Most patients with CFIDS refer to these as "good days" and "bad days." (People who are not ill must remember that a "good day" for someone with severe CFIDS may consist simply of getting out of bed.) Periods of remission and relapse can be entirely random, following no particular pattern, or can be cyclic, occurring at certain times of the year (fall and spring for many people) or, in women, may be influenced by hormonal cycles. Sometimes relapses can be attributed to a known cause, such as exertion, exposure to a toxin, or physical injury.

A final, but important, point concerning prevalence is that CFIDS is not restricted to any particular group. It can strike anyone at any time. It affects people of all ages, as we can see from Jeanette, who was 60 years old

CFIDS SIGNS AND SYMPTOMS CHECKLIST
(in order of frequency)

[ ] Severe, debilitating and disabling fatigue, usually made worse by physical exercise

[ ] Recurrent flu-like illness, often with chronic sore throat

[ ] Low-grade fever and feeling hot often, low body temperature

[ ] Random muscle and joint aches with "trigger points"

[ ] Nervous system problems
   [ ] Sleep disturbance
   [ ] Severe headache
   [ ] Changes in vision
   [ ] Seizures
   [ ] Numb or tingling sensations
   [ ] Loss of balance, dizziness
   [ ] Feeling "spaced out" or "cloudy"
   [ ] Frequent, unusual nightmares
   [ ] Depression
   [ ] Anxiety, panic attacks
   [ ] Personality changes (usually intensification of a previous tendency)
   [ ] Mood swings
   [ ] Difficulty moving the tongue to speak
   [ ] Tinnitus (ringing in the ears)
   [ ] Paralysis
   [ ] Severe muscle weakness
   [ ] Blackouts
   [ ] Photophobia (light sensitivity)
   [ ] Alcohol intolerance
   [ ] Changes in taste, smell, hearing
   [ ] Decreased libido
   [ ] Muscle twitches

[ ] Cognitive function problems
   [ ] Attention deficit disorder (inability to concentrate)
   [ ] Calculation difficulties
   [ ] Memory loss
   [ ] Spatial disorientation
   [ ] Word searching or saying the wrong word

CFIDS SIGNS AND SYMPTOMS CHECKLIST—cont'd
(in order of frequency)

[ ] Severe premenstrual syndrome (PMS) or exacerbation of symptoms before and during period

[ ] Weight changes, usually loss followed by gain

[ ] Painful, swollen lymph nodes (lymphadenopathy), especially on the neck and underarms

[ ] Abdominal pain, diarrhea, nausea, gas, irritable bowel

[ ] Thyroid pain or dysfunction

[ ] Severe new allergic reactions to medicines, food, and other substances

[ ] Night sweats

[ ] Heart palpitations

[ ] Uncomfortable or frequent urination

[ ] Rash of herpes simplex or shingles

[ ] Other signs and symptoms
    [ ] Rash
    [ ] Hair loss
    [ ] Chest pain
    [ ] Dry eyes and mouth
    [ ] Impotence
    [ ] Cough
    [ ] Temporomandibular joint (TMJ) dysfunction
    [ ] Mitral valve prolapse
    [ ] Canker sores
    [ ] Cold hands and feet
    [ ] Carpal tunnel syndrome
    [ ] Pyriform muscle syndrome causing sciatica
    [ ] Gum disease
    [ ] Endometriosis
    [ ] Shortness of breath
    [ ] Temperature and weather sensitivity

when she contracted CFIDS, and Maya, who was only 7 years old (see Chapter 10). CFIDS also affects men, though perhaps not in such high numbers as women (women are affected by all autoimmune diseases in higher proportions than men). Neither does CFIDS confine itself to a particular income group. Patients with CFIDS range from wealthy celebrities to school custodians, from doctors to construction workers. Contrary to the media myth that CFIDS primarily attacks white, middle-class women, CFIDS does not discriminate by race or ethnic origin. Results of a recent demographic survey conducted in San Francisco indicated a significant rate of CFIDS among African-American and Native American populations. The study also reported that the average yearly income of patients with CFIDS is about $15,000. Although CFIDS usually strikes sporadically, affecting only one member of a family or work group, it can also occur in epidemics. Since the 1930s more than 60 CFIDS epidemics have been recorded. At no time during these epidemics was there any indication that CFIDS was a particularly selective disease.

Historical Background

One of the most perplexing questions surrounding CFIDS is how it began. Like other questions about CFIDS, the answer remains elusive. Debate is ongoing among researchers as to whether CFIDS is a recent phenomenon or a disease with some history. Some argue that CFIDS has been around for several hundred years; others present compelling evidence that CFIDS is a relatively new disease, arising in the last few decades at best. Those who maintain that it has been with us for centuries point to accounts of other diseases with similar symptoms, such as muscular rheumatism in the 1680s or neurasthenia, first described in the late nineteenth century. Proponents of this position maintain that CFIDS, as it is currently described, is merely a new name for an old illness. In direct opposition to this viewpoint, many others believe that this is a true twentieth century disease, a product of the "cocktail effect" of an environment polluted by neurotoxins, new or mutated viruses, contaminated vaccines, and other factors.

The question of where the illness originated is as elusive as when. Outbreaks of CFIDS-like diseases were reported in Northern Europe and the United States as early as the 1930s. The first documented epidemic outbreak of CFIDS, or myalgic encephalomyelitis (ME), as the illness is known in Great Britain and Canada, occurred in 1934 in Los Angeles County Hospital and affected 198 health care workers, mainly doctors, nurses, and technicians. Because this outbreak followed on the heels of a poliomyelitis epidemic, in the first few weeks it was diagnosed as polio. However, this early diagnosis was revised when doctors noticed that, unlike polio, this new ailment did not cause paralysis or death. It also produced myriad symptoms: headache, easy fatigability (especially after exertion), loss of appetite, intestinal disturbances, sweating, chills, stiffness in the back and neck, weakness, pain, insomnia, impaired memory, mood swings, and hair loss. The disease tended to strike suddenly, with an incubation period of less than a week, although insidious onset over a few weeks was also observed, producing a set of symptoms that remained intense and variable over the first 6 months, then becoming chronic and relatively stable. Dr. Alexander Gilliam, the epidemiologist who chronicled the outbreak, remarked, "If the disease were not poliomyelitis, the epidemic is equally extraordinary in presenting a clinical and epidemiological picture, which, so far, is without parallel."

A second major outbreak occurred in Iceland in 1948 and 1949. Like the Los Angeles County Hospital outbreak, this epidemic also followed on the heels of a polio epidemic. An important difference was that the epidemic was not restricted to health care professionals but spread to the general population. The majority of the more than 1000 persons affected by "Iceland disease," as it came to be called, lived in three rural towns. Investigators were at first perplexed by this new disease, thinking it to be a form of polio. However, the symptom pattern did not match their expectations of polio. In all cases, those who came down with Iceland disease had muscle pain and tenderness, numbness, and twitching, but not paralysis. Doctors also noted an unusual and troublesome persistence of cognitive and emotional problems in the recovery phases.

A series of outbreaks occurred in the 1950s. One of the better documented was the 1955 outbreak in London at the Royal Free nurse's training hospital. Like other outbreaks, the attack rate was unusually high: 2.8% in men and 10.4% in women. Epidemic outbreaks also occurred in Adelaide, South Australia, from 1949 to 1951; in Kingston, New York, in 1951; in Coventry, England, and Denmark in 1953; and in Pittsfield, Massachusetts, and Punta Gorda, Florida, in 1956.

Very little is known about the incidence of CFIDS in non-European countries (with the exception of Japan where the illness is known as low natural killer cell syndrome, or LINKS). However, what is clear from a historical review is that, over time, the incidence of epidemic outbreaks has been matched, if not superseded, by increasing numbers of sporadic cases. Most people contract CFIDS individually, and it is to these people that current research efforts as to the nature, extent, and clinical outcome of the illness should be directed.

Contemporary Developments

One of the most significant outbreaks in recent CFIDS history occurred in Incline Village, Nevada, in late 1984. This outbreak propelled the illness into the public arena. Incline Village is a small resort town located on picturesque Lake Tahoe. In the fall of 1984, two local physicians, Dr. Daniel Peterson and Dr. Paul Cheney, began to see patients who seemed to have an unusually severe and debilitating flu. What was particularly puzzling to the doctors was that these patients did not recover. Months after the initial onset of the illness, patients still reported severe symptoms and, in many cases, there was no detectable improvement. As time went on, the doctors saw increasing numbers of patients with the same malady. Sometimes these patients were seen in clusters. In one instance, the members of a girl's basketball team became ill; in another, it was schoolteachers in the nearby town of Truckee, Nevada. By mid-1985 the number of patients with this mysterious malady topped 100.

The doctors were stymied by the illness. They had not previously encountered a disease process that reduced active, energetic individuals to bedbound invalids, with no identifiable cause. The symptoms they observed were unusual in both severity and range: exhaustion, pain, sleep disturbance, cognitive disorder, and a plethora of nervous system problems. Convinced that this was an outbreak of a new disease, the doctors contacted the Centers for Disease Control and Prevention (CDC), the government agency responsible for monitoring and controlling contagious diseases in the United States. Unfortunately, the CDC shed little light on the ailment and, in fact, ultimately presented a considerable obstacle for patients, subsequent researchers, and clinicians. Thereafter, in large part because of the CDC's casual treatment of the outbreak in Nevada, the illness became known as a figment of the overachieving young professional's imagination—the "yuppie flu," as dubbed by the press.

The dismissive attitude that characterized the government's response to the outbreak did little to help control the spread of the illness. Through the 1980s the number of patients with severe, unrelenting flu-like symptoms increased, prompting doctors to take notice. Dr. Carol Jessop in San Francisco noted that starting in the early 1980s patients began reporting a viral-like ailment that did not resolve over time. A Harvard University physician, Dr. Anthony Komaroff, first noticed patients with similar clinical symptoms in the late 1970s, but became even more attentive to the illness when he saw increasing numbers in his Boston practice in the early part of the next decade. During this time, Dr. Richard DuBois in Atlanta, Dr. James Jones in Denver, Dr. Irena Brus (now deceased) in New York, and Dr. Herbert Tanner in Beverly Hills all observed an increase in patients with this unique clinical picture. For these physicians the illness was indeed striking, and they puzzled individually about what was making their formerly healthy patients so ill that they were forced to leave jobs and schools and abandon so many of the activities previously important to them.

In 1985 another epidemic was reported, this time in a small rural community in upstate New York. Dr. David Bell, a pediatrician working in Lyndonville, began seeing patients with recurring flu-like symptoms, abdominal pain, dizziness, fatigue, headache, joint pain, and cognitive deficit in 1983. By 1987 more than 200 people, 44 of whom were children, had contracted the illness. Like Dr. Cheney and Dr. Peterson, Dr. Bell's attempts to draw attention to the outbreak met with little success. However, he continued in his search for an explanation and eventually joined with Dr. Peterson and Dr. Cheney to research the cause of this malady.

The persistence of a few doctors who refused to dismiss the suffering of their patients, combined with press coverage, however superficial, aroused public and professional interest in the illness. Medical journals such as the *Annals of Internal Medicine* began to publish articles that described a long-term flu-like disease with notable neurologic and immunologic components. At first the illness was attributed to the Epstein-Barr virus (EBV), which causes mononucleosis, because of the high titers of EBV antibodies in this group. At the time, EBV seemed to be a perfect candidate for a causative factor because many of the symptoms the patients had were similar to those of "mono." However, this theory was soon dismissed when it was shown that EBV antibody concentrations did not correspond to the severity of the illness, nor were high titers unique to patients with the illness. Over time, it was found that people with the mysterious ailment had high antibody titers to a number of viruses in the herpesvirus family: cytomegalovirus, coxsackievirus, and human herpesvirus 6. Nevertheless, the theory that EBV caused the new illness caught on, and the disease became popularized as "chronic Epstein-Barr" or just "Epstein-Barr."

In the late 1980s publicity about the illness began to gain momentum. Hillary Johnson, a journalist who contracted the illness, wrote an award-winning series for *Rolling Stone* magazine called "Journey Into Fear: The Growing Nightmare of Epstein-Barr Virus." The story attracted national attention. (Johnson later wrote *Osler's Web: Inside the Labyrinth of the Chronic Fatigue Syndrome Epidemic,* a compelling exposé of CFIDS history and politics.) In 1990 *Newsweek* ran a cover story on the illness, which was the bestselling issue of the year. Stories were aired on popular television programs such as "20/20." As a result, the CDC was flooded with calls from patients from all parts of the country who were desperately seeking information and advice. It seemed thousands more people had the illness than the agency had ever imagined.

From that point on, interest surged. Prodded into action by persistent patients and diligent doctors, in 1988 the CDC devised a case definition and gave the illness a name, chronic fatigue syndrome (CFS). Though many clinicians and patients considered the guidelines woefully inadequate and the name derisive, it did give physicians a uniform description and a place to begin in making a diagnosis. Patient groups also were formed. The end of the decade saw the birth of the first national organization, the National CFIDS Association, based in Charlotte, North Carolina. With a national organization came advocacy, representation at the national level, fund-raising for research, organized media campaigns, public awareness programs, and patient education. Local support groups sprang up all over the United States, providing information, assistance, and validation for hundreds of thousands of patients. In April 1990 the first international symposium was held in Cambridge, England, drawing clinicians and researchers from all over the world. It was a momentous event, providing doctors, epidemiologists, and medical investigators with the first opportunity to share their observations and knowledge about a disease that had puzzled observers for the better part of the century.

The current status of CFIDS is rapidly evolving. The CDC has recently placed CFIDS on its "Priority One: New and Emerging" list of infectious diseases, a list that also includes Lyme disease, hepatitis C, and malaria. Government research funds have increased 10-fold in 8 years, from a mere $1.2 million in 1988 to $13.5 million in 1996 and, although still far from sufficient, this funding has stimulated investigation into the nature and cause of the disease. Large patient organizations such as the 22,000-member CFIDS Association of America and the ME Associations of Canada and Great Britain have garnered considerable private support for CFIDS research and put pressure on government agencies and organizations. Through the efforts of these organizations, May 12 was declared International CFIDS Awareness Day. After 4 years of patient lobbying and activism, this day was formally recognized on the floor of both the U.S. House and Senate. Also in 1996 it was announced in San Francisco at the national conference of the American Association for Chronic Fatigue Syndrome that research at Temple University may have led to the discovery of a diagnostic test for CFIDS. And on the treatment front, Ampligen, a drug thought to be an important overall treatment for CFIDS, has finally become available in Canada and Europe and has achieved experimental status in the United States.

While the historical questions of how, when, and where CFIDS originated may be debatable, the question of its current status is not. Almost all reputable research institutions and clinicians agree that CFIDS has become a serious public health problem. The CDC estimates that CFIDS has affected around 500,000 individuals in the United States, a conservative estimate in most clinicians' opinion. Independent prevalence studies have estimated double or more this number, with figures reaching into the millions for the United States alone.

Although the definitive cause of CFIDS remains unknown, it is hoped that through the continued involvement of patient groups and increased funding for research some of the questions surrounding the cause of this elusive illness soon will be answered and a cure found.

In Search of a Cause

Although the enigmatic nature of CFIDS has inspired numerous scientific and popular publications, and millions of dollars (most would say not nearly enough) have been spent in research, relatively little is known about the mechanisms of the illness, and nearly nothing of its cause. Debate about each of these aspects of CFIDS has raged for at least a decade, with most specialists falling into one of several camps.

The theory that currently holds sway is that CFIDS is caused by a virus. This point of view is supported by history (CFIDS epidemics have followed polio epidemics), incidence (correlation with a flu-like prodromic illness), symptoms (swollen lymph nodes, low-grade fever, sore throat), and similarities with other viral ailments, notably mononucleosis and post-polio syndrome. A viral cause is also indicated by research. In the mid-1980s, Dr. Cheney and Dr. Peterson, the two clinicians who reported the 1984 outbreak in Incline Village, Nevada, found high titers of EBV in their patients. At the time, they believed the illness was caused by chronic activation of the virus. However, the presence of high titers in most of the healthy population made that theory untenable. Nevertheless, the idea that a virus was at the root of the problem persisted. In 1986 Dr. Michael Holmes, a researcher in New Zealand, found evidence of a retrovirus. This finding was supported by research conducted in 1990 by Dr. Elaine De Freitas of the Wistar Institute in Philadelphia. She found viral fragments in the mitochondria of cells from patients with CFIDS, which seemed to indicate the presence of a retrovirus.

Not all researchers agree that a retrovirus is implicated. Dr. John Richardson, a British physician who has been treating patients with CFIDS for four decades, believes an enterovirus much like that which causes polio may be at the root of the illness. He draws on the remarkable similarity and incidence of polio-related problems and CFIDS. Dr. Peter Behan and his team of researchers in Glasgow, Scotland, have also found indications of a persistent enteroviral infection in about 60% of patients with CFIDS they have tested. Dr. Behan speculates that the virus is a mutated form of poliovirus that attacks the brain rather than the spinal cord, causing a "cascade effect." Other researchers in Great Britain believe coxsackievirus may be the culprit. Stealth viruses and spuma viruses have also been proposed. The disturbing reality is that no conclusive evidence of active viral infection by a single virus has been found, despite all the clues to the contrary. It is as though researchers can find only the tracks of the beast, while the quarry itself evades capture.

Environmental factors have also been implicated as possible causes, particularly in cases with gradual onset. Those who contend that CFIDS is the result of environmental contamination essentially consider CFIDS to result from the body's inability to rid itself of toxins. This is the perspective Dr. Sherri Rogers puts forth in her book, *Tired or Toxic?* Dr. Majid Ali, another physician who believes that CFIDS is caused by toxic overload, writes in his book, *The Canary and Chronic Fatigue,* that "chronic fatigue sufferers are human canaries—unique people who tolerate poorly the biologic stressors of the late 20th century." His point of view is that people with CFIDS are prone to injury from environmental causes, such as pollution, chemical injuries, and unmanaged allergies, much as canaries are to underground gases. In other words, the CFIDS population is a warning to all the rest that the environment is becoming dangerous.

A number of other clinicians and independent researchers have also pointed out that environmental factors may play a key role in how CFIDS develops. Joe Mangano, MPH, puts forth the theory that CFIDS could be a radiation-related disorder (*CFIDS Chronicle,* Winter 1994). He points out that the immunologic abnormalities found in patients with CFIDS (large numbers of cytokines such as interferon alpha and interleukins and reduced number of natural killer cells) could be attributed to constant exposure to low-level ionizing radiation from atmospheric tests conducted since the 1940s (a period that roughly corresponds to the major CFIDS outbreaks in the United States). Mangano proposes that the effect of atmospheric fallout, though not enough of a factor in itself to cause a large-scale health trend such as CFIDS, may operate synergistically with other environmental factors, such as industrial pollution, carcinogens in consumer products, and occupational hazards, to create "health effects."

A third proposed theory is that CFIDS may be genetic. Proponents of this theory maintain that people with CFIDS have a genetic defect that enables them to contract the illness. However, to date no genetic marker has been found and this theory remains in dispute. Of course, no virus has been found either. But in the case of the virus, there are numerous indicators that a viral infection is present. What most undermines the genetic argument is that CFIDS can occur in epidemic form, as it has with some frequency.

While the debate continues and theories proliferate, people continue to be struck down by this curious, undefinable malady. The lack of a known cause can be a stumbling block for doctors. It certainly complicates the process of diagnosis in this day and age of test results. However, as with other illnesses whose cause is not clear, a diagnosis can still be made and appropriate treatments devised.

Diagnosis

Contrary to popular belief, CFIDS is a distinct, recognizable entity that can be diagnosed relatively early in the course of the disease, providing the physician has some experience with the illness. It is by no means a "wastebasket diagnosis." Experience is, in fact, the main stumbling block that prevents many physicians from making the diagnosis. They simply don't recognize it. Physicians who have attended outbreaks of the illness and, as a consequence, have seen hundreds or thousands of patients with CFIDS have little difficulty recognizing the specific markers, indicators, and signs.

A first step in making a diagnosis is to compare the patient's history and symptoms with the CDC case definition. The CDC case definition is not always a useful tool for clinicians. It was developed to define uniform study populations for research purposes. However, if a patient meets the CDC criteria, at least the first step will have been made toward a diagnosis. Unfortunately, a significant proportion of patients with CFIDS do not meet these rather rigid criteria. In these cases, an in-depth examination of the history and symptoms is particularly important. Usually the time required to take the history for a patient with CFIDS will exceed the expected 1-hour initial appointment by an hour or more.

Taking a careful history is essential in making a diagnosis and is much more important than comparing the patient's symptoms with the CDC case definition. The physician should consider type of onset (acute or insidious), triggering mechanisms (exposure to chemicals, viral infection, physical trauma), and any other mitigating factors that might influence the severity or persistence of the illness. In general, symptoms that develop quickly after an initial trigger are indicative of CFIDS.

Most specialists also question their patients carefully about the type of symptoms they are experiencing. CFIDS is a syndrome, which means that multiple symptoms must be present. Many of these symptoms are reflective of an autonomic nervous system disorder; others are indicative of a persistent viral infection. What is important to the doctor is not necessarily that you have all of the symptoms, or even a certain percentage, but that they cover a spectrum. The symptoms most doctors consider particularly significant are relentless, persistent, or disabling fatigue, pain, sleep disorders, and cognitive problems. Other symptoms can occur in an astounding array. Even if the patient does not have all of the symptoms, it is highly unlikely that a diagnosis can be made on the basis of only one or two.

Finally, the physician should order all the necessary tests to rule out illnesses that produce similar symptoms and, in most cases, insurance coverage permitting, look for immune system deficiency and other abnormali-

---

CASE DEFINITION FOR CFIDS*
(Centers for Disease Control and Prevention: December 1994)

Chronic fatigue syndrome is defined by the presence of the following:

1. Clinically evaluated, unexplained, persistent, or relapsing chronic fatigue that is of new or definite onset (has not been lifelong)
   - Is not the result of ongoing exertion
   - Is not substantially alleviated by rest
   - Results in substantial reduction in previous levels of occupational, educational, social, or personal activities

2. Concurrent occurrence of *four or more* of the following symptoms, all of which must have persisted or recurred during 6 or more consecutive months of illness and must have predated the fatigue
   - Self-reported impairment in short-term memory or concentration severe enough to cause substantial reduction in previous levels of occupational, educational, social, or personal activities
   - Sore throat
   - Muscle pain
   - Multijoint pain without joint swelling or redness
   - Headaches of a new type, pattern, or severity
   - Unrefreshing sleep
   - Postexertional malaise lasting more than 24 hours

*For reprints call the Centers for Disease Control and Prevention (404-639-1338).

ties typical in the CFIDS patient population. In most instances, exclusionary tests are not expensive or difficult to perform. Depending on the symptoms, the physician may wish to rule out Lyme disease, lupus, rheumatoid arthritis, or other autoimmune disorders, parasitic infections, heart disease, specific neurologic disorders such as multiple sclerosis, endocrine disorders such as hypothyroidism, and systemic infections and inflammatory conditions (as indicated by a high erythrocyte sedimentation rate). In general, patients with CFIDS test negative for other conditions. However, as many specialists have noted, nothing prevents a person from having two conditions simultaneously or developing one after the other. Thus a positive test result does not necessarily rule out a diagnosis of CFIDS. In fact, weakly positive results are sometimes indicative of the illness. Weakly positive antinuclear antibodies, for example, are not at all uncommon in the CFIDS population.

Immune system tests are more useful to confirm a specific diagnosis of CFIDS. Immune system testing is still in its infancy, so results cannot be reliably interpreted by anyone other than an immunologist or CFIDS specialist. Even among specialists, there is tremendous dissent as to what these test results actually mean. The value of having these tests done is to determine whether the patterns seen in the test results are similar to those of

---

SPECIFIC TESTS THAT HELP CONFIRM DIAGNOSIS OF CFIDS

These tests are expensive and, in most cases, cannot be performed locally. A positive result does not necessarily confirm a diagnosis of CFIDS, but merely supports it. A diagnosis can be made without performing any of these tests, but for the more severely ill, some may be advisable.

- *Viral infection:* Positive for cytomegalovirus, Epstein-Barr virus, human herpesvirus 6, and coxsackievirus; negative for hepatitis A or B virus
- *Immune system:* Low natural killer cell counts, elevated interferon alpha, tumor necrosis factor, interleukins 1 and 2; T cell activation, altered T4/T8 cell ratios, low T cell suppressor cell (T8) count, fluctuating low and high T cell counts, low and high B cell counts, antinuclear antibodies, immunoglobin deficiency, sometimes antithyroid antibodies
- *Exercise testing:* Decreased cortisol levels after exercise, decreased cerebral blood flow after exercise, inefficient glucose utilization, erratic breathing pattern
- *SPECT scans:* Hypoperfusion in either right or left temporal lobe especially after exercise

other people with CFIDS. Many (but not all) people with CFIDS have reduced numbers of natural killer cells, increased numbers of circulating cytokines (such as alpha interferon and the interleukins). Immune cell function also may be measured. Patients with CFIDS generally have diminished T and B cell function. Reaction to pokeweed mitogen, total immunoglobulin production (IgG, IgA, IgM), and demonstrable anergy (lack of immune response) when tested with foreign proteins can help determine the effectiveness of immune cell responsiveness.

Along with immune system tests, most CFIDS specialists look for evidence of viral reactivation. People with CFIDS usually show evidence of reactivation of latent viruses, particularly in the herpesvirus family, such as Epstein-Barr virus, human herpesvirus 6, and cytomegalovirus. Reactivation of latent viruses (as indicated by high titers) provides further proof of immune system dysfunction because in a healthy person these viruses are controlled.

Neurologic examinations are also useful in making a diagnosis. The Romberg test, a simple test that can be performed in the doctor's office, can indicate neurologic impairment. For those who can afford it, a single-photon emission computed tomography (SPECT) scan can reveal areas of the brain with reduced blood flow, also a common finding in people with CFIDS. For patients with severe cognitive impairment, IQ tests and other neurocognitive examinations may be recommended. Not all of these specialized tests are necessary to make a diagnosis, although someone applying for disability insurance may need some of them to file.

Although there is not yet a test that, by itself, confirms a diagnosis of CFIDS, the combination of exclusionary, viral, neurologic, and immune system tests usually suffice for a diagnosis. However, undergoing all these tests can be both expensive and nerve-racking for the patient. A single diagnostic test would considerably lessen the financial and emotional burden of lengthy testing. It is hoped that such a test for CFIDS will be available soon. Dr. Robert Suhadolnik, a professor of biochemistry and member of the Temple University Fels Institute for Cancer Research and Molecular Biology in Philadelphia, has reported that people with CFIDS may possess a novel enzyme. In studies performed over the last several years, Dr. Suhadolnik found that people with CFIDS have a defect in their antiviral defense system that he believes is due to a faulty enzyme known as ribonuclease (RNase) L. No healthy controls tested positive for the faulty enzyme in a small pilot study. "This new enzyme," he states, "may not function as well as the normal RNase L found in healthy people. It may explain why CFS patients' bodies have a hard time maintaining the energy necessary for cellular growth." It would also explain the difficulty in con-

TESTS AND OBJECTIVE MEASUREMENTS FOR CFIDS

Initial Office Observations
- Blood pressure: usually low (orthostatic hypotension)
- Temperature: low (97° F) or slightly elevated (<100° F) or, more commonly, both over the course of a day (excessive diurnal variation)
- Heartbeat: tachycardia (hard to detect in an office visit; Holter monitor more efficient)
- Throat: irritated
- Lymph nodes: tenderness in nodes of groin and neck, particularly on left side
- Pallor: usually present
- Positive Romberg test (tandem stance)
- Stiff, slow gait

Routine Screening Tests
- Complete blood cell count with differential: decreased number of white blood cells (leukopenia), increased number of white blood cells, abnormal red blood cell membranes, low concentrations of zinc and magnesium, low uric acid concentration (<3.5 mg/dl), total cholesterol concentration slightly elevated
- Sedimentation rate: Low (<5 mm/hr); sometimes brief periods of elevated rate (>20 mm/hr)
- Urinalysis: alkaline; mucus or blood, or both, without bacterial infection

Exclusionary Tests
- Autoimmune system: negative for lupus, rheumatoid arthritis, Hashimoto's disease
  NOTE: Patients sometimes test positive on initial screening but not on more specific tests.
- Endocrine system: Addison's disease, Cushing's disease, hypothyroidism, diabetes mellitus
  NOTE: Warranted if patient demonstrates signs of hypothyroidism, such as enlarged thyroid gland (goiter). Although some patients with CFIDS with enlarged thyroid gland test negative on standard tests, more refined tests may reveal secondary thyroid deficiencies.
- Heart: negative for mitral valve prolapse
  NOTE: Warranted if patient reports tachycardia. Tests sometimes reveal elevated transaminase concentrations and angiotensin-converting enzyme.
- Liver: negative for hepatitis
- Neurologic system: negative for multiple sclerosis (MS)
  NOTE: Warranted if patient shows severe neurologic, cognitive, and muscle dysfunction. Although some patients with CFIDS may test negative for MS, more specific testing (brain function) may reveal abnormalities.
- Bacterial: negative for tuberculosis, brucellosis, Lyme disease
- Cancer: negative for lymphoma
- Parasites: negative for toxoplasmosis, giardiasis, amoebiasis
  NOTE: Patients with CFIDS can have multiple parasitic infections as part of a prodromal illness.
- Toxins: mercury, solvents, pesticides, etc.

trolling viral proliferation in patients with CFIDS. The university has filed a patent application for the test and is currently seeking a corporate partner to license it. However, further studies in a larger patient population will be required before the test can be used as a reliable diagnostic tool. To this end, the National Institutes of Health (NIH) has appropriated funds for an expanded study.

Recovering From CFIDS

Most people who are diagnosed with CFIDS want to know, first and foremost, when they will recover. Will CFIDS last 2 years? Ten years? Or is it a life sentence? Unfortunately, for people with CFIDS, the answer to this question is not usually forthcoming. Doctors with little experience with the illness may tell their patients anything from "Go home and rest and you'll be better in a few months" to "Nobody recovers from CFIDS." Doctors with more experience, however, tend to be more circumspect. The reason for their hesitation is that there is simply too much variation from case to case and far too little information to be able to predict outcomes.

CFIDS is a notoriously unpredictable illness. Some people recover completely within 1 or 2 years and can return to their former lives, others improve enough to live with only minor modifications of their former lifestyles, some must learn to plan their lives within the parameters of symptoms that wax and wane, a few must adjust to long periods of illness, or "plateaus," with little or no improvement, and, at the far end of the spectrum, some do not show improvement and may even worsen over time.

Recovery times vary from a few months (although these short-term cases go largely unreported and therefore never make it into statistical tables) to decades. Statistics reported by physicians are highly individualized, with the more renowned CFIDS specialists (who see the most severe cases) giving the longest recovery rates and general and family practitioners the shortest. However, most physicians tell their patients that CFIDS, generally speaking, is a lengthy proposition—a matter of years, not months. The prospect of a very long illness is always dismal, which is why a diagnosis is often received with profoundly mixed feelings. The only bright spot in the picture is that recovery does not necessarily correlate with duration of illness. Dr. Dedra Buchwald, a physician in Seattle, concluded after a 5-year study of local patients with CFIDS that duration of the illness does not correlate with outcome.

Significant improvement and perhaps recovery are possible even after many years of illness. There are documented cases of long-term sufferers who have recovered completely. Anne, a CFIDS patient from North Carolina, claims full recovery after 19 years of illness. Dean Anderson, in a personal account, says he did not even begin to see an improvement until after 5 years (*CFIDS Chronicle,* Winter 1996).

The only generalizations that can be made about prognosis are that people with milder cases seem to stand a better chance of recovery (a truism for all illnesses) and people with early diagnoses who seek appropriate treatment tend to improve more quickly. The fact that early diagnosis and treatment seem to correlate with recovery rate, at least in some cases, should be sufficient motivation for the recently ill to seek the proper specialist. However, even those who spend years searching for a diagnosis should not lose heart. Recognition and treatment *any time* during the illness can bring substantial improvement, if not full recovery. For most people with CFIDS, especially those with severe cases, the possibility of "substantial" or even "partial" recovery should not be cause for distress but for celebration.

It is the fervent desire of all people with CFIDS and those who are close to them that a cure be found. Already far too many years have been lost and far too many plans and dreams abandoned by countless children and adults affected by this illness. While we are waiting, it is important to bear in mind that, above and beyond finding a cure, a number of variables can affect the outcome of CFIDS. Each person is different. What each has in common though is the need for hope.

The purpose of this book is to provide a cause for hope; that is, information that may enable you to make choices to influence the course of your illness for the better. If you are a medical practitioner or caregiver, this book may help provide much needed information and insights from various sources. In any case, we hope this book will enable its readers to "hang in there" and not lose sight of the light at the end of the long CFIDS tunnel.

II

THE MULTIFACETED SYMPTOMS OF CFIDS

How to Assess
and Monitor Symptoms

One of the hallmarks of CFIDS is diverse, wide-ranging symptoms that wax and wane. Because symptoms vary so much, and because some symptoms eventually fall into patterns, it is important to keep track of them.

Keeping a good symptoms record not only helps identify patterns as an aid to treatment, but can help distinguish CFIDS symptoms from secondary problems (infections, for example). An additional benefit of keeping charts is that office visits to clinicians go more smoothly. You don't have to keep all your symptoms in your head or worry about how well you can express them that day.

To keep track of symptoms, you need a method. The accompanying chart will help keep track of symptoms, daily influences, and certain objective measures. The first section includes information useful to you and your doctor: temperature, to track fever and low temperature fluctuations; basal temperature, to indicate thyroid problems; weight, to track sudden gain or loss; blood pressure; for women, day in menstrual cycle (day 1 is the first day of your period; many symptoms worsen in the last 10 days of the cycle); and weather conditions, which sometimes can exacerbate symptoms. The next section of the chart lists types of symptoms: primary symptoms, which are very indicative of CFIDS and often present throughout the illness; and more transitory secondary symptoms. Rating symptoms with a rating scale (1 = mild, 3 = intermediate, 5 = incapacitating) can prove important in the event that if symptoms worsen over time, a doctor may want to order tests for other systemic disorders such as thyroiditis, anemia, or diabetes. If secondary symptoms are consistently severe or worsen out of pace with primary symptoms, you should see your doctor. An added benefit of tracking symptoms is that it is easier to identify some of their causes, or at least some of the things that exacerbate symp-

SYMPTOMS CHART

Date _____

Basal temp _____ Oral temp: Morning _____ Afternoon _____ Evening _____
Weight _____ Blood pressure_____
For women: Menstrual cycle (day no.) _____
Weather _____

Symptoms (specify)   (1 = mild; 3 = intermediate; 5 = incapacitating)

Symptom	1	2	3	4	5
Allergies _____	1	2	3	4	5
Bladder _____	1	2	3	4	5
Cognitive (type) _____	1	2	3	4	5
Digestive _____	1	2	3	4	5
Dizziness _____	1	2	3	4	5
Ears _____	1	2	3	4	5
Emotional swings _____	1	2	3	4	5
Eyes _____	1	2	3	4	5
Faintness _____	1	2	3	4	5
Fatigue _____	1	2	3	4	5
Headache _____	1	2	3	4	5
Heart _____	1	2	3	4	5
Lymph nodes _____	1	2	3	4	5
Mouth _____	1	2	3	4	5
Nasal _____	1	2	3	4	5
Respiratory _____	1	2	3	4	5
Pain (where) _____	1	2	3	4	5
Skin _____	1	2	3	4	5
Weakness (where) _____	1	2	3	4	5
Other: _____	1	2	3	4	5
_____	1	2	3	4	5
_____	1	2	3	4	5

Sleep disorder: How many hours slept _____
Quality of sleep (awakenings, nightmares, etc): _____
_____

Medications/Treatments/Supplements

WHAT	WHEN	REACTIONS
_____	_____	_____
_____	_____	_____
_____	_____	_____
_____	_____	_____
_____	_____	_____
_____	_____	_____

toms. It is also easier to prove to yourself that you are, indeed, recovering if you keep good track of symptoms over an extended period. The third section of the chart lists medications, treatments, and supplements you are using.

In the beginning you may want to complete a symptoms chart daily for several months. Later, during recovery, you may make an entry only when trying new therapies, during relapses, or occasionally just to keep a record of your progress. *Remember, having CFIDS does not exempt you from other illnesses.* If you notice new or unusual symptoms, especially after CFIDS has been stable for awhile, make sure you bring these to the attention of your doctor.

In addition to rating your symptoms, you may want to rate your illness overall. Many people with CFIDS rate their illness on a scale of 1 to 10. The following scale will help you gauge your overall symptoms and energy level. For example, if you rate your condition at 8, you can do 80% of your normal workload, and it will take you perhaps 20% longer; at 5 you can plan on being able to do about 50% of what you would normally expect of yourself, and it will take you twice as long; at 2, you can do 20% of what you could do formerly, and it will take you five times longer; at 1, you can't do anything. When setting tasks for yourself, this rating scale will help you to be realistic and make allowances for your limitations. By making allowances for your limitations, you will accomplish more and with less frustration than if you set out with previous expectations in mind.

You can also use this scale to help evaluate treatments. Doctors often observe that people who are moderately to mildly ill respond much better to various treatments, whereas those who are severely ill have fewer options.

1 (Severe)   I am in bed all day. Getting up for more than 10 minutes makes me feel awful. My symptoms are incapacitating. I don't leave the house except for trips to the doctor.

2 (Severe)   I can get up for almost an hour, but I still can't move around much. I don't leave the house except for medical appointments and emergencies. I need help for household chores. I am always sick.

3 (Severe)   I have a "window" of time, maybe 2 or 3 hours, when I don't feel too bad, but I usually still have to rest during that time. If I do too much, I have a relapse. I can do some light housekeeping chores. Symptoms are always with me, though sometimes they lighten up.

4 (Severe-Moderate)   I can get up for 2 or 3 hours at a stretch, but I absolutely *must* rest for as much time as I am up. I can prepare simple meals and do light housekeeping. I can drive short distances, but prefer to have others do the driving. I can cope with my symptoms.

5 (Moderate)   I can get through the day, but I need a long rest or a nap. I can do nearly all my housekeeping chores. Symptoms are tolerable, though with relapses they can sometimes become severe. I can get out during the day to run errands or visit with friends if I rest afterward.

6 (Moderate)   If I take short, recuperative rests, I can get through the day. Sometimes I need to nap. By dinnertime, I am often quite tired, and I need to get to bed by 9:00 PM. I can drive short distances. I can work a little at home. Sometimes symptoms seem to vanish altogether for short periods of time.

7 (Moderate-Mild)   I can get through the day without needing a rest, but I need more sleep than I used to. I can work part-time on a flexible schedule, allowing for relapses. I have longer periods of feeling almost normal.

8 (Mild)   I can get through the day with no problem, provided I don't skimp on sleep or overdo it. I can work full-time, although I don't have much energy for anything else. Relapses are usually short and, with a little rest, I recover well.

9 (Mild)   My stamina is much improved. I can hold a full-time job. Provided I get enough rest and watch myself, I don't have relapses. I can go out in the evening without "paying for it later," although I'm still more tired than usual the next day. Symptoms are few and far between.

10   I am completely recovered. I have lots of energy, with no sign of symptoms. I am back to climbing mountains on weekends.

Obviously, the above criteria are not ironclad. Many people who rate their illness at a 5 or 6 still manage to force themselves to go to work. Others, because of their particular array of symptoms, may be able to get out more or perform more physical work. Children, for example, may have greater energy levels than adults with the same degree of illness, and some men may recover physical stamina faster than women, which allows them to work even when other symptoms are debilitating.

Becoming familiar with your symptoms and understanding their causes is one of the biggest challenges of CFIDS. Nevertheless, it is a challenge that, if met, can help open the way to choosing treatments and coping strategies that will be most effective for you.

3

Specific Symptoms and Treatment Tips

Allergies	Muscle Problems
Candida	Oral Problems
Cardiac and Cardiovascular Symptoms	Pain
Cognitive and Emotional Problems	Premenstrual Syndrome
Digestive Disturbances	Secondary Infections
Dizziness and Vertigo	Seizures and Seizure Activity
Endocrine Disturbances	Shingles
Fatigue	Sinusitis
Flu-Like Symptoms	Skin, Hair, and Nail Problems
Headaches	Sleep Disorders
Hearing Problems	Urinary Tract Problems
Hypoglycemia	Vision and Eye Problems
Joint Pain	Weather Sensitivity
Loss of Libido	Weight Loss or Gain

ALLERGIES

New onset of allergies or worsening of existing allergies is a widespread problem in patients with CFIDS. According to Dr. James Jones, 75% of people with CFIDS have allergies, compared with 25% in the general population. Allergies can be triggered by airborne agents, chemicals, or foods. The most frequent airborne allergies in CFIDS are to molds, dust, and pollens. Chemical odors (perfumes, hairspray, gasoline, household cleaners, plastic outgassing) can also produce allergic reactions. Food allergies and sensitivities are common and comprise the full spectrum of anything that can be ingested.

Allergy can be described as an overresponse of the immune system in which immune cells mistakenly identify an innocuous substance as a potentially harmful one. The immune response involves the production of histamine, a chemical that causes inflammation by increasing cell permeability and localized blood flow (histamine is a vasodilator). Normally, inflammation fulfills a positive role in combating infection. It serves to isolate a wounded area and draw fluid to it, thereby enabling white blood cells to identify and kill invading microorganisms. The increased permeability of cell membranes allows for the release of heparin and zinc, which are needed for connective tissue repair after injury. If the mucous membranes are involved, the resulting inflammation produces cold symptoms, stomach pain, and diarrhea. If the skin is affected, the inflammation produces itching or rash. When the allergic response is systemic, the inflammation can occur in any soft tissue (throat, joint area, gums, brain) producing an astonishingly wide array of symptoms.

It is not surprising, given the huge overlap between allergic reactions and CFIDS symptoms, that some allergists have mistaken CFIDS for allergy. The difference is that CFIDS usually occurs suddenly and is prolonged, whereas allergies generally run in families, are short-lived after provocation, and manifest themselves gradually, often over the course of a lifetime. Neither are they (generally) accompanied by fevers. To confound matters, many clinicians have noticed that, although people with CFIDS demonstrate clear evidence of allergic reactions on standard tests, their allergies seem to fluctuate with the severity of the illness. This has led a number of clinicians and researchers to propose that many of the allergic reactions experienced by people with CFIDS should better be classified as sensitivities. Despite this debate, there are some significant commonalities between the two phenomena.

The immune system hyperresponse brought about by CFIDS uses the same mechanism as an allergy—the action of inflammation-mediating chemicals. Lucy Duchene, Ph.D., proposes that histamine overproduction can substantially contribute to the development of CFIDS' most significant effects (*CFIDS Chronicle*, Summer 1993). Chief among these are increased excretion of electrolytes, leading to dehydration and alteration in cell function; binding to acetylcholine receptors, causing insufficient nervous system responses in muscle and brain function; increased delta waves, leading to daytime lethargy and disturbed sleep; stimulation of the vagus nerve, contributing to activation of the parasympathetic nervous system and general metabolic slowing; irregularities in heart rate; gastrointestinal disturbances from histamine-induced release of gastric juices,

---

ALLERGY SYMPTOMS

Allergies can affect any organ, with symptoms that may include the following:

Skin: Pallor, itching, burning, tingling, flushing, warmth or coldness, sweating behind the neck, hives, blisters, blotches, red spots, pimples, dermatitis, eczema

Eyes: Blurred vision, itching, pain, watering, eyelid twitching, redness of inner angle of lower lid, drooping or swollen eyelids

Ears: Earache, recurring ear infections, dizziness, tinnitus, imbalance

Nose: Nasal congestion or discharge, sneezing

Mouth: Dry mouth, increased salivation, stinging tongue, itchy palate, toothache

Throat: Tickling or clearing, difficulty in swallowing

Lungs: Shortness of breath, air hunger, wheezing, cough, mucous or recurrent bronchial infections

Heart: Chest tightness, pounding or skipped heartbeats

Gastrointestinal tract: Burping, heartburn, indigestion, nausea, vomiting, abdominal pain, gas, cramping, diarrhea, constipation, mucus in stool; frequent, urgent, or painful urination, bedwetting (in children)

Muscular system: Muscle fatigue, weakness, pain, stiffness, soreness

Central nervous system: Headache, migraine, vertigo, drowsiness, sluggishness, giddiness

Cognition: Lack of concentration, feeling of "separateness," forgetting words or names, anxiety, tension, panic, overactivity, restlessness, jitteriness, depression, premenstrual syndrome (PMS)

leading to acid stomach and other gastrointestinal problems; release of adrenal hormones, leading to activation of the sympathetic nervous system, speeding up of heart rate, increased glucose metabolism, and, when prolonged, eventual adrenal exhaustion and hypoglycemia; changes in gonadotrophin and prolactin levels, causing hormone imbalance; changes in immune system function; and last (but not least) *both* stimulation and depression of certain parts of the hypothalamus. As the brain appears to be one of the main sources of the syndrome's many myriad effects, the ability of histamine to cross the blood-brain barrier, affect the metabolism of serotonin and acetylcholine, and ultimately alter functioning of the hypothalamus makes it a prime culprit for causing CFIDS symptoms.

Airborne Allergens

When most people think of allergies, what comes to mind is the sneezing, wheezing, itching eyes, sinus headaches, and runny nose that are the typical responses to airborne allergens.

POLLEN. The strongly scented, bright-colored flowers typical of heavy-pollen plants do not usually cause problems for people with hay fever because they are usually cross-pollinated by insects. Plants that produce light, abundant, widely wind-distributed pollen create problems for allergic individuals. When these small, light pollens are inhaled, the grains pass into the bronchi, where they can cause the wheezing of an allergic response. To complicate the picture, some pollens contain as many as 15 allergenic compounds, which can stimulate a variety of other systemic reactions. You should suspect an allergy to pollens if you have the following symptoms during spring and fall:

- Your eyes itch and you have a thin, watery nasal discharge.
- You feel worse outdoors between 8:00 AM and noon, when most plants release pollens.
- You feel worse on clear, windy days.
- Your symptoms improve after a heavy rainstorm, when pollens are washed out of the air.
- Your symptoms improve after the first frost in fall.

MOLD. The principal activity of mold is to break down organic matter to make it available for other life. As nature's greatest recycling force, molds can hardly be avoided. They can be found on farms, in houses, at work, in factories, outdoors and indoors, in showers, refrigerators, food, under rugs, and any place it is warm and humid. Molds can also colonize the body, as in systemic or local Candida overgrowth, athlete's foot, ringworm, and various other fungal infections. Molds cause special problems because the frequent overgrowth of Candida experienced by people with CFIDS can produce an allergy to molds in general (see Candida). In contrast to pollen and food allergies, mold symptoms do not include itchy eyes. Symptoms include severe fatigue, dizziness, vertigo, rashes, and cognitive problems. Suspect an allergy to molds if you have the following symptoms:

- You feel worse in humid weather.
- You feel worse outdoors between 5:00 and 9:00 PM.
- You feel worse when mowing or raking leaves.
- You feel much worse from August to the first heavy frost.
- You feel worse in damp places, basements, and bathrooms.
- You feel worse after eating mushrooms, seaweed, fermented products, aged cheeses, beer, tofu, pickles, or vinegar.

ANIMAL DANDER, FUR, AND FEATHERS. Many people are sensitive to animal hair and react to fur coats and trimmings, feather pillows, stuffed toys, wool clothing, yarn, felting, carpets, and wigs. Allergies to animal dander can also produce an allergic reaction to serum from those same animals. For example, to avoid an allergic response, people with horse dander allergies need to be careful about receiving horse antiserum (tetanus shots). Suspect allergies to animal dander if you feel worse when you are exposed to animals or animal hairs in items such as bedding or clothing.

DUST. Dust is a complex mixture composed of breakdown products of airborne allergies plus inorganic matter from synthetics, smoke, soot, cellulose, dead skin cells, and mite or other insect droppings. You can be allergic to any component of dust, and it is impossible to pinpoint exactly what causes symptoms without testing. If you feel worse indoors, after dusting or vacuuming, or first thing in the morning, you may have an allergy to dust.

TREATMENT TIPS

- Dust with a damp sponge to avoid spreading dust.
- Avoid vacuuming or emptying vacuum bags (which harbor molds).
- Eliminate under-the-bed storage.
- Use easy-to-wash curtains, bed covers, pillows, rugs, and clothing.
- Empty and clean drawers. Use drawers only for storing clean clothes.

- Avoid keeping knickknacks, books, or dust-catching clutter in your room.
- Do not allow pets in the bedroom.
- Replace furnace and air-conditioning filters often; check for mold.
- Use an air filter in your room; high-efficiency particle arresting (HEPA) filters are best ($109 from Real Goods; 800-762-7325).
- Use nonsedating antihistamines (Claritin) or steroidal nasal sprays (Nasalcrom) for symptom relief.
- Take natural antihistamines (quercetin, bromelain) and vitamin C for nutritional support.
- Avoid eating moldy or mold-laden foods, inhaling old dust (such as in attics and used-book shops), and make sure bathrooms and kitchens are free of mold and mildew.

Food

Allergies and intolerance to various foods are common in people with CFIDS. Dr. Robert Loblay, lecturer in immunology and Director of Allergy Service at the Royal Prince Alfred Hospital in Sydney, Australia, estimates that food intolerance is a "significant factor in 20% to 30%, and may be the principal trigger in perhaps 5% to 10%" of the CFIDS population. In some of these individuals, allergies to other substances (pollen, dust) may have predated the onset of CFIDS; in others, food sensitivities are a new problem brought on by CFIDS itself (see Chapter 9 for a more in-depth discussion of food intolerance).

The distinction most clinicians make between food allergy and food intolerance is subtle. Currently, most allergists agree that food allergies are mediated by immunoglobulin E (IgE), an antibody that attaches itself to histamine-releasing mast cells. Allergens, because they produce antibodies, provoke an immune response even in the tiniest amounts. They often occur in groups, for example, citrus fruits, fungi, or milk products. The most common allergies are to corn, eggs, milk, soy, sugar, wheat, and yeast. Allergies can be tested for with a radioallergosorbent test (RAST), which measures the amount of IgE antibodies a person produces in response to specific substances.

Intolerance to certain foods, on the other hand, is not IgE modulated and cannot be measured with the RAST. It often results from increased permeability of the small intestine lining (leaky gut), a problem that can arise after infections from viruses or Candida and treatments with certain drugs (e.g., antiparasitic agents, antibiotics, chemotherapy). When the intestinal wall is compromised, molecules derived from food digestion pass through the membrane before they are completely broken down. The oversized molecules now circulating in the blood stream provoke an immune response, although this may be delayed by several hours or even days. In the case of food intolerance, the less you eat of a food the less likely it is to bother you. And whereas true allergies usually last throughout life (the immune system "remembers" the offending protein), sensitivities are often transient.

The conditions that lead to food sensitivities are multifold. An initial viral trigger can affect the gut mucosa, making the intestinal wall more permeable. In addition, negative responses to certain foods could be a result of low amounts of T suppressor cells, the immune system cells that modulate immune responses to food molecules. Parasites, Candida, and alterations in intestinal flora after antibiotic intake are also possible factors contributing to food sensitivities. Needless to say, people with CFIDS can experience all these conditions so it should not be surprising that food sensitivities are common in the CFIDS population.

Reactions to food allergies and sensitivities are fairly similar. Suspect food sensitivities if you have the following symptoms:

- You feel excessively thirsty after eating.
- You experience bloating within 20 minutes after eating.
- You experience bowel problems, dizziness, heart palpitations, fatigue, insomnia, depression, or anxiety after eating certain foods.
- You have any symptoms after eating citrus fruits, milk products, wheat, solanaceous foods (nightshade family, such as potato, tomato, eggplant, peppers), or artificial colorings or preservatives.

TREATMENT TIPS

For food allergies and sensitivities, the first order of business is to identify and avoid the offending foods. A record should be kept of symptoms that arise, such as heartburn, increased heart rate, bloating, headache, or diarrhea after eating certain foods, and those foods should be avoided. Note whether symptoms decrease after a few days. (In some cases, however, symptoms increase for a few days when the offending item is withdrawn.) Foods should be isolated as much as possible. Don't mix too many at a single meal to better judge their aftereffects.

Second, diet should be rotated. In the rotation diet, no food is eaten more than once in 4 days. Not only does this diet allow you to identify foods that may be causing trouble, it helps prevent the formation of allergic responses from overexposure. Because people with CFIDS have a strong tendency to have allergies, this last point is crucial. Of course, many people with food reactions find that they eat too few foods to rotate them. In that case, alternate as best you can. When reactions occur, the best immediate course of action is as follows:

- Drink a glass of water with a half-teaspoon of baking soda or trisodium compound (Tri-Salts) to increase alkalinity (allergic reactions are acidic).
- Take nonacid vitamin C.
- Take over-the-counter sinus allergy medication (Alka-Seltzer Plus) or antihistamines if the reaction is severe.
- Drink plenty of water.

An interesting new drug approach to food allergies that has been reputed to have some success in Sweden is the use of orally administered cromolyn (Gastrocrom). In severe cases, judicious use of systemic anti-inflammatory agents (hydrocortisone, cortisol) can be lifesaving. Cortisol is the body's most powerful anti-inflammatory chemical and can stop inflammation cold. However, it also depresses the immune system and, over time, can depress adrenal function. It should be used sparingly and only in cases in which immune system hyperreactivity threatens to create malnutrition. GLA (evening primrose oil) and Cytotec, a synthetic prostaglandin, are also helpful in treating food sensitivities and leaky gut. (For information on how to heal leaky gut, the source of most food sensitivities, see Digestive Disturbances.) Zinc deficiency can lead to excess histamine production; thus increased dietary zinc may help control food sensitivities.

Chemical Sensitivities

Sensitivities to synthetic chemicals are fairly common in people with CFIDS, although many may not be aware that their symptoms are attributable to chemical exposure. People who experience fatigue, dizziness, anxiety, or other symptoms after shopping in furniture or dry goods stores, sitting in a new car, strolling through a mall, or filling the tank at a gas station are probably chemically sensitive.

Chemical sensitivities were first described in 1951 by Dr. Theron Randolph, the pioneering physician who discovered that people who demonstrated allergies to fruits (all fruits in this case, not just specific families) were actually reacting to the pesticide residues left on them. Dr. Randolph observed that even in small doses, chemicals can cause severe reactions in sensitive individuals. In 1962 Dr. Randolph published a landmark book, *Human Ecology and Susceptibility to the Chemical Environment,* in which he identified the chemicals responsible for a wide range of human ailments.

Chemical sensitivity usually develops over a long time. Small amounts of chemicals continually enter the body through the skin, nasal passages, or digestive tract and can eventually induce sensitivities, with symptoms that for all intents and purposes are identical to those of common allergic reactions (though not all chemical sensitivities are IgE-mediated). IgE-mediated chemical reactions include hives, rashes, and skin eruptions. Delayed responses can include any of the symptoms common to other allergies, such as confusion, respiratory problems, fatigue, diarrhea, excessive thirst, tinnitus, runny nose, cramps, and itching. Chemical sensitivities can also surface as the result of massive exposure to a contaminant, such as a chemical spill or fire, pesticide spray, or general anesthesia. In these cases, the massive exposure overwhelms the body's normal detoxification mechanisms or damages the regulatory systems (in the brain) that normally direct endocrine and immune functions.

INDOOR CHEMICAL AIR CONTAMINANTS. Building materials, carpeting, glues, paints, plastics, deodorants, tobacco, insecticides, and disinfectants are common sources of indoor pollution found in most homes. Of particular concern is the outgassing of contaminants such as formaldehyde from sources such as pressboard, found in most recently built homes. Low-level exposures, even though they can induce symptoms, originate from sources that are not easily detected and thus remain hidden. Other common sources of indoor pollution are copy machine inks, correction fluid, carbon paper, solvents used in the workplace, and gas leakage from stoves and heaters.

OUTDOOR CHEMICAL AIR CONTAMINANTS. Traffic exhaust, smog, paving and resurfacing of roads, industrial fumes, and the indiscriminate spraying of lawns are the most common sources of outdoor pollution. Of these, exposure to gasoline and diesel fumes presents the biggest problem for the chemically sensitive because they are ubiquitous and virtually unavoidable.

DRUGS AND MEDICATIONS. People with chemical sensitivities frequently develop sensitivities to drugs as well. Many drugs are synthetic, that is, they are derived from petroleum, a common source of sensitivity for many people. In addition, the excipients, preservatives, colorings, and inactive ingredients found in many medications may provoke reactions. Many people with drug sensitivities are unable to tolerate antibiotics or local anesthetics.

CLOTHING AND PERSONAL CARE PRODUCTS. Synthetic fabrics, as well as the detergents, finishers (such as formaldehyde), sizing, dyes, and plastic residues found on many natural fabrics, can provoke topical or systemic reactions in many people. The harsh chemicals often included in body lotions, skin cleaners, cosmetics, and deodorants are also common sources of irritation for the chemically sensitive.

TREATMENT TIPS

In a 1995 survey conducted by a DePaul University research team, 305 patients with multiple chemical sensitivities (MCS) were asked to rate treatments on the basis of personal experience. Of these patients, 93% rated "adopting a practice of avoiding exposures to chemicals which could cause MCS reactions" as a "major" or "enormous help" (*CFIDS Chronicle*, Winter 1996). It is clear from this report and from testimonies of numerous people with chemical sensitivities that effective control of chemical reactions hinges on avoidance. Clean, filtered water and air, and organic foods help cut down the chemical load and remove all sources of contamination from the home (see Chapter 8 for more information on alternatives to toxic household chemicals).

Nutritional support can also be of help, particularly those nutrients that help mediate allergic symptoms and provide support for the liver and kidneys. Vitamins C and B_{12} are especially important. The entero-hepatic resuscitation program is a nutritional program supposed to help with chemical sensitivities. Alpha ketoglutarate and glutathione are two of nature's most potent natural detoxifiers, as are all antioxidants.

MORE INFORMATION

American Academy of Allergy and
  Immunology
611 East Wells Street
Milwaukee, WI 53202
800-822-2762 (toll-free telephone)

Asthma and Allergy Information Line
PO Box 1766
Rochester, NY 14603
800-727-5400 (toll-free telephone)

Food Allergy Network
10400 Eaton Place, Suite 107
Fairfax, VA 22030-5647
800-929-4040 (toll-free telephone)

Human Ecology Action League (HEAL)
PO Box 49126
Atlanta, GA 30359
404-248-1898 (telephone)

FURTHER READING

Krohn, Jacqueline. The Whole Way to Allergy Relief and Prevention: A Doctor's Complete Guide to Treatment and Self-Care. Washington, D.C.: Hartley and Marks, 1991.

Loblay, Robert H, and Swain, Anne R. The Role of Food Intolerance in Chronic Fatigue Syndrome. In Hyde, Byron M, ed. The Clinical and Scientific Basis of ME/CFS. Ottawa, Ontario: Nightingale Research Foundation, 1992.

SEE

- Digestive Disturbances.
- Chapter 4: Antihistamines, Cytotec, Hydrocortisone.
- Chapter 5: Alpha Ketoglutarate, Amino Acids (glutathione), Bioflavonoids, Entero-Hepatic Resuscitation Program, Minerals (zinc), Vitamins.
- Chapters 8 and 9.

CANDIDA

Candida albicans is a yeast-like fungus found in the moist mucous lining of the intestines, genital tract, mouth, and throat. A certain level of Candida in the body is normal; some conditions, however, can cause rampant overgrowth. The overgrowth, manifested in easily observed "yeast" infections of the vagina and mouth, as well as less apparent systemic infections, can lead to serious health problems.

People with compromised immune systems often have both topical and systemic infections. The stubborn, recurring local infections such as athlete's foot, vaginal yeast infections, and thrush are indications that the immune system is not operating fully. The immune system is simply too weak to combat the rapid proliferation of yeast throughout the body. When the immune system is compromised, Candida can spread from the mucous linings of the mouth and intestines to other organ systems, as well as the blood stream, causing a systemic infection with wide-reaching effects. In fact, a number of clinicians believe that systemic Candida infections may contribute to some of the more troubling and persistent long-term symptoms of CFIDS.

As a case in point, a number of common digestive problems are believed to be caused or exacerbated by yeast overgrowth. Yeast can adhere to the intestinal walls, causing loss of integrity of the mucous lining. This damage results in greater permeability of the lining, allowing undigested food particles to pass through (leaky gut). When these undigested food molecules reach the blood stream, many systemic allergic reactions can occur. Bloating, gas, diarrhea, and food, drug, and chemical sensitivities owe their origins, in many cases, to this problem. In addition to symptoms related to increased intestinal permeability, people with yeast overgrowth experience fatigue, headaches, cognitive problems, and endocrine imbalances (hypothyroidism and hypoglycemia).

Many researchers believe that a combination of immunosuppressive factors contributes to the likelihood of yeast infections developing. Dr. Carol Jessop, an internist in California who has treated systemic yeast infection in thousands of patients with CFIDS, has noted that 84% of her patients have undergone repeated and prolonged antibiotic treatment, 70% have taken oral contraceptives, and 10% have taken prescribed steroid drugs (*CFIDS Chronicle,* Spring 1991). All of these drugs can be immune system inhibitors and may be linked to Candida overgrowth. Dr. Jorge Flechas has also addressed the problem of Candida overgrowth as it is related to immune system disregulation in patients with CFIDS. Dr. Flechas proposes that Candida overgrowth may be linked to a specific immune defect (*CFIDS Chronicle,* Summer/Fall 1989). He has noticed that patients with CFIDS commonly demonstrate T cell abnormalities, such as T suppressor cell depletion and reduced number of natural killer cells. Because the T cells are largely responsible for controlling viral and fungal infections, a defect in the system may allow reactivation of latent viruses and fungal overgrowth.

Due to the fact that so many of the symptoms caused by overgrowth of Candida are the same as CFIDS symptoms, it can be difficult to differentiate the two. To make a diagnosis, a careful medical history must be taken, with particular attention to courses of antibiotics, steroid therapy, or oral contraceptives taken in the past. In addition, the presence of certain symptoms may be highly suggestive of candidiasis. Oral thrush, recurrent vaginitis, topical fungal infections, such as athlete's foot, chemical and food sensitivities, and gastrointestinal problems may warrant further investigation. Vertigo, sinusitis, and premenstrual syndrome (PMS) may also be indicative of a systemic Candida infection. If a patient has these signs and symptoms, laboratory testing for Candida may be recommended. A quantitative stool analysis can reveal Candida overgrowth and imbalances in intestinal flora (Great Smokies Diagnostic Laboratory; 800-522-4762). Blood tests to detect the presence of Candida antibodies in the blood stream are also available (Immunosciences Lab; 800-950-4686).

Few physicians believe that Candida overgrowth is the underlying cause of CFIDS, but many agree that yeast overgrowth can greatly exacerbate symptoms. As Dr. Flechas states, "[Candida] can take a bad situation and make it worse." And, as many people with CFIDS have found, the reduction in yeast overgrowth can lessen the general overload on the body, allowing for greater overall improvement over time.

TREATMENT TIPS

- Prescription antifungal medications are normally recommended for systemic Candida infection. The most commonly prescribed drugs are nystatin and Diflucan. Nizoral, while effective, is used less often because of the potential for liver toxicity. Sporanox, a newer antifungal agent, is also used for systemic infections. Your doctor may recommend a 3- to 6-week trial to help determine which of your symptoms are yeast related.

- Nonprescription antifungal agents, including garlic (liquid, capsule, or fresh), caprillic acid, pau d'arco, and tea tree oil, can also be effective. These can be applied topically or taken orally (except for tea tree oil, which can only be applied topically). Grapefruit seed extract is also a potent antimicrobial agent, but is extremely caustic and should not be used by anyone with a sensitive stomach or esophagus. It can be purchased in health food stores and from nutritionists and some chiropractors.

- Probiotics such as acidophilus and bifidus bacteria are usually recommended to treat yeast problems. Health food stores generally carry a wide array of different strains and combinations. Many people prefer the enteric-coated varieties because they are not destroyed by stomach acid.

- Most physicians recommend dietary modifications to help control the infection. Yeast thrives on sugar so a mainstay of the diet is to avoid sweets. Alcohol, refined carbohydrates, milk (because of the lactose), and fruits may also be eliminated in the early stages of treatment. Specialists also recommend avoiding fermented products (soy sauce, moldy cheeses) and pickled products because these contain yeast and mold. Although Candida does not need molds to grow, the Candida overgrowth often creates allergies to all mold and fungus. As a consequence, eating moldy foods provokes allergic symptoms. A good rule of thumb is to emphasize whole grains, high-quality proteins, and lots of vegetables. If possible, foods should be purchased fresh and without additives, hormones, or antibiotics, which exacerbate the condition. Some supermarket chains are beginning to carry "natural" meats.

- Vaginal and throat yeast infections should be treated when they occur. Over-the-counter antifungal creams can now be purchased, but many women still prefer prescription drugs for insurance reimbursement. The main problem that may arise from using these creams, however, is allergic reaction (characterized by burning and itching). You may want to discuss some of the single-treatment options (such as Vagistat) with your gynecologist or other doctor if this is a problem. Throat infections (thrush) can be treated with an oral nystatin preparation and with any kind of acid gargle (vinegar, lemon) because molds and fungus will not grow in an acid environment. If you can tolerate yogurt, a yogurt "swish" (around the mouth and down the throat) also helps.

- Supplements recommended (mainly for their immunity boosting qualities) include vitamin C, zinc, vitamin B complex, essential fatty acids (evening primrose oil, borage seed oil), and fish oils.

- It is important to avoid breathing molds, chemicals, and other irritating inhalants. If you need to take antibiotics for any reason, it is wise to supplement with acidophilus or bifidus bacteria to replace helpful bacteria that have been destroyed. These friendly bacteria will keep the yeast under control during treatment.

MORE INFORMATION

Candida Research Foundation
1638 B Street
Hayward, CA 94541
510-582-2179 (telephone)

FURTHER READING

Crook, William. Chronic Fatigue Syndrome and the Yeast Connection. Jackson, Tenn.: Profesional Books, 1992.

Rosenbaum, Michael, and Susser, Murray. Solving the Puzzle of Chronic Fatigue Syndrome. Tacoma, Wash.: Life Sciences Press, 1992.

SEE

- Chapter 4: Antifungal Agents.
- Chapter 5: Essential Fatty Acids, Herbs, Minerals, Probiotics, Vitamins.

CARDIAC AND CARDIOVASCULAR SYMPTOMS

Heart-related symptoms are among the most worrisome for patients with CFIDS because of the serious nature of cardiac problems. Although many patients with CFIDS have chest pain, blood pressure fluctuations, and periodic increases in heart rate, few (less than 5%) experience any notable cardiovascular problems. Dr. Byron Hyde has noted that among his patients, and in many of the epidemic outbreaks of CFIDS, cardiovascular problems tend to appear early in the illness—in the first month—and disappear by the third to twelfth month. In some cases, however, heart problems will either resurface or even appear for the first time after some years have passed. Abnormalities such as premature atrial and ventricular contractions, increased tendency for mitral valve prolapse (especially in children), pericarditis, myocarditis, palpitations (skipped heart beats), tachycardia (rapid heart beat), various arrhythmias, ectopic heart beats, edema (swelling in the hands and feet), nasal stuffiness (not due to allergies), and unusual readings at electrocardiography (ECG) or Holter monitoring are not unusual.

Palpitations (Tachycardia)

A sudden increase in heart rate (up to 150 bpm) either while resting or upon standing is fairly common, especially in severe or acute cases. Heart rate alterations can occur at random or follow fairly regular patterns. Times of day in which adrenal output is low (4:00 AM and 4:00 PM) may produce conditions for erratic heart rate. Sudden heart rate increases can also occur after exercise, lifting, and, in the severely ill, after changing position in bed. Pounding of the heart is also a common heart problem and, although frightening, is rarely dangerous.

Low Blood Pressure (Hypotension)

Sudden decreases in blood pressure, occasionally manifested as "blackouts" or periods of sudden faintness, are common in patients with CFIDS. Dr. Luis Leon-Sotomayor, the cardiologist who recorded the 1965 CFIDS epidemic in Galveston, Texas, observed that hypotension was common in his patients with CFIDS, particularly after activity or upon standing. (Normally, the systolic component of blood pressure rises after standing.) The apparent disregulation of blood pressure in CFIDS is not, as it would appear, directly connected to cardiac problems but is the result of hypothalamic dysfunction since the hypothalamus, among its many other functions, is responsible for maintaining arterial pressure.

Studies performed at Johns Hopkins University have recently confirmed Dr. Leon-Sotomayor's observations. The Johns Hopkins' researchers concluded that some patients with CFIDS have a condition known as neurally mediated hypotension (NMH) (*Lancet*, 1995). The condition is characterized by fainting (syncope) and, in CFIDS, periods of faintness. NMH represents a flaw in neuroendocrine coordination. Normally when blood pressure falls, the brain sends a signal for the adrenal glands to release adrenaline (epinephrine). The adrenaline signals the heart to beat more vigorously, raising blood pressure. Once the heart rate increases and blood pressure is restored, the nerves within the left ventricle send a message to the brain that blood pressure is too high and the brain in turn sends a signal to lower blood pressure.

In people with NMH, this well-coordinated system for maintaining blood pressure goes awry. People with NMH have low blood pressure, causing blood to settle, or pool, in the lower extremities. When the heart starts to beat more vigorously to compensate, the nerves in the left ventricle send the erroneous message that pressure is already too high, forcing blood pressure to drop even farther. The result is a feeling of faintness. In NMH, any excess release of adrenaline can produce the same result, which is why some people feel faint at the sight of blood or after having a fright.

NMH can be treated with drugs that regulate heart rate (beta blockers) or increase blood volume (Florinef). Norpace, an antiarrhythmic drug, while sometimes recommended, is used less frequently because of its side effects. Midodrine, a newly approved drug, may also be prescribed for NMH. An interesting nondrug alternative used by some alternative practitioners is licorice, an herb with steroidal properties but without the many side effects of steroids. Increasing the intake of salt and liquids (to increase blood fluid volume) is a recommended adjunct to all medications.

Shortness of Breath (Dyspnea)

Shortness of breath, particularly after exertion, is common in patients with CFIDS. Many people experience the phenomenon of "air hunger" even if they are not moving. It is not uncommon to wake up with it. In CFIDS, researchers have found that the heart does not speed up quickly enough to meet the extra demands placed on it by exercise. Although the body's need for oxygen is increased, the heart fails to deliver. The result is chest pain and shortness of breath. In severe illness, even getting out of bed too quickly can produce this effect.

•   •   •

Heart attacks are not generally associated with CFIDS, but anyone with a history of heart problems needs to be conscientious about following up on cardiac symptoms. If symptoms are severe or persistent, wearing a Holter monitor for a day or having a test for mitral valve prolapse might be recommended. Inasmuch as many of the symptoms produced by mitral valve prolapse (breathlessness, fatigue, edema) are common in CFIDS, a thorough doctor may wish to investigate the possibility of mitral valve prolapse just to be on the safe side.

TREATMENT TIPS

Sometimes pharmaceutical treatments such as beta blockers (propranolol, atenolol) are used to regulate heart beat and blood pressure. Doctors who prescribe these drugs generally prefer to confirm a cardiac abnormality first because of the risks involved in long-term usage. CFIDS clinicians almost always recommend restricting aerobic exercise in the acute stage to avoid any potential risk of virally induced cardiac problems. Calcium channel blockers and magnesium are also sometimes used to control heart problems, although these, like other heart medications, must be carefully monitored by a cardiologist. Two nutritional supports noted for strengthening and improving heart function are CoQ10 and omega-3 essential fatty acids.

MORE INFORMATION

Society for MVP Syndrome
PO Box 431
Itasca, IL 60143-0431

FURTHER READING

Hyde, Byron M, and Jain, Anil. Cardiac and Cardiovascular Aspects of ME/CFS, A Review. In Hyde, Byron M, ed. The Clinical and Scientific Basis of ME/CFS. Ottawa, Ontario: Nightingale Research Foundation, 1992.

SEE

• Chapter 4: Beta Blockers, Calcium Channel Blockers, Florinef.
• Chapter 5: CoQ10, Essential Fatty Acids, Herbs (licorice), Minerals (magnesium).

COGNITIVE AND EMOTIONAL PROBLEMS

Cognitive, emotional, and perceptual problems affect nearly every person with CFIDS at one time or another during the course of the illness. They are, in fact, so prevalent that many doctors consider them to be as great an identifying feature of the illness as fatigue. In some cases these problems are evident at onset; in others they develop after a few weeks or even months have passed. Although not, perhaps, as obvious to the casual observer as some of CFIDS' more overt symptoms (muscle weakness, pain, fever), cognitive and emotional problems can be just as disabling. Indeed, in some cases cognitive problems form the nexus of disability, making it impossible for the more severely affected to hold a job, read a book, or even carry on a coherent conversation. The cumulative effect of these symptoms (most notably, lack of concentration combined with short-term memory loss) results in what most people with CFIDS call "brain fog."

Researchers agree that many cognitive, emotional, and perceptual changes that arise as a result of the illness are organic; that is, they are due to alterations in normal brain function rather than to secondary psychological factors (such as being upset about having CFIDS). Many people with CFIDS have observed that distortions in emotional and mental states seem to correlate with the degree of severity of their other symptoms (usually, but not always, fatigue). This seems to point to a similar, if not the same, origin for both. Dr. Jay Goldstein, Dr. Ismael Mena, and others have suggested that physiologic symptoms, such as muscle weakness, temperature fluctuation, and decreased blood pressure, as well as emotional and cognitive symptoms, all can be caused by abnormalities in an area of the brain that roughly corresponds to the limbic system and adjacent regions of the temporal lobe.

The limbic system is a ring of structures located at the center of the brain. It is composed of a number of small but vitally important components that affect nearly every aspect of physical and psychological function. The hypothalamus, a thumb-sized assembly of about 20 nuclei located just below the thalamus (the brain's sensory processor), is responsible for regulating the autonomic nervous system, the endocrine system (through the pituitary gland), certain emotions relating to the "fight-or-flight" response, and sleep. It has a central role in mediating immune system responses and is a virtual thoroughfare for fibers connecting the higher cortical centers governing thought with structures in the midbrain and limbic system that regulate motor activities, the senses, memory, and emotion. Alterations in hypothalamic function can result in sleep disturbances (insomnia, hypersomnia), loss of homeostasis (the body's ability to maintain itself within constant parameters of temperature, blood pressure, and so on), eating disorders (anorexia, gorging), and mood disturbances (panic, rage, anxiety), as well as cause disturbances in distant areas of the brain that rely on communications from the nerve fibers passing through the hypothalamus. Other structures in the limbic system (basal ganglia) affect motor function. If these are functionally impaired, tremors and difficulty sequencing complex motor coordination (such as speech) may result. The amygdala and hippocampus, two closely related limbic structures embedded in the temporal lobe, play an important part in learning and processing short-term memory. Damage to these results in learning and information retention problems, as well as difficulty with visual and aural comprehension.

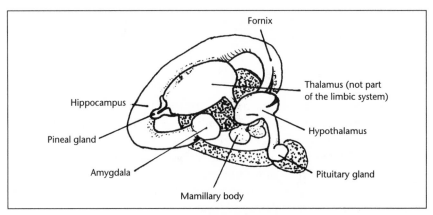

The Limbic System

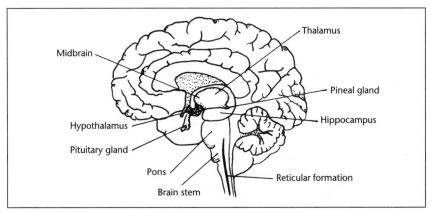

Mid-Sagittal Section of the Brain

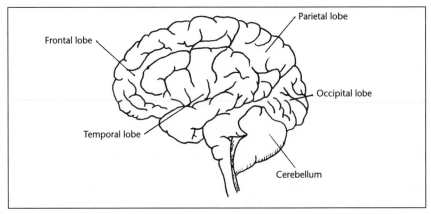

The Principal Lobes of the Brain

Given the wide range of neurologic symptoms experienced by people with CFIDS, it is not surprising that radiologic examinations, such as single-photon emission computed tomography (SPECT), positron emission tomography (PET), and magnetic resonance imaging (MRI), of the brains of patients with CFIDS have revealed low blood flow (hypoperfusion), small lesions, and lowered glucose absorption in the areas of the brain around the hypothalamus. The juncture between the temporal and parietal lobes (roughly above and slightly behind the ear) is also an area frequently found to be deficient in adequate blood supply. (This area corresponds to the part of the brain responsible for correlating complex sensory information.) Deficiencies and abnormalities have also been noted in the motor cortex, frontal lobe, and limbic system. Impairment of these areas of the brain produces a wide range of cognitive, emotional, and perceptual problems in people with CFIDS.

Cognitive Problems

LOSS OF CONCENTRATION. Loss of concentration is one of the most common—and serious—cognitive problems affecting people with CFIDS. Problems in this area can significantly affect work performance. One source of concentration problems is a loss of comprehension of either aural or visual information. The brain lags and either processes new information slowly or misses it entirely. When the input is aural, there seems to be loss of the initial orienting information. The person may be listening, but the information simply does not register; as a consequence, the person cannot focus or make sense of what follows. Sometimes a delay in processing results in longer pauses than usual before a verbal response is made. Processing delays can also produce a mistiming of conversational turn-taking resulting in interruptions and apparent non sequiturs. Often, information must be repeated several times before it registers.

Visual processing can also be significantly delayed. Material may have to be read many times before it is absorbed, and sometimes words in a sentence do not make sense, especially if the syntax is complicated or the meaning ambiguous. Reaction times may also be slowed. People may run red lights or disobey other traffic signs because the information does not register as fast as is required to act on it. Dr. Byron Hyde believes the loss of comprehension associated with CFIDS is due to a dysfunction in the area of the angular gyrus in the region of the left posterior (rear) parietal lobe, an area of the brain that processes and interprets both visual and aural information. However, dysfunction in the posterior temporal lobe also has been noted with some frequency.

SHORT-TERM MEMORY LOSS. The loss of short-term memory can present serious difficulties. People who forget why they came into a room may also forget where they are driving. People simply forget what they were doing and why. The problem can become so severe that people will not be able to finish a sentence. Memory loss can also manifest itself in loss of the ability to remember people's names or faces (facial agnosia). People with these problems may find it hard to identify friends, relatives, students, or coworkers, especially if they are called on to come up with an identification quickly; even the best known people and places can suddenly seem strange and unfamiliar. Problems with memory and learning are traditionally associated with dysfunction of the hippocampus, though other structures in and around the limbic system may also be involved.

MULTITASKING. Multiple-task sequencing is related to word sequencing. People with problems in multitasking may find it difficult to follow step-by-step instructions, prepare food from a recipe, or perform tasks that require a series of separate actions. Putting away objects held simultaneously, for example, a saltshaker and a stick of butter, may be impossible if the impairment is severe. People may also lose the ability to look up numbers in a telephone book or words in a dictionary. Children with CFIDS may be particularly shy of doing these tasks, forgetting alphabet order easily and finding it difficult to remember numbers in sequence. Younger children may experience significant problems in school as a result. Adults may also experience a similar decrease in learning ability, particularly if the information is complex. People with multitasking and simultaneous processing problems are, as a rule, easily distracted and need to keep input at a minimum when doing required or necessary tasks. They should not listen to the radio while driving. They should avoid conference telephone calls or meetings with several people. If crowds, malls, big events, and parties trigger symptoms, these environments should be avoided or a small area should be created in which the person can remain stationary while others circulate.

LINGUISTIC REVERSALS (PSEUDODYSLEXIA). People with CFIDS routinely structure linguistic elements backward. They commonly reverse word order, letter order (when typing or writing), initial sound order (when speaking), and even sentence order in a paragraph, resulting in a series of seemingly disconnected digressions rather than a logical flow of ideas. Any of these problems can stem from disruptions in the final stage of linguistic output, which are thought to occur in the supplemental motor area of the brain. This area, located deep within the central fold separating the two hemispheres, acts as a kind of holding area for final linguistic assembly. Problems there result in word, letter, and short-term ordering problems. Dysfunctions in the left temporal lobe (roughly above the left ear) also cause significant problems in linguistic production. True dyslexia and aphasia are the result of permanent damage to this area, which is why the temporary problems arising from CFIDS are referred to as "pseudo."

WORD SEARCHING (PSEUDOAPHASIA). Another linguistic problem for CFIDS patients is word searching. Commonly used words are hard to retrieve and, when they finally are uttered, may sound or even be wrong. Often a similar sounding word is substituted incorrectly for the "missing" word or a response may be completely inappropriate. The person speaking may not catch these errors, in some cases resulting in significant loss of communicative ability. Most of these retrieval problems are related to lack of blood flow to the left temporal lobe, the part of the brain responsible for most language-oriented tasks.

MATH PROBLEMS (DISCALCULIA). Problems with math are rife in the area of cognitive dysfunction. People have difficulty balancing checkbooks, following timetables, adding columns of figures, and especially subtracting. As a consequence, work that requires a lot of calculating, such as preparing taxes, can become so stressful that it can induce a relapse. People with CFIDS frequently wobble or fall during the Romberg test if they are also required to subtract by sevens from 100. Discalculia is associated with dysfunction in the temporal lobe.

TREATMENT TIPS

A number of approaches can be taken to improve cognitive symptoms. Drugs can be taken that act directly on neurotransmitters and the central nervous system (Klonopin, naphazoline, antidepressants). Another approach is to remedy the mechanical problem of low blood flow to the brain by increasing circulation. Drugs used for this purpose are primarily vasodilators, calcium channel blockers, and the beta blockers (nitroglycerin, nimodipine, atenolol). Pentoxifylline (Trental), a drug used to lower blood viscosity, can also increase blood flow to the brain, and reputedly helps alleviate short-term memory loss. For some cases of CFIDS, central nervous system stimulants such as Cylert or Ritalin can be helpful, as can Prozac or Wellbutrin. Herbs that increase blood flow, such as gingko, gotu kola, and bilberry, have also been used to enhance cognitive capacity. An important nutritional support is CoQ10.

An alternative approach involves enhancing brain function through cognitive rehabilitation. The brain's neurons are remarkably capable of regenerating dendrites. In other words, when individual cells are destroyed, others can take over their function, given the proper stimulus. Working with new or different learning techniques can restore much of the cognitive function lost in the acute stage of CFIDS. Biofeedback and meditation techniques are also reported to be effective in alleviating cognitive dysfunction.

SEE

- Chapter 4: Ampligen, Antidepressant Drugs, Beta Blockers, Calcium Channel Blockers, Central Nervous System Stimulants, Pentoxifylline.
- Chapter 5: CoQ10, Herbs, NADH, Vitamins.
- Chapter 6: Biofeedback, Meditation.

Emotional Problems

For people with CFIDS, emotional changes can be just as unsettling as the physical symptoms produced by the illness. The emotional swings that are typical in all stages of the illness can be difficult for both the person experiencing them and for the people around them. In the acute stages of CFIDS, strong, sometimes overwhelming, feelings can seemingly appear out of nowhere. Most people find these intense emotions highly disturbing, particularly when they are accompanied by severe physical and cognitive symptoms. In many cases, the emotions that accompany exacerbations of the illness are complicated by sensory and perceptual alterations, such as changes in vision and hearing, which may lend an air of unreality to the outside environment. Some people even report feelings of dissociation or a sense that they are watching themselves, as though in a movie.

When patients report these symptoms, it is all too common for the attending physician to recommend that the patient see a therapist or psychiatrist. Because people with CFIDS are already struggling with a disease that has just barely gained acceptance in the medical community, they are often offended by the suggestion. They may feel stigmatized or blame themselves for "creating" their illness. Many find that unless the sessions are conducted by a therapist who is knowledgeable about chronic illnesses, they are not particularly helpful. In some cases, an incorrect diagnosis such as depression or bipolar disorder may result. The reason therapy often fails is that the emotional roller coaster produced by the onset of CFIDS is as organic as the fever, swollen glands, low blood pressure, or any other measurable physiologic signs or symptoms attributable to an illness. Contrary to popular notions that "negative" emotions produce illness, CFIDS demonstrates the reverse (see Chapter 7).

The intense emotions characteristic of acute CFIDS, which include rage, terror, overwhelming grief, anxiety, depression, and guilt, are the result of the same mechanism that produces cognitive difficulties; that is, alteration in the normal functioning of the limbic system and related structures. It has long been known by neuroscientists that stimulation of one part of the hypothalamus produces rage, and electrical stimulation of the other side produces profound calm. This experiment was the impetus for Dr. Herbert Benson's landmark treatise, *The Relaxation Response,* a book that provides the foundation for many of the stress management techniques currently practiced by psychologists. The brain is not limited to these two rather primitive responses, however. Changes in neurotransmitter activity can cause depression (low serotonin levels), irritability (low followed by high serotonin levels), euphoria (high norepinephrine levels), and jitters or acute anxiety (excitatory neurotransmitters). High levels of vasopressin (a hormone produced by the hypothalamus) have been associated with the continual review of unpleasant experiences or memories typical of depression. The areas of the brain most affected by alterations in neurotransmitter activity are the limbic system, which functions, in part, as a processor of emotions, and the temporal lobe, in which emotion is joined to experience to facilitate memory formation. These are, of course, two of the areas most commonly affected by CFIDS.

That many of these emotional states are generated by the brain itself does not indicate that all emotions experienced by people with CFIDS can be attributed to neurologic dysfunction. Disturbances in the endocrine system that lead to hypoglycemia and hypothyroidism can also produce severe depression, and lethargy. Adrenal disturbances can cause panic and extreme anxiety. Irritation is often produced by the hormonal imbalances that accompany premenstrual syndrome (PMS), as are uncontrollable outbursts of rage and grief. Accompanying these psychophysiologic causes are the inevitable emotional upsets and frustrations that result from not having a functioning mind or body, losing a career or family, worrying about loss of income, and the threat of mortality. These may result in secondary, or reactive, depression, a mood disturbance due to a traumatic life event. Secondary depression can be just as devastating as primary (physiologic) depression and should be treated with the same seriousness.

Although it is important to remember that emotional states can be generated by purely organic (chemical) disturbances, it is equally important to keep in mind that the line between physiologic and psychological disturbance is not well established. In reality, the two are intertwined, each feeding into, supporting, and providing the basis for the other. Both need to be attended to in order to maintain a sense of emotional equilibrium.

TREATMENT TIPS

For the many fears, anxieties, and doubts that accompany any long-term illness, a situational counselor can be of great benefit. In general, someone who has had experience working with people with CFIDS will be more helpful than someone who has not. Psychologists who are unfamiliar with the illness will sometimes attribute the strong emotions produced by neuroendocrine disturbances to suppressed childhood events, such as abuse, neglect, or other stressful life experiences, and insist on psychotherapy. While these problems may occur coincidentally with CFIDS, it is important to remember that they are not the cause. During periods of acute or ongoing illness, advice on how to cope with the illness itself is much more useful. Support groups can alleviate much of the feeling of isolation that accompanies the illness and can provide comfort and solace. Severe depression should be treated with counseling, medication, or both. Drug treatments for depression usually center on antidepressants. While not everyone responds well to these drugs, some find them useful for alleviating depression and panic. Low doses of Prozac have been effective in treating the depression that accompanies PMS and hypersomnia. Zoloft and Paxil are two other antidepressants that have been recommended for treatment of CFIDS. Anxiety states are usually treated with very low doses of a benzodiazepine (Xanax or Valium) or other anxiolytic agents (BuSpar), always taking care to monitor for depression.

Herbal treatments include skullcap (for anxiety and jitters) and valerian (for anxiety). An important supplement for emotional stability is vitamin B complex. Patients with CFIDS have reported that vitamin B complex helps stabilize their mood, enabling them to handle stressful situations without so much upset. The amino acid arginine, sometimes recommended as a mood enhancer, should not be used to treat CFIDS because herpesviruses are replicated by arginine. Deprex, a homeopathic remedy for mood disorders and depression is also available (Vaxa International; 800-248-8292). Other remedies that have been effective in some people with CFIDS are controlled hyperventilation (deep breathing exercises, to assuage panic), meditation, autohypnosis, Bach remedies, and biofeedback.

Avoiding upsetting or stressful situations is also a good strategy to use whenever possible, especially in acute stages of the illness. Support from other people who have had CFIDS is invaluable for learning to cope with emotional swings and upsets. Once we begin to share our experiences with others, most of us find that we are not alone in what we feel. That, in itself, is one of the best therapies of all (see Chapter 7).

FURTHER READING

Courmel, Katie. A Companion Volume to Dr. Jay A. Goldstein's Betrayal by the Brain. Binghamton, N.Y.: Haworth Medical Press, 1996 (an easy-to-read companion guide and interpretation of Dr. Goldstein's work for the layperson).

Goldstein, Jay A. Betrayal by the Brain. Binghamton, N.Y.: Haworth Medical Press, 1996 (gives some valuable insights into the limbic system dysfunction characteristic of CFIDS).

Restak, Richard. The Brain. New York: Bantam, 1984.

Restak, Richard. The Receptors. New York: Bantam, 1994 (authoritative, insightful, and highly informative examination of the workings of neurotransmitters in the brain).

SEE

- Chapter 4: Antidepressant Drugs, Antihistamines, Benzodiazepines.
- Chapter 5: Amino Acids, Butyric Acid, Herbs, Vitamins.
- Chapter 6: Bach Remedies, Biofeedback, Hypnosis, Meditation.
- Chapter 7.

DIGESTIVE DISTURBANCES

The gastrointestinal tract is composed of a series of organs, all of which are involved in the processing of food. These include the esophagus, stomach, gallbladder, liver, and small and large intestines. For the most part, the actions of these organs are regulated by the nervous system.

Although the main function of the digestive system is food processing, the digestive tract has also been referred to as the "second brain" because of its broad interface with the nervous system. This involvement is so extensive that gastroenterologists have referred to the enteric nervous system as a separate facet of the autonomic nervous system. Neurotransmitters such as serotonin, which were formerly thought to be produced exclusively in the central nervous system, have been found in abundance in the intestines. The action of these neurotransmitters, along with other neurohormones, regulates the peristaltic action of the digestive organs, organizes the timing of the opening and closing of interorgan valves, determines the strength and frequency of contractions, and controls the release of digestive juices. Because the network of nerves (found on the inside of mucous membranes throughout the digestive tract) is responsible for the smooth functioning of these organs, any error or defect in the nervous system will lead to multiple problems, from the esophagus all the way to the rectum.

It is likely that many of the gastrointestinal difficulties manifested in people with CFIDS stem from nervous system problems. Because the stomach and intestines rely on the subtle interaction of the parasympathetic (mediated by the vagus nerve and the action of acetylcholine) and sympathetic (mediated by noradrenaline) nervous systems, any imbalance

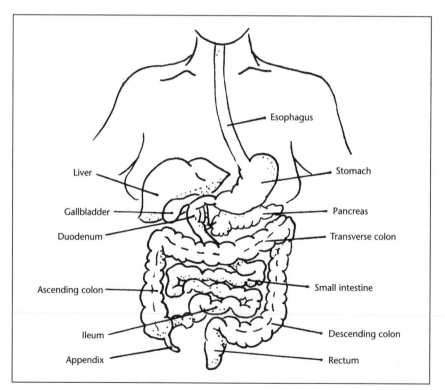

The Gastrointestinal Tract

in these systems inevitably results in faulty digestion. Indeed, as research has shown, people with CFIDS seem to have both poor vagus nerve tone and a disregulated sympathetic nervous system (as demonstrated by the irregular output of the adrenal glands). This may explain both the persistence and extent of gastrointestinal symptoms that plague more than 60% of the CFIDS population.

Esophagus

The esophagus is an 8- to 9-inch long tube that extends from the base of the throat, just below the Adam's apple, to the stomach. Its function is to transport food from the throat to the stomach by means of peristaltic action. The upper third of the esophagus consists of striated muscle, and the lower two thirds of smooth muscle. The two valves at the upper and lower ends of the esophagus (upper and lower esophageal sphincters, respectively) allow food to pass first into the esophagus, then out to the stomach. The lower valve also prevents reflux of corrosive stomach acid to the esophagus and throat. Problems with the esophagus can arise from faulty valve operation or from difficulties in the muscles responsible for peristalsis.

SPASM. One of the most distressing esophageal problems in CFIDS is the esophageal spasm. Because the spasm usually occurs in the center of the chest, the pain is often mistakenly attributed to the heart. An esophageal spasm can feel like a tight, pressure-like pain that sometimes radiates to the stomach or mid-back. Unlike cardiac pain, however, the pain does not radiate down the arms or increase after exertion. Esophageal spasms in the striated muscle portion of the esophagus produce a painful cramping sensation. Often spasms in the lower portion are painless but nonetheless disturbing. Spasms in this area are generally thought to be caused by an exaggerated motor response to peristalsis; that is, the esophagus contracts too much. Repeated spasms of this nature are referred to as diffuse esophageal spasms and are not uncommon in people with CFIDS.

Treatment of esophageal spasms is somewhat limited because the problem is usually not chronic. Muscle relaxants may help some who experience spasms in the upper esophagus, to diminish the force of the spasm. Avoiding foods that irritate the stomach also helps. Spasms in the lower part of the esophagus are sometimes caused by reflux. Carbonated drinks, acid foods, foods that are too hot or too cold, or indeed any food to which there is sensitivity may cause esophageal spasms. Even sudden changes in temperature, (for example, a hot shower) can trigger esophageal spasms in the sensitive individual. Emotional upset and stress can exacerbate this problem. Avoidance of esophageal stressors and general stress management programs (see Chapter 7) can help reduce the frequency and severity of esophageal spasms.

DIFFICULTY SWALLOWING (DYSPHAGIA). Dysphagia frequently is experienced in the acute or initial stage of CFIDS and during relapses. It is characterized by a complete inability to swallow, even if there is food in the mouth. The inability to swallow, although sometimes misdiagnosed as "anorexia," is not due to an aversion to food but, in most cases, can be attributed to sympathetic nervous system arousal typical of severe or acute CFIDS. The peristaltic action of the esophagus is governed by the vagus nerve, which acts in response to the release of acetylcholine through nerve endings in the esophageal muscle, resulting in the regular muscle contractions involved in swallowing. The sympathetic nervous system, mediated by the adrenal hormone noradrenaline (norepinephrine), produces the opposite effect, inhibiting the peristaltic action of the esophagus. When large amounts of adrenal hormones are released, as a result of stress or any other sympathetic nervous system arousal, it becomes difficult to swallow.

TREATMENT TIPS

People who have difficulty swallowing can benefit from any measure that calms the sympathetic nervous system (specifically, the adrenal glands). Sometimes a mild tranquilizer (see Chapter 4: Benzodiazepines) can help if the problem is severe. A calming tea, such as skullcap or valerian, can be used if tranquilizers are not tolerated (see Chapter 5: Herbs). A CFIDS specialist and gastroenterologist, Dr. Thomas Steinbach, recommends drinking 2 oz of warm water mixed with 1 teaspoon of apple cider vinegar to ease dysphagia caused by esophageal spasms.

Stomach

Heartburn and reflux can be caused by a lax lower esophageal sphincter or excess stomach acid. Heartburn associated with reflux can be prevented by changing posture, altering diet, and reducing stomach acidity. An extra pillow placed under the upper back while lying down tilts the stomach downward, preventing its contents from sloshing against the sphincter. Sitting up straight or bending slightly backward accomplishes the same function. Bending over or forward should be avoided when the stomach is full. In addition, products that relax sphincter pressure and relax smooth muscles, including alcohol, tobacco, coffee (even decaffeinated), peppermint, chocolate, garlic, and onions, should be restricted. Spicy, acid, and excessively sweet or salty foods can also irritate the esophagus and should be avoided. Fatty meals delay gastric emptying, which can lead to heartburn. Large meals can also aggravate the condition. Certain drugs and medications may also exacerbate heartburn. Among these are progesterone-containing oral contraceptives, aspirin, nonsteroidal anti-inflammatory drugs (NSAIDs), tricyclic antidepressants, and beta blockers.

Treatment with cholinergic drugs such as bethanechol (Urecholine) and methacholine (Mecholyl) can help increase peristaltic action and sphincter tone, but tend to produce small bowel and colon contractions, nausea, and diarrhea, and therefore should be used only if the problem is severe. In addition to preventive measures, most doctors recommend taking antacids after a meal (Tums or the laxative Milk of Magnesia, provided diarrhea is not a problem). If these are not available, small amounts of bicarbonate of soda (baking soda) in water can be taken, although intake should be limited to no more than a teaspoon a day to avoid upsetting the body's pH balance. Prilosec, a prescription medication that acts to reduce stomach acid, may also be recommended.

Conversely, it appears that heartburn symptoms can also be caused by too little stomach acid. Dr. James Balch, in *Prescription for Nutritional Healing,* notes that a number of people with chronic heartburn problems have found that taking a small amount of apple cider vinegar diluted in a little water actually helps relieve symptoms. If antacids do nothing to relieve symptoms or if they worsen them, a little apple cider vinegar might be helpful.

Excess stomach acid can also lead to heartburn, but of more concern is the possibility that the excess acid can lead to ulceration of the stomach lining. The initial treatment for excess acid is the same as for heartburn— avoid irritating or acid foods and take antacids. A bland diet consisting of easily digested, nonacidic, cooked foods and avoiding drugs that produce gastric irritation (aspirin, NSAIDs, opiates) are the usual recommendations. If the problem is severe, a drug that limits gastric secretion, such as cimetidine (Tagamet) or ranitidine (Zantac), will probably be prescribed. These work by blocking the effects of histamine in the stomach, thereby limiting gastric acid and pepsin secretion. If there is no evidence of ulcer, however, these drugs should be used cautiously because they interfere with digestion by limiting gastric secretion and may cause various side effects. For this reason, another drug, sucralfate (Sulcrate) is often prescribed for ulcers. Instead of limiting gastric secretion, it works to heal the damaged tissue of the ulcer. A derivative of licorice, DGL (available in health food stores), has been shown to be effective in healing stomach ulcers as well. Control of allergies can often help if excess acid production is due to allergies (histamine promotes gastric secretion) (see Allergies).

NAUSEA. Many people with CFIDS feel continually nauseous for months, regardless of what they eat and in the total absence of any easily recognizable infection.

Although nausea can arise spontaneously from factors associated with improper digestion, other causes should also be considered. Antibiotics, which radically alter intestinal flora, can produce severe nausea, as can antimicrobial agents (metronidazole), beta blockers, and other drugs commonly prescribed to treat CFIDS. Vertigo, carsickness, eye strain, migraine headaches, and systemic Candida infection also can produce nausea in CFIDS. Disruption of neurotransmitter levels can lead to nausea as well. Serotonin, one of the most versatile and widely distributed of the neurotransmitters, controls gastrointestinal smooth muscle contraction and the emesis reflex (vomiting).

TREATMENT TIPS

For quick relief of nausea, acupressure is sometimes helpful. A point on the inside of the wrist is used by acupuncturists to increase appetite and control nausea. To find it, place three fingers across the inside of the wrist, with the top finger placed just below the crease where the hand joins to the arm. The pressure point is at the middle of the arm, on the line where the bottom finger rests. Sometimes holding a thumb there can relieve nausea. Ginger is an herb that is effective for most cases of nausea. It can be chewed raw or in candied form or taken as ginger ale. Acidophilus bacteria may help relieve nausea related to Candida infection or intestinal flora imbalance. When nausea is accompanied by upset stomach, activated charcoal tablets can sometimes help (though these should be taken judiciously because they slow the absorption of nutrients from the intestines). The herb lemon grass, taken in a tea, is also excellent for calming the stomach. The antihistamine Antivert is also effective for treating nausea.

Small Intestine

The small intestine, which attaches to the stomach on one end and the large intestine on the other, is composed of three main segments: the duodenum, jejunum, and ileum. Bile from the liver and pancreatic enzymes enter the duodenum through their respective ducts, assisting in the further breakdown of food that stomach processes have begun. The jejunum is the longest segment of the small intestine and the most important as far as nutrient absorption is concerned. Water, minerals, and other nutrients are absorbed into the blood stream through the jejunum. Vitamin B_{12} and bile salts are absorbed through the ileum. The ileum, the distal portion of the small intestine, ends at the cecum, in the lower right quadrant of the abdomen.

PERMEABLE INTESTINE ("LEAKY GUT"). The small intestine, unlike the stomach, has a permeable mucous lining that serves as both a screen for unwanted material (notably, toxins) and a sieve for acceptable nutrients. If the mucosa becomes inflamed as a result of damage from bacterial or viral infection, allergic reactions, parasitic infections due to *Giardia lamblia*, chemotherapy, radiation, or environmental insults, the membrane becomes too permeable, allowing larger molecules to pass through. These larger molecules in turn excite the immune system, creating an allergic-like response to what would normally have been innocuous food by-products. Indeed, many researchers believe the faulty action of leaky gut is responsible for most food allergies. According to Dr. Paul Cheney, the vast majority of his patients with gastrointestinal symptoms have leaky gut as the primary underlying problem. The diagnosis of leaky gut is easy to make, requiring nothing more than a urine test performed after the patient has ingested a special sugar solution (Great Smokies Diagnostic Laboratory; 800-522-4762). The amount of sugar that passes into the urine is an indication of the permeability of the intestinal mucosa.

TREATMENT TIPS

- Secretory immunoglobulin A (IgA), the most abundant immunoglobulin in external secretions, is essential to maintain the normal function of the intestinal lining as an immune barrier. The synthesis of secretory IgA requires the amino acid L-glutamine. People with leaky gut can take L-glutamine as a supplement to support the production of secretory IgA or, if the amino acid is not tolerated (the side effect of depression counterindicates its use in some people), secretory IgA can be taken orally (Probioplex).

- *N*-acetyl-D-glucosamine (NAG) is a precursor in the synthesis of the proteins that form the outer layer of the mucous lining of the small intestine. Synthesis of NAG starts with L-glutamine, However, in some persons the conversion of L-glutamine to NAG is abnormal, resulting in a deficiency. In addition to serving as an important element in formation of the mucosa, NAG promotes development of beneficial bacteria and inhibits binding of Candida to the intestinal wall.
- Gamma-linoleic acid (GLA), found in borage seed oil and evening primrose oil, is an essential fatty acid that serves as a precursor to prostaglandin E_1 (PGE_1), an anti-inflammatory agent. In both animal and human studies, GLA protected the intestinal lining from damage caused by aspirin and other toxins. Most health food stores carry evening primrose oil and borage seed oil. A PGE_1 analogue can also be taken directly, in the form of the prescription drug Cytotec, which protects the mucous lining of the stomach and small intestine.
- Gamma-oryzanol (rice bran oil) is another well-tested product effective in treating many gastrointestinal disorders, including duodenal ulcers, chronic gastritis, irritable bowel syndrome, nausea, heartburn, abdominal pain, eructation, and diarrhea. Researchers have proposed that the broad action of gamma-oryzanol is a result of its function as a potent antioxidant as well as its ability to normalize vagus nerve stimulation of gastric secretion.
- Permeability Factors (Tyler Encapsulations; 800-869-9705) combines L-glutamine, NAG, GLA, and gamma-oryzanol. This product must be ordered by a health care professional.

Large Intestine

The colon is that part of the large intestine that extends from the cecum to the rectum. It is divided into three main segments: the ascending colon, located along the right side of the body; the transverse colon, which travels along the top of the abdomen; and the descending colon, which follows down the left side and then curves in to form the rectum. The hepatic and splenic flexures, named after the organs they are closest to (liver and spleen), form the "angles" of the large intestine; the rest is relatively straight, unlike the convoluted small intestine.

The large intestine is responsible for final stages of digestion, removal of excess water from digested food, and the formation of feces. All of these functions are aided by the presence of friendly bacteria, without which food could not be assimilated and processed. By the time the waste products (the remains of ingested food) are ready to be expelled, all that remains is water, bacteria, and undigested cellulose.

Problems in the large intestine are typified by the symptoms of irritable bowel syndrome and are rife in people with CFIDS. It is generally thought that these problems stem from faulty gut motility (that is, the rate at which the intestines propel food along is somehow out of sync), resulting in cramping, gas, bloating, nausea, increased appetite, constipation, or diarrhea. In CFIDS, symptoms like those of irritable bowel syndrome can be caused by sympathetic nervous system arousal, Candida overgrowth, viral infections, or food sensitivities.

GAS. Gas, which accumulates as a result of faulty digestion, is common in CFIDS. In the large intestine, gas tends to accumulate at the hepatic and splenic flexures, sometimes causing severe pain that radiates to the shoulders. Gas trapped at the hepatic flexure may cause such sharp pain that it precisely mimics a gallbladder attack or even a heart attack.

TREATMENT TIPS

Treatment of gas is, for the most part, preventive. Foods that cause gas, such as onions, cabbage, broccoli, cauliflower, brussel sprouts, milk (for those with lactose intolerance), and foods that are hard to digest (beans) or to which there are sensitivities should be avoided. Food should be chewed carefully and liquid should not be gulped with meals. If bloating and acidity occur immediately after eating, a little baking soda can help dispel gas before it descends to the intestines. Peppermint tea or peppermint products are also effective as are over-the-counter treatments for gas and indigestion.

DIARRHEA. Many people with CFIDS experience diarrhea. In some, it can be severe, requiring medical interventions such as cortisol injections. Diarrhea is basically caused by intestinal dysmotility. Intestinal motility consists of two kinds of contractions: segmental contraction, which mixes food, and propulsive contraction, which helps move the contents of the intestines forward. When propulsive contractions are too frequent or strong, food is passed along rapidly, resulting in diarrhea. Anything that causes the small intestines to become inflamed will produce diarrhea, as will a number of toxins (cholera, typhoid), viruses, parasites (Giardia, amoebas), and nervous system or endocrine disorders. Food sensitivities, particularly lactose (milk sugar) intolerance, can produce mild or intermittent diarrhea.

TREATMENT TIPS

If diarrhea is severe, a doctor may prescribe an antispasmodic medication to slow intestinal motility. Less severe cases may respond to over-the-counter antidiarrheal medications, but these are only stopgap measures, at best. If food sensitivities are suspected, an elimination diet may be helpful, avoiding the most common symptom-causing foods, such as milk, wheat, fructose and sorbitol (two sweeteners that often cause effects similar to lactose intolerance), citrus, and eggs. Certain drugs and medications can also cause diarrhea, so the medicine cabinet should be checked if diarrhea has started suddenly or worsened recently.

Hydration is essential during episodes of diarrhea. If you become dehydrated, check with your physician regarding rehydration with electrolye solutions. In the interim, liquid intake can be supplemented with water in which a little sugar has been dissolved or Pedialyte can be used.

CONSTIPATION. It is common for people with CFIDS to experience constipation at one time or another during the course of the illness. In many cases, the constipation is related to irritable bowel syndrome (implying that segmental contractions predominate over propulsive contractions). Limited diet, dehydration, and hypothyroidism also can lead to constipation.

Diet restrictions that limit the intake of fresh fruits and vegetables can result in a decrease of dietary roughage The absence of sufficient roughage creates a situation in which the bowel is not stimulated enough to produce regular contractions, resulting in slowed bowel motility, or constipation. Another common source of constipation in CFIDS is dehydration. The alteration in cell metabolism common in people with CFIDS (*CFIDS Chronicle,* Spring 1995) results in an increased tendency for anaerobic cell metabolism. Anaerobic cell metabolism requires more water than aerobic cell metabolism. If the extra water is not available, whether due to inadequate intake or mineral imbalances, dehydration results. As a person becomes dehydrated, more water is removed from the feces and stools become smaller, more compact, and more difficult to expel.

Constipation from diet restrictions or dehydration should improve with a small increase in dietary fiber. Psyllium husk can be taken in water or high-fiber cereals (such as Nutri-Grain) and whole grains can be eaten. Water intake should also be increased (a gallon a day is not too much). For those who can tolerate dried fruit, the old home remedy of a few prunes (or prune juice) is effective. Laxatives are generally not recommended by physicians for long-term use because they ultimately lead to dependence.

Gallbladder

The gallbladder is a small organ that hangs, like a partially blown up balloon, between the liver and duodenum. It acts as a receiving station for bile produced by the liver. Its main function is to release the bile so that fats may be digested. Problems with gallbladder function (such as obstructive stones) result in faulty processing of fats and the ensuing symptoms of nausea, belching, and intense pain in the upper right quadrant of the abdomen that radiates outward toward the side and back.

People with CFIDS, although rarely prone to gallstone development, do experience classic gallbladder pain. Radiographs, however, seldom show any mechanical or structural problem, even when attacks are severe. In some cases hyperkinesis is diagnosed, indicating only that the gallbladder seems to be producing spasms, with unclear cause. Gallbladder contractions are ultimately regulated by the autonomic nervous system. It is interesting to note that in several cases of gallbladder attacks in people with CFIDS in the Lake Tahoe epidemic, human herpesvirus 6 was found in gallbladder biopsy specimens.

TREATMENT TIPS

Gallbladder attacks can be alleviated somewhat by avoiding foods that stimulate the gallbladder (fatty meals and cold drinks). Pain can be alleviated by applying moist heat (compresses or hot water bottle) to the affected area. Some drugs can help regulate gallbladder spasms as well. Apple juice or olive oil flushes, two home remedies for gallstones, usually worsen the condition in people with CFIDS. In the case of severe or persistent symptoms, a consultation with a gastroenterologist is highly recommended.

Liver

The liver is a large organ that spans the region from the right inner ribs to the side of the rib cage, reaching nearly down to the waist. It produces bile, which breaks down fats, carbohydrates, and proteins; stores glycogen for the body's immediate energy needs; metabolizes toxins, drugs, and metabolic waste products such as ammonia; and aids in immune system function, in part by acting as a cleanup crew. Immune system complexes that have been engaged in battling invading viruses are transported through the blood stream to the liver. In the liver, macrophages devour what is left of the invaders, helping to escort immune-activating proteins from the body. In this way the liver serves two functions. It cleans out debris and helps the immune system downregulate itself.

Because of its intimate involvement in all facets of digestion, toxin elimination, and immune system function, the liver frequently suffers strain in CFIDS (although it should be mentioned that liver function tests usually yield normal results). Many people who experience pain or tenderness over the area of the liver (upper right quadrant) notice that a number of substances tend to aggravate it, including fats, alcohol, chocolate, allergens, and many pharmaceutical agents.

In addition to pain or discomfort over the liver, many people experience a peculiar malaise often described as feeling "poisoned." Even at its mildest, most people find this sensation intensely uncomfortable. In CFIDS, the poisoned feeling may be closely related to ischemic pain; that is, pain generated when the blood supply to an area is cut off. Metabolic waste products (such as ammonia and carbon dioxide) produced as a result of muscle use are normally removed through the circulatory system. When circulation is impaired, toxins build up and irritate nerve endings. The result is the tingling, uncomfortable sensation felt when circulation is restored to an area that has been temporarily cut off from normal blood flow. It has been proposed by Dr. Paul Cheney, Dr. Scott Rigden, and other clinicians that people with CFIDS generate greater quantities of metabolic waste products because of faulty carbohydrate metabolism (*CFIDS Chronicle,* Summer 1995). To compound the problem, elimination of these extra waste products proceeds slowly in people with sluggish liver function, leading to a state of general autointoxication, or self-poisoning.

TREATMENT TIPS

Milk thistle (or Silymarin) is an herb that possesses the unique quality of stimulating liver regeneration. A number of people with CFIDS report taking this herb to both protect the liver and enhance sluggish liver function. Dandelion root tea, a mild diuretic, can also be taken as a liver tonic. Sufficient intake of water is also recommended to flush toxins from the liver. Keeping the liver warm (warm baths or a hot water bottle) helps the liver function at greater efficiency. As in all bodily functions, heat speeds metabolic processes. Antioxidants (vitamin C, vitamin A, superoxide dismutase) and glutathione also help to reduce free-radical damage to liver tissue. The entero-hepatic resuscitation program may be helpful in restoring liver function in moderate to mild cases of CFIDS.

Resting definitely helps alleviate the "poisoned feeling," as does avoiding liver irritants. Activated charcoal can also be useful to absorb toxins. Any dietary or supplement regimens that help elimination would be beneficial. Drinking a lot of water most certainly helps. Remedies for leaky gut (butyric acid, Cytotec, and glutamine) are useful, as is alpha ketoglutarate, the citric acid cycle metabolite that aids in removing ammonia.

FURTHER READING

Guillory, Gerard. IBS: A Doctor's Plan for Chronic Digestive Troubles. Washington, D.C.: Hartley and Marks, 1991.

Thompson, W Grant. Gut Reactions: Understanding the Symptoms of the Digestive Tract. New York: Plenum Press, 1989.

SEE

• Chapter 4: Antihistamines, Cytotec, Tagamet and Zantac.
• Chapter 5: Alpha Ketoglutarate, Amino Acids, Antioxidants, Butyric Acid, Entero-Hepatic Resuscitation Program, Herbs (milk thistle), Vitamins.
• Chapter 6: Acupressure, Acupuncture, Aroma Therapy, Bed Rest.

DIZZINESS AND VERTIGO

Vertigo can add a very unsettling element to CFIDS. When the world suddenly turns sideways, starts spinning, or will not hold still, you cannot adjust. Simply lying in bed can be a Herculean task for people with severe vertigo, which, along with spatial disorientation, can produce nausea, headache, sweating, faintness, and feelings of panic. Many people with CFIDS experience vertigo as an inability to watch television or read. Others merely feel mild, transient dizziness.

Vertigo is thought to be caused by an inner ear problem. The function of the labyrinth, the part of the inner ear that controls balance, can be altered as a result of viral or bacterial infection (labyrinthitis), reduced blood supply to the ear, or conditions that affect the brain (such as stroke or migraine). Balance disorders can also be caused by eye problems. Optometrist Dr. Roderic W. Gillilan says motion sickness can be caused by sensitivity to rapid eye movements, particularly when seeing motion. His patients undergo a process of desensitization called "dynamic adaptive vision therapy," in which they relearn how to use their eyes. The problem of vertigo in CFIDS is probably related to viral labyrinthitis. According to Dr. Samuel Whitaker, an otologist at the University of California at Irvine, patients with CFIDS may have a viral infection of the inner ear that causes a balance defect. Dr. Whitaker examined 11 CFIDS patients with vertigo and found that all had a viral condition called "endolymphatic hydrops" (*CFIDS Chronicle,* Summer 1993). Patients with this condition are unable to adjust to the difference between what they are seeing and what their inner ear is telling them about their balance. They may *feel* their bed is on its side and clutch it so as not to fall off, even though they can see it is upright. This condition is probably caused by the reactivation of viruses found in most patients with CFIDS. Other causes of vertigo in CFIDS may be alterations in inner ear fluid pressure caused by allergies, Candida, infection, low blood pressure (neurally mediated hypotension), and sinus problems. Hypoglycemia can also cause light-headedness because it reduces glucose supplies to the brain. Some medications commonly prescribed to treat CFIDS (tricyclic antidepressants, for example) can cause vertigo. Patients who experience dizziness after starting a new medication should check with their doctor.

TREATMENT TIPS

Diamox, a diuretic normally used to treat cognitive disorders in CFIDS, may help alleviate inner ear problems because it reduces fluid pressure. Other blood pressure medications sometimes used in CFIDS (such as nitroglycerin and calcium channel blockers) may also help when ear problems are caused by excessive pressure. Antivert, an antihistamine, is commonly prescribed to treat vertigo. Dramamine or scopalamine may be prescribed if Antivert is not effective. It should be noted, however, that because medications containing scopalamine affect neurotransmission in the brain, they may produce unwanted psychological and neurologic side effects in people with CFIDS.

Herbs that increase blood circulation (gingko) may be beneficial for those who experience dizziness as a result of low blood pressure, poor circulation, or hypoglycemia. Vitamin B can often be helpful.

Dietary changes may help in some cases of vertigo. Too much salt or sugar can create pressure fluctuations in inner ear fluid. Reduction of salt has been helpful in treating Meniere's disease, an inner ear disorder characterized by vertigo, balance problems, and tinnitus. Reducing sugar helps alleviate hypoglycemia and Candida overgrowth.

MORE INFORMATION

Vestibular Disorders Association
1015 NW 22nd Avenue
Portland, OR 97201-3079
513-229-7705 (telephone)

FURTHER READING

The Doctor's Book of Home Remedies. Emmaus, Pa.: Rodale Press, 1990.

SEE

- Candida, Hypoglycemia.
- Chapter 4: Antihistamines, Calcium Channel Blockers, Diamox, Nitroglycerin.
- Chapter 5: Herbs, Vitamins.

ENDOCRINE DISTURBANCES

Thyroid

The thyroid is a butterfly-shaped gland located at the base of the neck just under the Adam's apple. It is directly regulated by the pituitary gland, which in turn receives instructions from the hypothalamus. Like those of the other hormone-secreting glands of the endocrine system, the thyroid's effects are far-reaching. The basic function of the thyroid gland is to regulate body metabolism (the rate at which the body uses calories to produce energy), which it accomplishes by secreting regulatory hormones. If the thyroid secretes excessive amounts of these hormones (hyperthyroidism), the body's metabolic rate increases, resulting in weight loss, nervousness, rapid heart beat, heat intolerance, rapid growth of hair and nails, and frequent bowel movements with soft stool. If too little of these hormones is secreted (hypothyroidism), the metabolic rate slows, resulting in weight gain, lethargy, cold intolerance, rough, dry skin and brittle nails and hair, and constipation.

Dr. Thomas Steinbach, a CFIDS specialist practicing in Houston, Texas, has found that 30% of his patients demonstrate thyroid dysfunction (as indicated by blood tests). The chief problem encountered in this group is decreased thyroid function, or hypothyroidism. The symptoms of hypothyroidism so closely match those of chronic CFIDS that in most cases patients have already undergone thyroid testing—a number of times in some cases—long before the diagnosis of CFIDS is considered. Symptoms of hypothyroidism typically include lethargy, weight gain, hair loss, constipation, edema (facial edema creates the puffy eyes characteristic of hypothyroidism), muscle soreness (due to water retention), memory loss, reproductive problems (infrequent ovulation, miscarriage, short menstrual cycles), and, in some patients, balance problems and difficulty walking. Although hypothyroidism can also result from viral infections, excessive iodine intake, certain medications (lithium), and radiation, the most common cause of hypothyroidism is chronic lymphocytic thyroiditis, or Hashimoto's disease. In Hashimoto's disease the thyroid becomes underactive as the result of an autoimmune response in which the immune system attacks thyroid gland tissue. The resulting inflammation (thyroiditis) impairs thyroid function. If thyroid dysfunction is the suspected cause of symptoms, blood tests can be performed to determine concentrations of thyroid-stimulating hormone (TSH), triiodothyronine (T_3), and thyroxine (T_4). Thyroid antibody testing is performed if Hashimoto's disease is suspected (confirmed by the presence of antibodies). In most people with CFIDS, test results are normal, which is not surprising because the thyroid problems are not due to primary thyroid failure but to disregulation of hypothalamic hormones, which control activity of the thyroid gland.

In *The Doctor's Guide to Chronic Fatigue Syndrome*, Dr. David Bell speculates that the excess cytokine production brought about by CFIDS could create functional impairment of the thyroid, not by altering the amounts of thyroid hormones but by blocking their effect. This type of hormone problem would not be detected by standard thyroid tests (nor would impairment of hypothalamic hormones that regulate thyroid function). When thyroid dysfunction is not the real cause of symptoms, the disorder is referred to as secondary (rather than primary) hypothyroidism. It appears that this is true in many people with CFIDS, especially those with either inconsistent hypothyroid symptoms or symptoms that fluctuate between those of hypothyroidism and hyperthyroidism (characterized in CFIDS by weight loss, insomnia, nervousness, intolerance to heat, rapid heart beat, tremor, and muscle weakness).

TREATMENT TIPS

Diagnosed hypothyroid conditions are usually treated with a thyroid hormone substitute (Synthroid or Levothroid). A naturopath may recommend kelp, thyroid gland extracts, or Armour thyroid. Certain foods should be avoided, such as kale, rutabaga, cabbage, and turnips, because they contain goitrogens (chemicals that can interfere with thyroid hormone production).

FURTHER READING

Wood, Lawrence. Your Thyroid: A Home Reference. Boston: Houghton Mifflin Co., 1982.

Adrenal Glands

The adrenal glands are small, almond-shaped glands located at the top of the kidneys. Their main function is to produce hormones that respond to and regulate the body's reaction to stress. The adrenal hormones produced in the inner part of the adrenal glands (medulla), adrenaline (epinephrine) and noradrenaline (norepinephrine), speed up the nervous system to produce the well-known "fight-or-flight" response. Those hormones produced by the outer part of the adrenal glands (cortex), the corticoid hormones, control water retention, inflammation, and immune system function.

The symptoms produced by adrenal dysfunction are among the more troublesome in CFIDS because they carry a sense of urgency or panic. Typical adrenal, or catecholamine, symptoms are rapid heart beat, chest pain, hyperventilation, and panic attacks. This set of symptoms indicates that too much adrenaline is being released into the body, overstimulating the sympathetic nervous system. Most acutely or severely ill people experience these symptoms frequently, particularly when under any kind of stress. Curiously, the opposing set of symptoms, or those related to underactive adrenal function, are also common in people with CFIDS. These include intolerance to cold and heat; lowered resistance to infections, toxic drugs, trauma, fatigue, and stress; hypoglycemia; low blood pressure; and eventually disturbance of electrolyte metabolism (excess excretion of sodium and retention of potassium).

Although these two problems seem very different, they are actually part of the same type of dysfunction that besets the thyroid. Like the thyroid, the adrenal glands are controlled by the pituitary gland and hypothalamus. By extension, the adrenal symptoms found in CFIDS do not really represent primary failure of the adrenal glands (as in Cushing's disease or Addison's disease) but are a consequence of brain signal abnormalities. Studies performed by Dr. Mark Demitrack and associates confirm that the main problem with adrenal hormone production in CFIDS arises from the hypothalamus (*Journal of Clinical Endocrinology and Metabolism,* 1991). It seems that the adrenal glands either underreact or overreact to stimuli, producing too much hormone when the stimulus is slight and none when the stimulus is great.

TREATMENT TIPS

Meditation, stress reduction exercises, and self-hypnosis can all be effective treatments. The hypothalamus responds to all kinds of input (psychological, emotional, sensory) and can be calmed or stimulated using these techniques. Other types of adrenal support include vitamin B_{12}, vitamin C, vitamin B_5 (pantothenic acid), zinc, and adrenocortical extract. The herbs astragalus and licorice have been used with some success to support adrenal function as well. Cortisone is sometimes administered to severely ill patients, although its use in CFIDS is controversial. In less severely ill patients, low doses of beta blockers may be recommended, accompanied by careful monitoring of blood pressure. Adrenal stimulants are usually recommended in mild cases only because they cause worsening of symptoms in the acutely ill.

SEE

- Chapter 4: Beta Blockers.
- Chapter 5: Herbs, Minerals, Vitamins.
- Chapter 6: Aroma Therapy, Biofeedback, Hypnosis, Meditation.
- Chapter 7.

FATIGUE

Virtually every person with CFIDS suffers from fatigue. The term "fatigue," however, does not do justice to what people with CFIDS actually experience. People with CFIDS often find themselves at a loss for words when it comes to describing how exhausted they feel. Patients come to doctors saying they feel "crushed," "totally wiped out," "comatose," or "paralyzed" or use descriptive phrases such as "I feel like I've been hit by a truck," "I can't get out of bed," or "I can't lift my toothbrush." The truth is that CFIDS fatigue is unique. In its severe form it can be all-encompassing, which can be devastating. It can rob a person of livelihood, family, career, hope, will, and feeling. In its mild form, fatigue is manifested as loss of energy or stamina. In either case, the terms currently available do not convey the profound loss of vitality produced by CFIDS exhaustion. More than an understatement, however, the word "fatigue" is misleading because its widespread use has led to a dismissive attitude on the part of the medical establishment, which views fatigue as a normal part of modern life.

There is nothing normal or natural about the fatigue experienced by people with CFIDS. Unlike the state of tiredness a person might feel after a busy day, the fatigue produced by CFIDS is not relieved by a good night's sleep, a workout, a protein snack, a change in lifestyle, a vacation, or any of the other measures that normally help the healthy person "recharge." The reason none of these measures work is self-evident. CFIDS fatigue is not the natural product of exertion. It is a reflection of the profound metabolic, neurologic, and immunologic dysfunction wrought by illness.

The definitive cause of CFIDS fatigue has not yet been established because the cause of the disease itself remains undetermined. However, there is ample evidence that the mechanisms of CFIDS, which are largely associated with immune system disregulation, contribute to the exhaustion that is the hallmark of CFIDS. The normal immune system response to disease that produces cytokines (especially, interleukin-1) not only generates fever and flu-like symptoms but also promotes slow (delta) wave activity in the brain. (Delta waves are normally found during deep sleep.) This type of immune activation leads to exhaustion in CFIDS, as in any illness. People with CFIDS also experience metabolic disregulation at the cellular level. With disturbance of the body's energy-producing processes, in particular, disruption of adenosine triphosphate (ATP) production, the body cannot recuperate, no matter how much will power is exerted.

Considering the lack of adequate terminology to describe CFIDS fatigue, it is incumbent on the CFIDS community—clinicians and patients alike—to find new terms and expressions to convey what is meant by "fatigue."

Postexertional Fatigue

Fatigue directly generated by exertion is one of the distinguishing features of CFIDS. In severe cases, any exertion (a shower, a trip to the store, or balancing the checkbook) can trigger fatigue. Although exercise is normally recommended to help alleviate tiredness, in CFIDS exercise not only exacerbates fatigue, it can bring on a general worsening of all symptoms. It is this distinctive feature that should alert the attentive physician to the presence of CFIDS.

The excessive fatigue that comes after exercise, or indeed any activity (usually peaking a day or two later), is directly related to metabolic responses that in CFIDS have gone awry. Normally, metabolic processes increase after exercise. Blood circulates faster; heart rate increases, providing more oxygen to muscle tissue; and cortisol is released. In CFIDS exercise seems to produce quite the reverse. Heart beat does not increase sufficiently to provide extra oxygen, leaving a person out of breath, tired, and, more crucial, without sufficient blood supply to the brain. Laboratory tests conducted on people with CFIDS have confirmed this deficit. Single-photon emission computed tomography (SPECT) scans obtained a day after exercise in people with CFIDS show widespread hypoperfusion of brain tissue. Endocrine tests reveal that cortisol concentrations also decrease, inhibiting release of glycogen stores from the liver. The resulting lowered oxygen levels prompt a switch from aerobic to anaerobic metabolism, creating lactic acid buildup and tissue acidosis. This will be felt a day later as stiff, aching muscles and general malaise.

It is likely that the subjective impression of having "hit the wall" that most people with CFIDS feel after even a little exercise is accurate. The body's energy needs are met through metabolic processes at the cellular level (in mitochondria for the most part). Citric acid is broken down by a long series of enzyme-mediated reactions (the Krebs cycle) to produce ATP, the cellular source of energy. If the Krebs cycle is interrupted, ATP is not formed and enough energy simply is not available. Interruptions in the Krebs cycle can be verified with a urine test (Organic Acids Test, Meta Metrix Labs; 770-446-5483). This test costs about $150 and can be ordered by a doctor. The results of the test indicate the point of disturbance in the Krebs cycle and identify the type of support specifically needed.

A number of therapies can alleviate fatigue. Some patients find that vitamin B_{12} and magnesium therapy help alleviate postexertional fatigue. CoQ10 and branched-chain amino acids also help increase energy and stamina. Primary therapies such as Kutapressin, Ampligen, and gamma globulin also improve postexertional fatigue. Above all, it is crucial to establish limits. In severely ill patients, any activity (visiting with friends, taking a shower, walking around the house) can produce the same symptoms as vigorous exercise. These patients should not attempt any exercise and should carefully monitor all activity. In milder cases, exertion should be curtailed (done for less time and interspersed with rest periods), modified (walking or swimming instead of running), and rigorously monitored for negative effects. In short, patients need to adjust their lifestyle according to the level of illness. It is of no benefit for people with CFIDS to push themselves beyond their limits. Quite the contrary, "push" inevitably leads to "crash," in many cases producing unnecessary relapses. During recovery, activity levels can be increased judiciously with rate of improvement, while making allowances for the ups and downs of CFIDS.

Lethargy

People with CFIDS often describe a kind of tiredness characterized by a feeling of heaviness, lassitude, sleepiness, slowness, and inability to do things. People who experience lethargy generally feel worst in the late afternoon or have trouble waking up in the morning. The feeling of lassitude or lethargy may be due to endocrine disturbances that create decreases in blood sugar (as indicated by lethargy before or shortly after meals or after not having eaten for several hours). Treatment for this type of fatigue includes chromium, Krebs cycle supports (such as alpha ketoglutarate, vitamin C, essential fatty acids, carnitine, CoQ10), a hypoglycemic diet (especially if fatigue or sleepiness is felt after meals), adrenal support, and rest.

Lucy Duchene, Ph.D., also points out that these symptoms can be caused by the edema and hypotension brought on by increased amounts of histamine released during allergic reactions (*CFIDS Chronicle,* Summer 1993). If you notice that fatigue increases during allergy seasons (fall, spring), treatments geared toward relieving allergies (antihistamines, vitamin C) may help relieve allergy-related fatigue. A feeling of weariness can also result from changes in blood pressure, cardiac arrhythmias, water retention, electrolyte imbalance, and, at the neurologic level, increased delta wave activity, all of which can be generated by excess amounts of histamine or by neurologic and endocrine disturbances (see Allergies, Cardiac and Cardiovascular Symptoms, Endocrine Disturbances).

Agitated Exhaustion

The term "agitated exhaustion" is used by Dr. David Bell in his book, *The Doctor's Guide to Chronic Fatigue Syndrome,* to characterize the type of fatigue typical of the acute stage of CFIDS and it describes very well the inability to "turn off" that the severely ill suffer. It is often described as a "tired and wired" feeling. A person with this type of fatigue does not feel sleepy, although the desire for rest is overwhelming. This type of exhaustion is usually accompanied by insomnia and catecholamine-related symptoms such as rapid pulse, hyperventilation, panic, and loss of appetite. The cause of this type of fatigue is thought to be neurologic. Dr. Paul Cheney puts forth a possible explanation for many of the neurologic upsets experienced in CFIDS (*CFIDS Chronicle,* Spring 1995). He proposes that toxins that accumulate in the brain as a result of cell dysfunction, liver toxicity, or excess cytokine production can lead to alterations in the normal firing pattern of neurons in the brain, resulting in a state of sustained neuronal arousal. In the state that Dr. Cheney describes, even small stimuli spark strong responses from the nervous system. The continued state of arousal characteristic of acute and severe CFIDS results in agitated exhaustion. Dr. Cheney points out that nearly every treatment that slows nervous system responsiveness aids in controlling neurologic symptoms, including benzodiazepines (Klonopin), magnesium, taurine, nimodipine (Nimotop), melatonin, calcium channel blockers, butyric acid (Butyrex), and gamma-aminobutyric acid (GABA). Meditation, hypnosis, acupuncture, and biofeedback can also provide help.

TREATMENT TIPS

Treatment for all kinds of fatigue should include lifestyle changes and adequate rest. Nutritional supplements that support the Krebs cycle give the body more energy at the cellular level. These include alpha ketoglutarate, essential fatty acids, carnitine, NAC, vitamin C, vitamin B complex, vitamin B_{12}, magnesium, CoQ10, branched-chain amino acids, and all food-based supplements. Other useful supplements include NADH, royal jelly, zinc, blue-green algae, DMG, and herbs such as astragalus.

For stable CFIDS, the occasional use of stimulants can be of benefit. Central nervous system stimulants (Ionamin, Cylert, and Ritalin) are sometimes recommended, as are antidepressants (Prozac, Zoloft, and Wellbutrin). Stimulants should be used with care, however, as overdose will only exacerbate the problem.

In essence, treating fatigue is treating CFIDS. Dr. Paul Cheney has noted that, in his experience, fatigue is the most difficult symptom to treat because it is so central to the disorder. He also makes the astute observation that fatigue may represent a defense response in sicker patients. "In this instance, excessive attention to the treatment of fatigue may actually worsen the patient's condition" *(CFIDS Chronicle,* Spring 1995). It might be well to keep this statement in mind before embarking on an aggressive program to combat CFIDS fatigue.

SEE

- Allergies, Candida, Cardiac and Cardiovascular Symptoms, Endocrine Disturbances, Hypoglycemia, Pain, Sleep Disorders.
- Chapter 4: Ampligen, Antihistamines, Benzodiazepines, Calcium Channel Blockers, Central Nervous System Stimulants, Gamma Globulin, Kutapressin.
- Chapter 5: Amino Acids, Blue-Green Algae, CoQ10, DHEA, Essential Fatty Acids, Herbs, Melatonin, Minerals (magnesium, zinc), NADH, Royal Jelly, Vitamins (vitamin B_{12}).
- Chapter 6: Bed Rest, Biofeedback, Exercise, Meditation.

FLU-LIKE SYMPTOMS

CFIDS has often been described as the flu that never ends. Flu symptoms such as achiness, sore throat, tender lymph nodes, fever, chills, and malaise have appeared in national and international case definitions of CFIDS and figure prominently in most doctors' descriptions of typical CFIDS. In some people, flu-like symptoms appear early in the illness and decrease markedly over time; others may manifest few or mild flu symptoms. However, in people who have a strong viral onset and an increased susceptibility to colds and flus, flu-like symptoms predominate throughout the illness. This seems to be especially true in young people. Flu symptoms can be confusing for people who catch "every bug that's going around." It is hard for them to determine whether they have a new ailment, such as strep throat, a cold, or flu, or are merely experiencing a relapse of CFIDS.

The presence of flu symptoms has been one of the primary motivations for attributing a viral cause to CFIDS. Even though researchers have so far been unable to isolate a single viral source for CFIDS, antiviral treatments have been used with success in some cases in which viral symptoms persist.

Sore Throat

Throat pain, scratchiness, and tenderness are typical of CFIDS. In children, sore throat tends to be most pronounced in the morning; in adults, it can appear at any time, but tends to worsen after exercise, exertion, or before relapses. Sometimes, even though the throat is not sore, it may feel "clogged" and require constant clearing. Many people take this as a sign of impending relapse and scale down their activities accordingly. Even when sore throat is severe, bacterial or viral cultures rarely reveal any infection. The throat itself may appear red or have characteristic "crimson crescents" around the tonsillar membranes of the upper throat at examination, but there is rarely pus or mucus. Dr. Burke Cunha suggests that the presence of these singular deep red crescents may be diagnostic of CFIDS because they have been noted in up to 90% of his patients (*CFIDS Chronicle*, Summer 1993).

Sometimes the more severely ill show signs of thrush, an oral Candida (yeast) infection. Thrush appears as a white lace-like coating of the tongue and cheeks that is hard to scrape off. Thrush is treated with prescription antifungals and home remedies such as lemon gargles and yogurt oral "swishes." (Candida, like fungus, will not grow in an acid medium, and the acidophilus in yogurt replaces Candida in its growing environment.)

Irritated, scratchy throat that results from dry mouth (dry eyes may also accompany this symptom) can be relieved by herb teas (slippery elm, mullein, sage) taken with honey. A simple home remedy if herbs are not available is hot lemon and honey tea to help coat the throat. Zinc lozenges, available at health food stores and some pharmacies, can help nip a sore throat in the bud. (Zinc should be consumed in very small quantities with food.) Sambucol, an herbal extract made from black elderberry, is also effective against sore throat. Vitamin C drips and gargles have been reported effective in relieving sore throat. Some people have reported cessation of sore throat after Kutapressin, gamma globulin, or acyclovir therapy.

Tender Lymph Nodes

Although lymph node tenderness was included in the original CFIDS case definition from the Centers for Disease Control and Prevention, Dr. David Bell in his book, *The Doctor's Guide to Chronic Fatigue Syndrome*, reports that only about 50% of his patients have tender lymph nodes. The lymph nodes in the front and back of the neck, armpits, elbows, and groin seem to be most frequently affected. Although the lymph nodes are rarely enlarged, they feel tender to the touch or sore on movement (for example, rolling the head back produces a tight tender feeling under the jaw). Dr. Paul Cheney has found that the left side is usually affected more than the right (*CFIDS Chronicle*, Spring 1995). The fact that most people with CFIDS can accurately identify most of the nodes in these areas (even if they are completely unaware of what they are identifying) should be enlightening to doctors who consider this symptom imaginary. The presence of lymph node pain, especially at onset, when it is most prominent, seems to indicate active involvement of the lymphatic system in CFIDS; that is, an infection is present. Lymph system involvement is typical in bacterial and viral infections (notably mononucleosis). The lymph system carries protein messages, or cytokines, which are released by T cells in an immune-activated state to aid in the mobilization of T and B cells. (These cells combat invading pathogens.) When lymph production is accelerated, the fluid backs up, causing tissue swelling (edema). It is significant that most of the lymph-related edema in CFIDS (including ear, tooth, and jaw pain; pain on the side of the neck; and tenderness of the lymph nodes) occurs on the left side because 90% of the lymph flows into the blood stream at a point just below the left collar bone (supraclavicular area). Dr. Cheney suspects that backup from the congested lymph system is responsible for these symptoms.

Fever and Chills

Low-grade fever (temperature, 100° F or less), often occurring in the afternoon or after exercise, is not unusual in people with CFIDS, although subnormal body temperature perhaps is more common. A resting temperature of 97° F or below, although rare in the general population, is quite common in severe CFIDS. Even more typical, although not commented on as often as fever, is abnormal daily temperature fluctuation, with a low of 97° F in the morning and a high around 99° F by afternoon. What is most unusual about these temperature variations is that the accompanying sensations are so exaggerated. A slight fever of less than a degree produces a feeling of intense heat. Temperature drops can produce a bone-chilling sensation of cold that no warm bath, hot tea, or pile of blankets can remedy. Most researchers agree that the variations in temperature experienced by people with CFIDS are typical of hypothalamic disregulation. Temperature variation tends to normalize during recuperation and can be one of the signs that recovery is under way.

Sweats

Night sweats and spontaneous daytime sweats unaccompanied by fever are typical of acute CFIDS, although they also can accompany relapses, hormonal changes, and even fluctuations in barometric pressure. Night sweats are a particular problem because they result in insomnia. It is difficult to sleep through night sweats. Many people have to get up in the night simply to change their nightclothes. Unlike the sweating associated with flu, both day and night sweats tend to be localized; that is, they affect only a limited part of the body, typically the upper torso and neck, although the legs, arms, and rib cage may also be affected. Some people also break into sweats when exposed for any length of time to electric lights, televisions, computer screens, or telephones. Sweating, like body temperature, is controlled by the hypothalamus and in all likelihood represents an aspect of the same neural disregulation that produces temperature fluctuations.

Night sweats are generally difficult to treat (although one CFIDS patient reports that the Bach flower remedy, scleranthus, helped her considerably). It helps to equip the bed with many light layers that can be easily thrown off and to wear absorbent cotton nightclothes. Some people find that a fan or opening a window at night is helpful.

TREATMENT TIPS

Primary antiviral and immunomodulatory therapies seem to have the greatest effect on flu-like symptoms. Many people who have persistent flu-like symptoms or repeated viral infections have reported success with Kutapressin, gamma globulin, and hydrotherapy.

SEE

- Chapter 4: Ampligen, Antiviral Agents, Cytotec, Gamma Globulin, Kutapressin.
- Chapter 5: Alpha Ketoglutarate, Amino Acids, Butyric Acid, Entero-Hepatic Resuscitation Program, Herbs, Vitamins.
- Chapter 6: Bach Remedies, Hydrotherapy.

HEADACHES

Headaches are common in CFIDS. Dr. Jay Goldstein estimates that some 75% of his patients with CFIDS experience headaches. Most of these patients report either worsening of previously experienced headaches or onset of a new type of headache, often described as "like nothing I've ever had before." As the brain has no pain receptors, the pain of a headache must be generated in the structures in and around the brain. These include the meninges (the membranes that encase the brain), the large arteries and venous sinuses of the brain, the cranial and cervical nerves that enervate the brain, and the scalp, face, and neck muscles. Headaches are the direct result of pressure, inflammation, traction, or displacement of any of these structures. Headaches can arise from a variety of sources, such as endocrine disturbances, neurologic disorders, and physical trauma, among others.

Migraine Headaches

A sudden change in arterial dilation produces the intense, throbbing pain of a migraine. The migraine headache is produced when a spasm develops in the carotid artery and the blood that is normally metabolized by the brain is released directly into the veins. The initial constriction of the artery produces the characteristic "aura," the zone of flashing, shining, or shimmering lights, that can precede a migraine by 15 to 30 minutes. The subsequent release of blood can cause severe pain, sometimes accompanied by nausea and vomiting. Migraines are usually one-sided (left or right) and can last for hours, sometimes days. The underlying cause of migraine is now considered to be neurologic. The muscles that control the shunt arteries responsible for releasing blood into the veins are controlled by the neurotransmitter serotonin. Changes in serotonin concentrations or function can lead to mistiming of the muscle contractions around the arteries. Migraines can be triggered by bright lights, strong odors, eye strain (from reading or watching television), emotional stress (which releases serotonin), changes in weather, and certain foods. Foods high in tyramine, a breakdown product of the amino acid tyrosine, can cause migraines, although the mechanism is not clear. Patients with headaches should take note if they have cystitis since the list of foods implicated in both disorders is the same (see Urinary Tract Problems). Some doctors suspect that tyrosine in food acts to initiate the release of norepinephrine (see Urinary Tract Problems for a list of foods high in tyramine). It is theorized that the release of norepinephrine (a vasoconstrictor) leads to reduced blood supply, but as the amount of circulating norepinephrine wanes, the blood vessels compensate by excessive dilation, producing headache. Other researchers believe that people who have migraines have difficulty metabolizing amines (amino acids, monoamines such as serotonin, nitrites, and MSG) due to deficiencies in the enzymes responsible for breaking down these substances. Because amines influence blood vessel diameter, their incomplete or slow breakdown can lead to problems in blood vessel control. All of these theories are relevant in CFIDS because neurochemicals (serotonin, norepinephrine, and amines) are related to many other CFIDS symptoms.

A preventive measure for migraines is to avoid triggering events and, at the first sign of an aura, to retire to a dark room and apply ice. Dr. Goldstein mentions that although Prozac can trigger headaches, it is sometimes also helpful to treat migraine, as are calcium channel blockers and tricyclic antidepressants (which increase levels of circulating serotonin). Imitrex and Diamox both are reported to be helpful in relieving the symptoms of migraine and pressure-type headaches. A new migraine medication, lidocaine drops (an inhalant), reportedly provides relief for some. (It should be noted, however, that many people with CFIDS do not find relief in the medications usually prescribed for migraine.) Some find meditation, stress-reduction exercises, and biofeedback useful tools for warding off impending migraine. Magnesium supplements may lessen the severity of premenstrual migraine, according to some researchers. In these cases it may be helpful for women to take magnesium supplements (360 mg three times a day) during the week before their period begins.

Sinus Headaches

Sinus headaches are common in people with allergies, but can also be caused by a cold, flu, or other secondary infections in people with low resistance. The sinus headache results from excessive mucus that is generated in the sinuses to either combat viral or allergic infection. When the sinuses are blocked, stuffed, or inflamed, the pressure creates a headache, with localized pain in the forehead accompanied by runny nose or postnasal drip. If neither of these last two symptoms is present, the sinus pain may not be due to sinus congestion but to nerve irritation. Because neurologic pain can run the entire length of a nerve, the source of this referred pain may be as far away as the back of the neck (see Sinusitis).

Tension Headaches

Dull, continual headaches are referred to as tension headaches, although they are not caused by anxiety, as the name might suggest. In CFIDS they seem to originate in the back of the neck or at the base of the skull and can travel around to the temples in a band of pain. Sometimes the pressure can be so intense that it feels as though the head is in a vise. In his book, *Could Your Doctor Be Wrong?*, Dr. Jay Goldstein states his belief that this type of headache is not generated by muscle tension, as has been previously thought, but by trigger points. The aggravation of the headache, he contends, is the result of the spreading pain brought on by the irritation of the trigger point, not by muscle contraction. Dr. Goldstein recommends that with this type of headache the patient should try to locate the trigger point. There may be two or three points on the edge of the trapezius muscle (which rises along the top of the shoulders when they are shrugged) that are tender to touch. The point implicated in headaches is the one closest to the neck. It can generate pain that spreads up the neck, along the side of the head, and around to a point just behind the eye. Other headache trigger points are located on the shoulder blades (levator scapulae) and jaw (masseter) muscles. Pain that seems to originate in the teeth and course up the side of the face may be mistakenly attributed to temporomandibular joint (TMJ) dysfunction when masseter trigger points are involved. (The masseter muscle is located about an inch in front of the earlobe and runs up to the top of the head, producing multiple trigger points.) Treatments for pressure headaches include localized heat or ice on back muscles (when trigger points are in the shoulder blades and trapezius muscle), use of a transcutaneous electrical nerve stimulator (TENS) unit, local gentle massage, acupuncture, and saline solution injections into trigger points, followed by stretching of the surrounding muscle. Some physical therapists have also recommended putting two tennis balls in a sock and resting the back of the neck on it to treat headaches associated with neck pain. One patient with serious headaches reported good results from using this technique. Drug treatments effective for tension headache include ibuprofen (Advil), Flexeril, and some of the benzodiazepines (Valium and Klonopin). Omega-3 and omega-6 essential fatty acids found in fish oils are good dietary supplements to help relieve muscle tension.

·   ·   ·

It should be noted that headaches can also be brought on by a decreased glucose supply to the brain (low blood sugar). This type of headache is characterized by a generalized, prickly ache over the top of the head, often accompanied by sleepiness. Hypoglycemic headaches can be relieved by eating and lying down (see Hypoglycemia).

TREATMENT TIPS

Although most people simply take aspirin or acetaminophen (Tylenol) to relieve the immediate pain of a headache, the usual over-the-counter oral medications do not seem to provide as prolonged or immediate relief in patients with CFIDS as they do in the general population. Some headache sufferers have mentioned that ibuprofen works best. Ice packs placed at the back of the neck seem to relieve eye pain associated with headaches. Gentle massage may be helpful, although deep or vigorous massage can make migraine worse. Pain management techniques such as meditation, hypnosis, relaxation methods, and breathing exercises, which have some effect in controlling vascular headache, have limited effect on muscle tension or trigger-point headache.

MORE INFORMATION

National Headache Foundation
800-843-2256 (toll-free telephone)

Migraine Trust, United Kingdom
071-278-2676 (telephone)

Migraine Foundation of Canada
416-920-4916 (telephone)

FURTHER READING

Rapoport, Alan, and Sheftell, Fred. Headache Relief. New York: Simon & Shuster, 1990 (discusses all types of headaches, their causes and effective treatments).

Wyckoff, Betsy. Overcoming Migraine. Barrytown, N.Y.: Station Hill Press, 1991 (a short, concise compilation of vascular headache treatments, including specific drug information, alternative treatments, and a list of headache clinics in the United States, Canada, the United Kingdom, and Australia).

SEE

- Allergies, Hypoglycemia, Pain, Sinusitis, Urinary Tract Problems.
- Chapter 4: Antihistamines, Calcium Channel Blockers, Diamox, Nitroglycerin, Pain Relievers.
- Chapter 5: Essential Fatty Acids, Minerals (magnesium).
- Chapter 6: Acupuncture, Biofeedback, Hypnosis, Massage, Meditation, TENS.
- Chapter 7.

HEARING PROBLEMS

Problems in the auditory system tend to be not as frequent or severe as visual problems, but can be very distracting. As many auditory problems are neurologic in origin, routine ear examinations nearly always yield normal findings.

Hyperacuity

One of the most frequent auditory problems reported in CFIDS is an intolerance to normal sound volume and range, particularly in the upper frequencies. Loud noises can generate a startle response in the acutely ill as well, producing rapid heart beat and flushing. People with CFIDS also find that multiple sound inputs become intolerable. A radio, television, and conversation occurring at the same time can produce profound discomfort.

Tinnitus

Ringing, buzzing, humming, clicking, hissing, popping, and squeaking noises generated in the ear rather than from any outside source are not unusual in CFIDS. Tinnitus can be caused by blocked eustachian tubes, which during periods of sinus congestion and colds become filled with fluid. People with allergies may find that they experience tinnitus during allergy season. Fluid retention in premenstrual syndrome (PMS) also can exacerbate tinnitus, as can increased blood flow to the area from exercise or vasodilators. Tinnitus can be caused by salicylates, notably aspirin, as well. Allergy-related tinnitus is usually treated with antihistamines. For other types, acupuncture and massage to release excess fluid sometimes provide relief. For some people, hypnosis can be effective. In most cases, however, tinnitus is so mild and transitory that it is left untreated.

Hearing Loss

Some people experience hearing loss in CFIDS. Sounds become muffled and indistinct. Sometimes only the high register is affected, making music sound curiously flat, as though a stereo channel were missing. The loss of auditory function, in most cases, is not related to ear problems, whether neurologic or mechanical, but to sinus congestion.

Pain

Sharp transient pain in the ears is not uncommon in CFIDS. Although the pain is severe, it rarely lasts more than a few seconds. Like many other ear symptoms, pain can be generated by increased pressure due to blocked fluid.

Itching

The left ear, in particular, seems to be susceptible to deep itching, which, because of its location, cannot be relieved. The itch and occasional accompanying pain do not, in most cases, signal the presence of an ear infection. The likeliest source of the itch is lymphatic fluid congestion. The lymph system drains at a point just above the left collar bone. If the fluid backs up, it can produce swelling along the left side of the neck, left-sided jaw and molar pain, and itching in the left ear.

TREATMENT TIPS

For pressure-type ear pain and associated headache, massaging a point about an inch in front of the earlobe seems to help. Placing a drop of a 50-50 mixture of hydrogen peroxide and alcohol in the ear canal (the home remedy for swimmer's ear) also helps relieve some of the pain associated with congested sinuses, as do antihistamines. Gingko, CoQ10, and some of the treatments used to alleviate dizziness can also be helpful in relieving some ear problems. Some people have reported success with "ear candles," an alternative treatment sold in some health food stores.

SEE

- Allergies, Dizziness and Vertigo.
- Chapter 4: Antihistamines.
- Chapter 5: CoQ10, Herbs (gingko).

HYPOGLYCEMIA

Hypoglycemia (low blood sugar) is fairly common in CFIDS patients. Our bodies need sugar to produce heat and energy. We normally obtain sugar from eating carbohydrates, such as grains, vegetables, potatoes, fruits, and beans. The complex carbohydrates found in vegetables and whole grains are slowly broken down to form simple sugar molecules (glucose), which are gradually absorbed through the wall of the small intestine and carried to the liver, where they are stored as glycogen. When the body needs sugar to increase energy output, operate muscles and organ systems, or produce warmth, the liver converts glycogen into its usable form, glucose, which is transported through the blood to any part of the body where it is needed. Because the need for glucose is almost constant (the brain is entirely fueled by glucose), blood sugar must remain fairly stable for the body to function normally. When glucose concentrations in the blood drop below the norm, the brain (via the pituitary and thyroid glands) signals the adrenal glands to release cortisol. Cortisol stimulates the liver to release more glycogen to raise the blood sugar level and keep it steady. If, however, a person experiences chronic or repeated dips in blood sugar levels, whether from excess intake of simple sugars or malfunction of any of the organs involved in glucose production and release, the adrenal glands become overtaxed and symptoms of low blood sugar develop. A sudden or prolonged decrease in blood sugar levels can cause sleepiness, faintness, muscle tremor, cold hands and feet, muscle pain, irritability, depression, anxiety, blurred vision, numbness, indigestion, vertigo, exhaustion, insomnia, hot flashes, carbohydrate craving, itching, nightmares, forgetfulness, ravenous hunger, moodiness, weakness in the legs, and heart palpitations. These could serve as a catalog of CFIDS symptoms were it not for the notable (and significant) absence of fever, sore throat, and lymph node tenderness.

In CFIDS, however, hypoglycemia is not the cause of the illness—although it may cause many symptoms—but the result of profound metabolic upset. If the normal functioning of the body requires adrenal hormones to keep the blood sugar level constant, reductions or excesses of these hormones will in themselves cause fluctuations in blood sugar levels. Because the adrenal glands rely on signals from the pituitary and thyroid, and ultimately the hypothalamus, a problem in any of these areas will affect renal production. The resulting fluctuations in blood sugar levels are the inevitable consequence of erratic adrenal function.

TREATMENT TIPS

For treating common hypoglycemia, doctors rely principally on dietary changes. In his book, *Hypoglycemia: A Better Approach,* Dr. Paavo Airola recommends frequent small meals high in complex carbohydrates and protein (to slow the metabolism of sugars) and avoidance of stimulants (coffee, tea, caffeinated drinks) and sweets (cookies, cakes, candies, alcohol, refined flour products, dried dates, juices, including carrot juice, and anything containing sugar). The flood of simple sugars into the system provokes a decrease in blood sugar levels. For people with CFIDS, following Dr. Airola's advice seems to help. During episodes of hypoglycemia, eat something as soon as possible and either sit or lie down until blood sugar level rises. Because homeostatic regulation is slow in CFIDS, this can take 15 to 20 minutes. Then get up and eat something substantial. In any event, do not go for more than 3 hours without eating something (carry food with you when you go out). Eat some whole grains and proteins at each meal. Avoid all sugars. *Do not fast.* Stress, emotional upset, and overexertion, because they stimulate adrenal output, exacerbate the symptoms of hypoglycemia. Thus, including stress reduction exercises as part of your daily routine will be helpful.

Supplements that can help include vitamin C (to normalize blood sugar and improve adrenal function), vitamin B complex (vitamins B_6, B_5, and B_{12}, in particular, are important to the adrenal, pancreas, and liver supports), magnesium (to aid in carbohydrate metabolism), calcium (for proper utilization of other minerals and vitamins), and chromium (to regulate blood sugar). An herb that is especially beneficial is licorice, long regarded by the Chinese as a powerful adrenal support and the "emperor" of all herbs.

SEE
• Chapter 5: Herbs (licorice), Minerals, Vitamins.

JOINT PAIN

In his book, *The Disease of a Thousand Names,* Dr. David Bell reports that some 65% of his patients with CFIDS experience joint pain (arthralgia). Joint pain for many is a prominent, recurring symptom. Arthralgia tends to affect the ankles, knees, elbows, shoulders, and sometimes hips. Arthralgia in CFIDS is migratory, transient, and can develop after many of the other CFIDS symptoms. Joint problems tend to predominate in children; some adults with CFIDS never experience them.

Because the pain is rarely accompanied by any swelling or redness, most doctors do not test for arthritic conditions or joint-related diseases. However, if pain and stiffness persist, the patient may be tested for any of a number of conditions that affect the joints, such as Lyme disease, rheumatoid arthritis, or lupus.

Lyme disease is a bacterial infection that, in its late stages, can produce inflammation in the large weight-bearing joints (knees and hips) as well as cause fatigue, problems with thinking, memory loss, and emotional changes. If results of the Lyme test are positive, the disease is treated with antibiotics.

Rheumatoid arthritis is an autoimmune disease that causes inflammation of the synovial membrane, the thin sheath that cushions and lubricates the joints. Rheumatoid arthritis tends to start in the small joints of the fingers (second and third), feet, and wrists and develops symmetrically, affecting both sides of the body similarly. Because rheumatoid arthritis is systemic, it can produce low-grade fever, fatigue, muscle achiness, weight loss, and depression, in addition to joint pain. In the early stages of rheumatoid arthritis there may be no visible swelling or redness. Therefore, patients with any of these symptoms should have a blood test for rheumatoid factor (RF), a test that is about 80% accurate in identifying rheumatoid arthritis. Rheumatoid arthritis is treated with anti-inflammatory drugs. It should be mentioned that a number of people with chronic infections (including CFIDS) also test positive for rheumatoid factor.

Systemic lupus erythematosus, an autoimmune disease that primarily affects women, causes joint pain in the hands, wrists, elbows, knees, and feet. Other characteristic symptoms include a red rash over the cheeks and nose, hair loss, photosensitivity, Raynaud's phenomenon, kidney problems, and depression. The initial test for lupus is the antinuclear antibody test (ANA), which, in 95% of all cases, will indicate whether an autoimmune process has developed. Lupus is treated with anti-inflammatory drugs. A few people with CFIDS also test positive for antinuclear antibodies.

Although true arthritis (involving swelling, redness, and heat around the joint) is uncommon in CFIDS, many of the symptoms that accompany arthritis are not.

Common Joint Problems

GELLING. Gelling is stiffness in the joints that develops after holding a position (usually sitting) for awhile. It is especially noticeable after sitting in positions that require bending of the joints, such as sitting cross-legged or holding a book up while lying in bed for more than 15 or 20 minutes without changing position. Gelling affects children as well as adults. The stiffness can be relieved with a few minutes of gentle movement of the affected joint.

PAIN. Joint pain tends to be sporadic and transitory and, in most cases, is asymmetric (occurs on one side of the body). The pain is most often felt in the soft tissue around the joint (knee pain, for example, is felt in the muscle above the knee and ankle pain in the top of the foot). Very rarely is the pain accompanied by swelling. However, any inflammation that develops should be examined by a physician (see Pain).

CARPAL TUNNEL SYNDROME. Dr. Jay Goldstein has noted that associated carpal tunnel syndrome is fairly common in CFIDS (*CFIDS Chronicle,* Fall 1992). In carpal tunnel syndrome the median nerve that supplies blood to half the hand is "pinched" by excess fluid accumulating in the area around it (the carpal tunnel). The pressure on the nerve causes tingling and numbness in the tips of the fingers and aching in the wrist that can spread up the forearm to the shoulder. The condition is exacerbated by putting any stress on the wrist. Dr. Karl Folkers, Director of the Institute of Biomedical Research at the University of Texas at Austin, believes that carpal tunnel syndrome is caused by a deficiency of vitamin B_6 and has observed that the symptoms nearly always disappear when vitamin B_6 supplementation is administered.

TREATMENT TIPS

Although many people do not treat joint pain specifically, those who do usually use over-the-counter nonsteroidal anti-inflammatory drugs (NSAIDs) and analgesics such as ibuprofen (Advil) or acetaminophen (Tylenol). More severe pain can be treated with narcotics (such as hydrocodone). Rheumatologists at Duke University Medical Center recommend that all of these medications should be used sparingly for joint conditions because of side effects and because the benefits of these drugs are usually so short-lived. Nutritionists recommend evening primrose oil (essential fatty acids), zinc, and vitamin B_6 for treatment of arthritic conditions. Gentle exercise such as rotation or other movement of the affected joint is also generally recommended for keeping good mobility. Acupuncture can sometimes ease the pain, as can transcutaneous electrical nerve stimulation (TENS). For people who suspect food allergies, a rotation diet and strict avoidance of offending foods (those of the nightshade family, in particular) can sometimes help prevent joint symptoms.

FURTHER READING

Pisetsky, David S. The Duke University Medical Center Book of Arthritis. New York: Fawcett Columbine, 1991.

SEE

- Chapter 4: Pain Relievers.
- Chapter 5: Essential Fatty Acids.
- Chapter 6: Acupuncture, TENS.
- Chapter 9.

LOSS OF LIBIDO

Although people with CFIDS rarely experience true sexual dysfunction (impotence, frigidity), loss of sexual desire is common, not just in severe cases but in mild cases as well. Loss of libido is a serious problem, not only because of curtailed sex life but because in some cases it leads to the loss of partners and spouses, which for many can be as devastating as the illness itself. Like most other symptoms, loss of sexual desire can be coped with, and even treated. Unlike every other symptom, however, coping with loss of libido requires the active involvement of two people.

In severe illness, the idea of lovemaking is simply beyond thought. Acute and severe CFIDS can produce such overwhelming physical effects (pain, especially) that the normal state of relaxation required for lovemaking is effectively eliminated. As one well spouse of a woman with CFIDS pointed out, "If my wife had advanced cancer, and I told the doctor that she had sexual problems because she didn't want to make love, he'd think I was nuts." The profound depression that often accompanies severe CFIDS also has the effect of limiting sexual accessibility. Even in mild CFIDS, in which physical symptoms are not incapacitating, the loss of sexual desire may represent a persistent, nagging problem.

Sexual desire, like all reproductive processes, is controlled by the sex hormones and neurotransmitters (dopamine, norepinephrine, acetylcholine, vasoactive intestinal peptide). Testosterone, the hormone that contributes to sexual "drive," is regulated by the endocrine system (which is adversely affected by the brain dysfunction typical of CFIDS). Testosterone is abundant in men but is also produced by women, especially around the time of ovulation. It is not surprising that many women feel the "urge" around that time of the month.

The neurotransmitters involved in sexual responses are numerous. In the early stage of arousal, acetylcholine and vasoactive intestinal peptide are released, signaling the parasympathetic nervous system to dilate blood vessels, decrease blood pressure, and, in men, start an erection. The vasodilating effects of early sexual arousal create a feeling of relaxation (which sometimes leads to sleepiness). Eventually dopamine and norepinephrine are released. These two neurochemicals stimulate the sympathetic nervous system. Heart rate increases, palms sweat, and blood vessels constrict. (Because of the excitatory effects of adrenal hormones, people with severe CFIDS usually find this stage of arousal overly stimulating and may feel ill as a result.) Histamine is also released, producing a flush. Release of oxytocin, a neuropeptide produced in the pituitary gland, is responsible for the muscle contractions that occur at climax. (Oxytocin is also credited with generating feelings of protectiveness, nurturance, and romance in people.)

It is not surprising that CFIDS causes disregulation of many of the hormones and neurochemicals that govern sexual responsiveness. The endocrine abnormalities discovered by Dr. Mark Demitrack and colleagues reveal both adrenal under- and overresponsiveness, resulting in altered production of adrenal hormones, in this case, norepinephrine (*Journal of Clinical Endocrinology and Metabolism,* 1991). Deficiencies in oxytocin and acetylcholine have also been found in people with CFIDS. With the general endocrine system upset and neurologic disregulation typical of CFIDS, problems with libido can be expected.

TREATMENT TIPS

Problems with libido are complex but can be effectively managed. The key to treating loss of libido is a thorough understanding of the problem. A firm belief on the part of both partners that the decreased sexual motivation is the result of illness rather than to loss of love can truly save a relationship. Counselors experienced with CFIDS may be able to offer invaluable help. A good counselor can help work out alternatives to previously established habits of emotional expression, appropriate ways to express sexuality during illness, and a means to open dialogue between partners in whom the frustration and despair of stymied intimacy may be long-standing.

Certain drugs can help increase libido. Most of these are stimulants and must be used with caution. Wellbutrin, an antidepressant, and the central nervous system stimulants Cylert and Ritalin all increase the amount of norepinephrine in the brain and concurrently act to increase sexual arousal. For those who are more severely ill, nondrug treatments may be effective. Vitamins, minerals (especially zinc), essential fatty acids, and the amino acids phenylalanine and tryptophan are vital in the formation and maintenance of the neurochemicals and hormones that produce sexual responsiveness. Look for foods high in these nutrients. Chocolate, the only food that contains a natural aphrodisiac, phenylethylamine, may be tolerated by some people with CFIDS. One patient with chronic CFIDS discovered that folic acid taken in combination with vitamin B_{12} alleviated libido problems.

The best remedy for loss of libido is recovery. Nevertheless, those still struggling with the illness need not despair. The best approach is to take advantage of it when it's there and not push things when it isn't. Sometimes just removing the stress of *having* to produce a response can act as a sexual stimulant. In all cases, remember there is no substitute for tender feelings, and these can be expressed any time when there is love and trust between two people.

MUSCLE PROBLEMS

Muscle-related problems are among the most frequently encountered symptoms in CFIDS, affecting approximately 80% of the CFIDS population. Although muscle pain, weakness, and tremor are common, their cause remains the subject of much debate.

Inflammatory muscle ailments that produce weakness and pain, such as polymyositis and polymyalgia rheumatica, although symptomatically similar, do not have much in common with the muscle problems generated by CFIDS. Some researchers have speculated that a virus affecting the nervous system, perhaps similar to poliovirus, may lie at the root of the overwhelming weakness characteristic of the acute stages of the illness. Although the similarity in muscle symptoms between post-polio syndrome and CFIDS is striking, no evidence of viral infection has been found in nerve or muscle tissue. Others have proposed that an alteration in protein metabolism in muscle cells may be at fault, yet there is very little evidence to support this view. The same is true for studies that examine enzyme levels and muscle tissue structure. Despite the lack of any definitive explanation for muscle problems, most CFIDS clinicians agree that the problem is either neurologic, like so many other CFIDS symptoms, or due to a mitochondrial dysfunction. Dr. Hirohiko Kuratsune and Dr. Audrius Plioplys have found in their own independent research that people with CFIDS demonstrate consistently depressed concentration of acylcarnitine (*CFIDS Chronicle,* Winter 1995). A deficiency in carnitine leads to the mitochondrial dysfunction that eventually causes muscle weakness.

Dr. Paul Cheney has proposed that in CFIDS, anaerobic cell metabolism predominates over aerobic cell metabolism (*CFIDS Chronicle,* Fall 1994; *CFIDS Chronicle,* Spring 1995). Unlike aerobic cell metabolism, which is fueled by circulating glucose (from carbohydrates) and oxygen, the much older process of anaerobic cell metabolism is fueled by stored glycogen and fructose. While the by-products of aerobic metabolism (carbon dioxide and water) are harmless, the by-products of the more inefficient anaerobic metabolism (lactic acid and ammonia) are not. Accumulation of these anaerobic toxins results in acidosis, which can produce a generalized deep ache and hard, stiff muscles.

Fibromyalgia

Dr. Dedra Buchwald, a physician from Seattle who conducted a long-term study of CFIDS patients, found that as many as 75% of these patients also had fibromyalgia. Fibromyalgia primarily affects women between the ages of 20 and 40 years. To date, this disorder has been diagnosed in 3 to 6 million patients in the United States, or 15% to 20% of all patients seen by rheumatologists. Of these, it is safe to conclude that many would also qualify for a diagnosis of CFIDS because of the similarity of symptoms. Despite the overlapping symptoms, however, it would be misleading to conclude that the two illnesses are the same because a subset of patients with fibromyalgia clearly suffer from a distinct illness.

Fibromyalgia, much like CFIDS, is a syndrome that has perplexed the medical community for decades. The cause of fibromyalgia has not yet been determined, but physicians have observed that it can be triggered by an injury or accident, infection, or sudden endocrine changes, such as childbirth. The predominant symptom in fibromyalgia is pain, although accompanying symptoms can include sleep disturbances, headaches, fatigue, and cognitive impairment. Typically, the pain waxes and wanes, but periods of physical exertion, illness, stress, and even changes in the weather may cause exacerbations. Pain is often localized in the muscles of the neck and upper back, although patients also report pain in the hands, lower back, thighs, shoulders, feet, and principal joints. A feeling of generalized achiness can accompany fibromyalgia, as can pain described as "burning," "stabbing," "throbbing," or "shooting." Prolonged periods of fibromyalgia pain can result in stiffness and exhaustion.

The diagnosis of fibromyalgia is based on a symptoms history and by the presence of tender points located on the surface of the body. There are 18 tender or "trigger" points that are commonly palpated to make a diagnosis, although the patient may feel pain in many other locations. Observable tenderness in 11 of 18 points can help confirm a diagnosis.

TREATMENT TIPS

The treatment of fibromyalgia is largely geared toward providing symptomatic relief. Rheumatologists commonly recommend nonsteroidal anti-inflammatory drugs (NSAIDs) for pain, as well as small doses of antidepressants or benzodiazepines to help with sleep disorders. (Often correcting an existing sleep disorder also diminishes pain.) Acupuncture, massage, and transcutaneous electrical nerve stimulation (TENS) are also effective, as are stress management techniques (meditation, self-hypnosis), to alleviate chronic pain. In severe cases, narcotics may be required to quell persistent pain. Many patients report success with supplements such as magnesium injections, malic acid, and essential fatty acids. Muscle relaxants can be used to help relax muscle knots and spasms associated with fibromyalgia.

MORE INFORMATION

Fibromyalgia Network
Box 31750
Tucson, AZ 85751-1750
800-853-2929 (toll-free telephone 8:00 AM to 5:00 PM Monday-Friday, Mountain time)
fmnetter@aol.com (e-mail)

FURTHER READING

Pellegrino, Mark J. The Fibromyalgia Survivor. Columbus, Ohio: Anadem Publishing, 1995.

Starlanyl, Devin, and Copeland, Mary Ellen. Fibromyalgia and Chronic Myofascial Pain Syndrome. Oakland, Calif.: New Harbinger Publications, 1996.

SEE

• Pain.
• Chapter 4: Antidepressant Drugs, Pain Relievers.
• Chapter 5: Essential Fatty Acids, Malic Acid, Minerals (magnesium).
• Chapter 6: Acupuncture, Massage, Meditation, TENS.

Spasm

Another type of muscle pain commonly found in CFIDS is the muscle spasm. Spasms commonly occur in the gluteal muscles (pyriform muscle spasm), producing what feels like sciatica; the diaphragm, esophagus, and intercostal muscles, leading to chest and rib cage pain; small muscles of the eyes and ears, resulting in eye and ear pain; and head, resulting in localized "spike" headaches.

TREATMENT TIPS

Muscle spasms are often relieved by taking magnesium supplements in elixir or injection form. Spasms also respond to Flexeril, supermalic, arnica gel, fish oil, evening primrose oil, and some of the benzodiazepines.

Weakness (Paresis)

The loss of muscle strength is common in severe cases of CFIDS and may persist well into recuperation. Sometimes the weakness may be so profound that a person is unable to get out of bed or must use a wheelchair. Weakness can be localized (arms, hands, legs, and neck) and can occur quite suddenly. Bouts of sudden weakness are often triggered by lifting (producing weakness in the legs), driving, or any form of weight-bearing exercise. In the very ill, even the amount of effort needed to maintain the weight of bedsheets, lift a toothbrush, or hold a telephone may be tremendous. Although some doctors have made the assumption that weakness in CFIDS is due to deconditioning, studies seem to indicate that in CFIDS muscle weakness is due to a malfunction in the nervous system. Muscle weakness comes on so suddenly in CFIDS, and so often in people who just days before becoming ill had been jogging, swimming, biking, hiking, dancing, and pursuing an active, healthy life, that it is irrational to attribute weakness to inactivity (although prolonged weakness may eventually result in deconditioning). Unlike poliomyelitis and other systemic illness, muscle weakness in CFIDS is not usually progressive. Doctors have noted that even people who have been bedridden or housebound for 1 or 2 years demonstrate a near-normal level of muscle strength, an observation that implies that CFIDS itself does not cause substantial muscle atrophy.

TREATMENT TIPS

Supplementation with carnitine has been reported to alleviate muscle weakness in many people with CFIDS. Other treatments for weakness include amantadine (Symmetrel), interferon, gamma globulin, magnesium, vitamin B_{12}, CoQ10, nitroglycerin, Prozac, antifungal agents, and Ampligen. It should be mentioned that, although antidepressants are commonly prescribed to relieve CFIDS symptoms, on occasion some of the tricyclic drugs can actually make muscle weakness worse. Patients who are taking antidepressants and experiencing increased muscle weakness should inform their doctor.

Tremor

Shaking of the arms, legs, and torso is not unusual in CFIDS, although it tends to pass within the first few months in most people. Tremor is most likely neurologic in origin. Even in those who do not experience overt shaking, a slight hesitation in movement, or "cogwheel" effect, has been observed by a number of physicians who attended CFIDS outbreaks in England and South Africa. Such hesitation is easily seen when a smooth, continuous motion is attempted, such as lowering an arm or leg from a raised position. As with twitches, disruption of normal basal ganglia function, whether from direct injury or disruption of the hypothalamus, causes tremor. Tremor is exacerbated by stress, tiredness, fasting, and decreases in blood sugar levels. A broad-spectrum nutritional supplement may help relieve this symptom considerably.

Loss of Coordination

Most people with CFIDS experience some aspect of coordination impairment. Unfortunately, people who drop things, break dishes, spill food on themselves, run into doorjambs, trip, or have difficulty negotiating stairs not only damage themselves, but have embarrassment to add to their long list of difficulties. A number of factors can contribute to clumsiness. Loss of muscle coordination is related to loss of strength. Sometimes the ability to coordinate muscles, which can lose strength suddenly and unpredictably, leads to dropping things. Impairment in depth-of-field vision and nervous system feedback (proprioception) can also lead to difficulty in judging distance, placement, and relative velocity. A person may underjudge the counter when placing a dish on it or overjudge a stair when placing a foot on it. Balance problems (ataxia), also quite common in CFIDS, may cause falling or tripping.

Twitches

Twitches (benign fasciculations) are common throughout the course of CFIDS. Twitches can occur in any body part (legs, arms, torso, face). They can occur continuously, sporadically, be widely distributed, or be confined to one area only (for example, the corner of an upper eyelid). Twitches increase with tiredness and decrease with rest. Research seems to indicate that twitches, like the loss of complex sequencing movements (as in speech), are due to a dysfunction of the basal ganglia. However, inasmuch as the nerve fibers that connect the basal ganglia to the cortex pass through the hypothalamus, disruption of hypothalamic function could just as well cause muscle symptoms. Twitches are also associated with a dysfunction of the cholinergic system. They are harmless in and of themselves and, although annoying, require no special treatment. Magnesium seems to reduce their frequency and extent.

SEE

- Hypoglycemia.
- Chapter 4: Ampligen, Antidepressant Drugs, Antifungal Agents, Antiviral Agents (amantadine), Benzodiazepines (Valium), Flexeril, Nitroglycerin, Pain Relievers.
- Chapter 5: Amino Acids (carnitine), Essential Fatty Acids (evening primrose oil, fish oils), Malic Acid, Minerals (magnesium), Vitamins.
- Chapter 6: Acupuncture, Hypnosis, Massage, Meditation, TENS.

ORAL PROBLEMS

Oral problems are common throughout the course of CFIDS. They can occur in the gums, teeth, joints, and muscles. Although oral problems can cause a great deal of pain, they are usually transient. Sometimes a toothache (particularly back molar) is so severe a person makes an appointment to have the tooth removed. Then the ache suddenly disappears completely (hopefully before the appointment is kept). Tooth pain, in particular, is notorious for coming and going, seemingly without reason. Its quixotic occurrence, however, is no reason to take it lightly. Dentists who count people with CFIDS among their patients have observed that gum problems are rife in this group. The many teeth complaints reported by people with CFIDS often are related to gum inflammation.

Fortunately, most common oral problems usually respond well to treatment.

Gums

Gingivitis is common in CFIDS. When food is chewed, small residues remain in the mouth and become trapped under the gums, causing them to become irritated. If the food particles are not removed, the gum becomes inflamed (gingivitis). Chronic inflammation can cause small pockets to form around the gums, leading to buildup of hardened plaque (tartar) under the gums. The gums respond to the tartar as they would to splinters. If the tartar is not removed, the gums eventually become diseased (periodontitis), and loss of teeth may ensue. Bad breath can be a sign of gum disease. If halitosis not related to sore throat, or upset stomach is a recurring problem, a trip to the dentist may be in order. In many cases, the inflammation can be caused by allergic reactions, viral infections, or poor circulation to the gums. Often gum inflammation is mistaken for a toothache. A person with frequent problems due to gum inflammation should keep his or her teeth and toothbrush clean and have teeth professionally cleaned every 3 months.

Teeth

Sensitivity to cold or heat is common in people with oral problems. This may be caused by increased nerve sensitivity. It is rarely a sign of incipient root problems, although the dry mouth experienced by many people with CFIDS can increase the risk of tooth decay. Tooth problems such as decay undermining a filling can exacerbate sore throat, headache, and jaw pain and should be attended to at once. Be aware, however, that people with CFIDS tend to react poorly to the epinephrine doctors and dentists add to anesthetics to make them last longer. Dr. Paul Cheney recommends requesting anesthetic without epinephrine, particularly for patients taking antidepressant medication (*Mass CFIDS Update,* Summer 1991).

Canker Sores

Canker sores are more the rule in children than in adults and can result from injury (a toothbrush or food scraping along the inside of the teeth) or infection in the mouth or throat. The sores look like small bumps with white heads. They can grow and are quite painful. To treat canker sores, sweets, starches, and milk products should be avoided and the mouth rinsed with hot salty water before and after each meal. With this regimen, canker sores usually disappear in a day or two. Lysine, an amino acid, and Zovirax, an antiviral agent, also are helpful in treating canker sores.

Temporomandibular Joint Syndrome

Temporomandibular joint (TMJ) syndrome in CFIDS is caused by muscle spasms or joint inflammation and only rarely by bite asymmetry. The muscles leading from the jaw to the top of the head are among the strongest in the body, a holdover from the days when our ancestors had to crack nuts between their teeth. When these muscles spasm, the result is severe, aching pain that extends from the jaw up the side of the head. The accompanying headache can be unbearable. People with this kind of pain often grind their teeth and may have nocturnal bruxism (teeth grinding during sleep). Sometimes opening the mouth wide stretches the muscles and helps relieve the pain of the spasm. Localized heat also helps relieve the pain. The lengthy (and expensive) bite readjustments recommended by dentists for TMJ are not usually helpful because the problem in CFIDS is seldom mechanical. Muscle relaxants, Flexeril, Klonopin, tranquilizers, herbal relaxants (valerian, skullcap), hypnosis, magnesium, massage, transcutaneous electrical nerve stimulation (TENS), and chiropractic are some ways in which TMJ has been alleviated in people with CFIDS.

Taste

The sense of taste is affected in CFIDS, making some foods taste bitter, metallic, or spoiled. Often the same foods eaten a few hours later taste fine. Alterations in taste are more frequent in the acute stage of CFIDS and during relapses. It has been speculated that changes in taste are largely due to limbic system disturbances, which affect the sense of smell. Children seem to be especially affected by alterations in taste and may become very picky eaters as a result.

TREATMENT TIPS

Oral hygiene is important to maintain healthy teeth. This is particularly relevant for people with gum problems. People with CFIDS should try to give their teeth a careful cleaning once a day with a toothbrush and dental floss. This can be accomplished in stages while sitting or even lying down. Using a soft, small-headed dry brush, gently rotate the bristles over and around the gum line of each tooth, about 10 times for each tooth. Start with the back molars and work around to the front. Then floss and rinse thoroughly. Even if you can only accomplish one cleaning a day, it will be sufficient to keep plaque from forming. Other times, rinsing with a warm saline solution after a brief brushing is all that is needed. After professional cleaning, it is wise to rinse the mouth and gargle three times a day with warm slightly salty water to help prevent infection. Frequent oral infections may be due to bacterial buildup on the toothbrush. Soaking the toothbrush in hydrogen peroxide kills any germs that may have collected in the bristles. After colds or other infections, it is best to replace the toothbrush with a new one. Natural cleaners that are good for the teeth and gums include baking soda (a mild abrasive; good for use by people sensitive to the ingredients in toothpaste), neem (a botanical gathered from the Neem tree in India; good for the gums), myrrh (an ancient herbal antiseptic available in health food stores; good for the gums). It should also be mentioned that the Japanese use CoQ10 to help cure gum disease.

Cautions
- Do not take antibiotics for gum problems unless a bona fide infection (with identified bacterium) can be verified. Antibiotics kill the bacteria needed for good oral ecology and may worsen gum problems in the long run (as will repeated rinsing with hydrogen peroxide).

- Try to avoid oral hygiene products that contain artificial colors, flavors, sweeteners, alcohol, or talc; these are often sources of gum irritation in people with CFIDS.
- Do not have all your fillings removed to eliminate potential leakage of mercury. While mercury poisoning resembles CFIDS in many ways, the two should not be confused. Elimination of numerous fillings is expensive, laborious, and thoroughly stressful, requiring use of anesthetics and other chemical substances that may cause harmful effects to a compromised immune system. Patients with silver amalgam fillings who believe their removal may be helpful should first have a hair test to check for elevated mercury concentration; then have the fillings removed over time taking care not to release mercury-containing filling fragments into the mouth (dentists use a rubber dam for this purpose). Be forewarned that, although mercury is certainly toxic, it is not likely that the small quantity of mercury that can leak from fillings will cause the myriad, persevering symptoms of CFIDS. The small number of people with CFIDS who have had fillings removed have not reported improvement. A few have felt worse for days to several weeks afterward because of the exhausting nature of extensive filling removal and replacement.

PAIN

Pain is nearly universal in CFIDS, although the frequency and degree may vary enormously. However, pain as a predominant symptom may overshadow all others. The deep, burning, relentless pain felt by so many people with CFIDS can be unbearable. Pain can also become a source of great frustration when its source is not clear. Doctors who do not see any cause for pain may dismiss the experience as "all in your head" or refer you to a psychiatrist, a situation deeply distressing for patients with chronic pain.

The experience of pain is completely subjective. Pain cannot be measured objectively, nor can pain levels be predicted by standard judgments of injury or trauma. The mechanism through which people feel pain is neurologic. Pain receptors in the skin (substance P, prostaglandins, bradykinin) respond to stresses such as heat, pressure, and tissue injury and relay pain messages to the brain through the nerves. The pain signal is eventually relayed to the thalamus, where it is differentiated into heat, cold, or pressure pain. The degree of pain a person feels after receiving the stimulus (the pain threshold) is completely individual and depends on the extent to which chemical messengers that relay the pain signals to the thalamus are counteracted by endorphins. Endorphins, which are chemically similar to morphine, are the body's own painkillers. When few endorphins are released, the experience of pain is much greater.

The origins of chronic pain in CFIDS are thought to be neurologic, either generated by increased irritability of the central nervous system, leading to overproduction of pain message chemicals (substance P has been implicated in fibromyalgia), to lack of counterregulation by endorphins, or excitement of the thalamus (damage to the thalamus can produce chronic burning pain). The increase in cytokine production (notably alpha interferon) that accompanies CFIDS further complicates matters because interferon binds to opioid receptors, making it more difficult for endorphins to block pain.

The principal areas in which chronic or recurring pain is experienced in CFIDS are muscles, joints, head, and digestive system organs (see specific discussions for additional information).

TREATMENT TIPS

Pain is such an essential and primeval part of our physiologic and emotional makeup that it is literally impossible to ignore. Chronic pain is incapacitating and may lead to the feeling that life is no longer worth living. Therefore, treatment of pain should not be neglected.

- Pharmaceutical pain treatments usually recommended for people with CFIDS include nonsteroidal anti-inflammatory drugs (NSAIDs), acetaminophen (Tylenol), Ultram, and narcotic agents. A number of people have also reported pain relief with use of antidepressant drugs, calcium channel blockers, nitroglycerin, Diamox, and Vistaril.
- Supplements that have been reported helpful in controlling pain in CFIDS include malic acid, magnesium, and evening primrose oil.
- Manual techniques for relieving pain include gentle massage, chiropractic, transcutaneous electrical nerve stimulation (TENS), low level laser therapy, and acupuncture.
- Effective mind-body techniques that alleviate neurologic pain include hypnosis, meditation and relaxation techniques, and biofeedback.

An interesting observation about an unusual treatment for protracted pain was made by a former marathon runner with CFIDS who experienced relentless, severe pain. A single shot of Demerol, given in the context of a medical procedure, relieved her pain for 8 months. She believes that the drug broke the neurologic cycle of pain. When strong measures are indicated, this type of treatment may be worth consideration.

SEE
- Digestive Disturbances, Headaches, Joint Pain, Muscle Problems.
- Chapter 4: Antidepressant Drugs, Calcium Channel Blockers, Diamox, Nitroglycerin, Pain Relievers.
- Chapter 5: Essential Fatty Acids, Malic Acid, Minerals (magnesium).
- Chapter 6: Acupuncture, Biofeedback, Chiropractic, Hypnosis, Massage, TENS.
- Chapter 7.

PREMENSTRUAL SYNDROME

Premenstrual syndrome (PMS) is a common hormonal disturbance that affects 70% to 90% of women in the United States at one time or another during their reproductive lives, according to Harvard professor and gynecologist Dr. Joseph Mortola. However, only 40% of women with PMS experience monthly symptoms. PMS can produce a plethora of symptoms, including weight gain, backache, acne, breast tenderness, sore throat, joint pain, swollen ankles, insomnia, cravings for sweets and starches, headache, irritability, anxiety, fatigue, lethargy, depression, and cystitis, among others. In some women, a few of these symptoms may predominate. For example, in some women PMS is manifested as profound depression or outbursts of temper. Others experience weight gain, breast pain, and edema primarily. Although PMS may constitute nothing more than minor aggravation for some, in about 10% of the women who experience PMS, symptoms can be overwhelming, necessitating treatment of some kind. In the CFIDS population this percentage may be higher. Many women with CFIDS report either new onset of PMS or a sudden worsening of symptoms. In addition, a number of women with CFIDS bear a double burden because they not only experience PMS symptoms but an exacerbation of CFIDS symptoms during this time as well.

There are three main patterns typical of PMS: (1) symptoms appear at ovulation (about 14 days before menstruation) and do not diminish until the end of menstruation; (2) symptoms appear at ovulation, then ease, only to reappear a few days before menstruation; and (3) symptoms appear a few days before menstruation and ease at onset. In all cases, the time after menstruation and before ovulation brings relief. For women with the first pattern this relief may occur for a scant week. PMS is not limited to one or another of these patterns, and women may experience several, depending on the severity of the illness.

PMS is generally attributed to an imbalance in the hormones responsible for the onset of the luteal (post-ovulation) phase of the menstrual cycle. The delicate orchestration of the hormones produced by the hypothalamus, pituitary gland, and ovaries enables the complex processes of fertility that occur at ovulation. At ovulation, a woman experiences a surge of luteinizing hormone (LH) from the pituitary gland, which signals an egg to make its journey from the fallopian tube to the uterus. At that point, the two primary female hormones, estrogen and progesterone, are released, signaling the pituitary to stop producing luteinizing hormone. Levels of these hormones remain high until just before the onset of menstruation, when their sudden drop allows the lining of the uterus to slough off and menstruation begins. In some women the levels of hormones responsible for the processes involved in ovulation and menstruation do not operate in concert. As noted earlier by Dr. Leon Israel (*Journal of the American Medical Association,* 1938) and more recently by Dr. Katherine Dalton, many women who experience the myriad symptoms associated with PMS have an inadequate amount of progesterone during the luteal phase. They believe the overabundance of estrogen in relation to progesterone causes PMS. However, hormonal deficiencies may not be the only precipitating factor. Sensitivity to some hormones, even in normal amounts, can cause symptoms in some women. And, it is important to remember that the endocrine hormones have effects on the immune system as well.

Estrogen receptors have been found in both animal and human thymus tissue, indicating a direct relationship between the immune system and the female sex hormone. Indeed, in a number of studies, estrogen generally depressed cell-mediated immunity (T cell function), even while elevating antibody responses to some antigens. This means allergic responses increase in the luteal phase, as cell-mediated immunity decreases. Estrogen also reduces natural killer cell activity, aids in the secretion of interleukin-1 and interleukin-6, and can influence the action of CD8 antigen, or T suppressor cells. These, in turn, have direct effects on hypothalamic and nervous system function. It is interesting that estrogen seems to be related to many of the prominent immune system abnormalities found in CFIDS.

In PMS, like CFIDS, the complex interaction between the immune, endocrine, and nervous systems has gone awry. In the light of these findings, it should not be surprising that autoimmune diseases predominate in women.

TREATMENT TIPS

PMS treatment varies according to the type and severity of symptoms.
- Vitamin supplementation is widely used for PMS in which depression and irritability predominate. Because vitamin B deficiency can cause overproduction of estrogen, supplementation with vitamin B complex accompanied by an additional dose of vitamin B_6 (pyridoxine) may be useful. Pyridoxine is usually administered in doses smaller than 100 mg to avert peripheral nerve injury (characterized by tingling in the extremities). The P5P form is the most easily absorbed. Vitamin A is reputed to be helpful for PMS-related agitation and insomnia, but as of yet no studies support these claims. Optivite, a supplement developed especially for women with PMS, is available in health food stores.
- Small doses of Prozac taken a few days before menstruation have been reported to ease PMS-related depression.
- Magnesium may be useful for alleviating mood swings, muscle aches, nervous tension, bloating, and breast tenderness. Dr. Guy Abraham and associates have directed studies in Los Angeles that show that women with PMS have lower levels of magnesium than those who do not. Whole grains, green leafy vegetables, legumes, seeds, shellfish, and mangoes all have high amounts of magnesium. Incidentally, so does chocolate, which may explain why so many women with PMS crave chocolate. Magnesium supplements of up to 360 mg can be taken.
- For sweet and carbohydrate cravings, edema, and hypoglycemia-type symptoms, a modified hypoglycemic diet seems helpful. Dr. Ronald Norris, senior consultant to the PMS Program, Inc., in Chapel Hill, North Carolina, recommends eating six small meals a day and limiting total protein intake to 20% of total daily calories. He also recommends increasing complex carbohydrates, eliminating sugar and refined carbohydrates, and reducing salt.
- Increasing intake of linoleic acid (found in safflower oil, evening primrose oil, borage oil, and linseed oil) can help reduce edema,

cravings for sweets, and blood sugar–related problems. Results are fairly rapid (1 to 3 months).

- Cutting back on salt and drinking diuretic herbal teas (cornsilk, for example) can help relieve edema.
- For severe PMS, Dr. Norris recommends a direct hormonal approach. He administers progesterone to women in whom deficiency of this hormone is implicated. He cautions that progesterone must be administered in its pure form (identical to the progesterone produced naturally in the body) to avoid side effects. The cream Progest (Transitions for Health; 800-888-6814) is also used by some alternative health care practitioners to the same end. Progest includes among its ingredients Mexican wild yam, a plant that contains a naturally occurring progesterone. Application of the cream, starting at ovulation, seems to help some women with PMS symptoms. Most alternative health care practitioners recommend taking evening primrose oil along with using the cream.
- The Chinese herb Dong Quai is reputed to have a positive effect in female hormone balance.
- Antihistamines seem to alleviate some PMS symptoms in women who are prone to allergies. It could be that, because allergies exacerbate PMS, antihistamines act to reduce the compounding effects of histamine on related PMS symptoms.
- Last, but not least, women with PMS should keep a calendar of their cycle. From ovulation to menstruation they are more susceptible to allergic reactions, less tolerant of stress, and much less capable of handling emotional upset. The second half of the cycle is not the optimal time to schedule stressful meetings, try new treatments, or make major changes in a relationship. An awareness of when PMS occurs makes it possible to at least avoid known pitfalls.

FURTHER READING

Lauersen, Niels H, and Stukane, Eileen. PMS and You: What It Is, How to Recognize It, and How to Overcome It. New York: Simon & Schuster, 1983.

Norris, Ronald V, with Sullivan, Colleen. PMS/Premenstrual Syndrome. New York: Rawson Associates, 1983.

SEE

- Chapter 4: Antidepressant Drugs, Antihistamines.
- Chapter 5: Essential Fatty Acids, Herbs, Minerals, Vitamins.
- Chapter 6: Acupuncture.

SECONDARY INFECTIONS

Increased susceptibility to secondary infections is a problem for a significant proportion of the CFIDS population. (About a third of CFIDS patients, however, report that they "never catch anything.") Some people find that during flu season they inevitably contract whatever "bug" is going around. In addition to catching the seasonal varieties of colds and flu, they also are more susceptible to other kinds of infections, such as upper respiratory tract or urinary tract infections, topical fungal infections, and recurring shingles. As if to add insult to injury, all of these infections last longer, occur more frequently, and, worst of all, may spark CFIDS relapses, usually concurrently or just after the initial infection. This is true even in cases in which prior immunity has been established. Different people tend to have different sensitivities. One may be plagued with recurring upper respiratory tract infections (particularly common in children) and another may have frequent bladder infections. Many infections seem to affect historically weak areas, that is, areas that have in the past been prone to infection or injury. Former smokers often develop respiratory tract infections, those with a history of allergies have an inordinate number of sinus infections, and those who have had many bladder problems may develop interstitial cystitis. The primary cause of recurring infections seems to be linked to immune system disregulation.

Researchers in this area agree that people with CFIDS suffer from a variety of immune system malfunctions. Most of the immune system testing that has been done over the past decade has revealed a number of immune system abnormalities, including low numbers of natural killer cells, excess cytokine production (alpha interferon, interleukins, and tumor necrosis factor), and lowered cell-mediated immunity. Unlike many other immune-related ailments, however, CFIDS does not seem to affect the immune system consistently. Dr. James McCoy, cancer and CFIDS researcher in Baton Rouge, Louisiana, has found that CFIDS patients tend to have fluctuating B and T cell proliferation rates; that is, immune system cells tend to multiply either faster or slower than normal (this type of measurement would relate to the actual function of the immune system more than to mere cell count). For example, B cells may replicate at an abnormally high rate during one stage of the illness, while T cells do not. The converse may be true at a different stage. It is not only possible, but likely, that a person with CFIDS will have several immune system changes over the course of the illness, at times with symptoms associated with lowered immunity (increased susceptibility to flu) and at other times with symptoms associated with a heightened immune system response (*CFIDS Chronicle,* Fall 1993).

Regardless of the specific immune system abnormalities a person may undergo at any given time, certain problems tend to occur repeatedly in the CFIDS population as a whole.

Viral Infections

Frequent occurrence of colds, flu, and upper respiratory tract infections is related to immune system disregulation and, as a consequence, these illnesses do not respond well to over-the-counter remedies (which, in any case, are not designed to alter the course of an illness). People with recurring viral infections report that injections of gamma globulin and Kutapressin have helped lessen the frequency and severity of these infections. People who have been exposed to measles or chickenpox for the first time, however, must work with their doctor to check the progress of the disease before it gets fully under way. Acyclovir taken within 72 hours of the first sign of chickenpox can check development of the disease. Large doses of vitamin A taken within 24 hours of onset also help lessen the severity of measles, flu, and other infectious viral diseases.

TREATMENT TIPS

A first course of action is to avoid situations or circumstances that may lead to greater risk for infection. For those who catch flu and colds, it is wise to avoid exposure to people who are ill, young children, crowded, confined areas (airplanes, movie houses), and other environments that might lead to greater exposure to germs. Because most colds are spread by hand-to-mouth contact, keeping hands clean (soap-and-water is sufficient) also reduces the risk of contagion. Sambucol, an herbal remedy, is reported to be effective against flu and colds. It can be purchased in liquid form or as lozenges. Unlike many pharmaceutical products, Sambucol is safe for use in children. Other herbal remedies include echinacea, goldenseal, and the antiviral agent St. John's wort. Some people find that high doses of vitamin C are helpful to limit the duration of a cold. The homeopathic remedy oscillococcinum has also been reported as helpful. For topical infections, the best course of action is to keep the affected area clean and dry and apply an over-the-counter antifungal ointment (such as Tinactin) once a day for 14 days. Tea tree oil, available in most health food stores, is also an effective topical antifungal agent. People with other kinds of infections should avoid anything that exacerbates symptoms and follow the treatment advice for the particular problem (see Candida, Oral Problems, Shingles, Sinusitis, Urinary Tract Problems).

SEE

• Chapter 4: Antiviral Agents, Gamma Globulin, Kutapressin.
• Chapter 5: Herbs, Minerals (zinc), Vitamins.

SEIZURES AND SEIZURE ACTIVITY

Although the incidence of seizures is rare in CFIDS, seizure-like episodes, especially during the first few months after onset, are not uncommon. These seizures do not usually involve loss of consciousness, however, and so may not be recognized. Often the seizure is described as starting with a "wave" of bad feeling accompanied by feelings of intense discomfort or fear. This last component may lead doctors to misdiagnose the patient's experience as a "panic attack."

Seizures and seizure activity are characterized by a sudden burst of electrical activity in the brain. The discharge can occur in both hemispheres, producing a generalized seizure (grand mal) with myoclonus (jerks), or localized in one area of the brain, producing a partial (focal) seizure. Seizures generally occur when the brain is either fully active (producing beta waves) or in a state of light sleep (producing theta waves).

The reasons for the sudden neuronal discharge are not entirely understood. However, many neurologists believe that seizures are caused by an imbalance in neurotransmitter activity. Neurotransmitters deliver only two types of message: fire or cease fire. The neuroexcitatory chemicals induce the neuron to release its electrical charge and the inhibitory chemicals prevent the neuron from firing. Seizures can be attributed to an imbalance in the two types of neurotransmitters leading to excess nervous system activity.

Dr. Paul Cheney has presented a hypothesis concerning neural activity in CFIDS. He believes people with CFIDS have excitatory neurotoxicity, or increased neuronal firing brought about by irritation of the nerve cells in the brain (due, in this case, to increased amounts of the cytokine alpha interferon). Dr. Cheney proposes that the overstimulation is caused by the predominance of the primary neuroexcitatory chemical N-methyl-D-aspartate (NMDA), which is normally in balance with the primary neuroinhibi-tor GABA (gamma-aminobutyric acid) (*CFIDS Chronicle,* Spring 1994; *CFIDS Chronicle,* Spring 1995). The imbalance can create many of the brain disturbances that produce some of the most debilitating symptoms of CFIDS, such as constant pain, insomnia, intolerance to stimuli of all kinds, and exhaustion. Given this explanation of how CFIDS affects the nervous system, it is easy to see how seizures might occur as part of the illness.

In accord with Dr. Cheney's hypothesis, seizures should be expected to be localized to one area of the brain (alpha interferon seems to primarily affect the limbic system). True to expectation, the type of seizure experienced by most people with CFIDS is partial, involving neuronal discharge in the limbic system or neighboring temporal lobes. However, some seizures do not fall into this category but seem to involve other parts of the brain. It is worth mentioning that even though a patient may experience seizure-like symptoms, electroencephalographic (EEG) findings are almost invariably normal. An EEG tracing shows only electrical signals from the outer portion of the cerebral cortex. Any unusual electrical activity in deep structures of the brain (such as the hypothalamus) is not recorded (as is the case with many types of epilepsy that demonstrate normal EEG findings).

Absence Seizures (Petit Mal)

Absence epilepsy, during which a person may be conscious but not aware of his or her actions, is common in CFIDS. Absence seizures generally do not last long, from a few seconds to a few minutes at most. In periods of absence, a person may continue with an activity (such as driving) as though partially asleep. One woman remarked that she often found herself in her driveway at home without the slightest recollection of how she got there. In general, absence seizures involve a lack of coordination between the part of the brain that controls awareness and the cortex.

Simple Partial Seizures

Simple partial seizures do not involve loss of consciousness, but produce altered sensations, perception, mood, or body function. Parietal lobe disturbances can be experienced as tingling in the face and extremities, jerking or stiffening in one area of the body, or feeling odd, crawling sensations. One can also see flashing lights or other visual disturbances or hear things (hallucinations). Changes in perception of time and memory result from temporal lobe imbalances.

"Sensory Storms"

Dr. Luis Leon-Sotomayor, the cardiologist who documented the 1965 CFIDS epidemic in Galveston, Texas, described a type of neurologic dysfunction that he called a "sensory storm." These storms affect the autonomic nervous system (regulated by the hypothalamus). A person experiencing a storm may first see an aura or sense that something very bad is about to happen. Storms produce sweating, pallor or flushing, elevated blood pressure, slowed respiratory rate, tachycardia, dizziness, and the feeling that one is about to lose consciousness. These autonomic storms are terrifying, but the effects generally pass within an hour. After such an experience, a person may feel lingering tiredness or malaise. Dr. Byron Hyde has observed that storms tend to occur spontaneously during the first few weeks of CFIDS (although they can repeat at specific times of day), then slowly pass as the illness progresses. A milder version may be experienced during relapses and after periods of stress.

Grand Mal Seizures

A small percentage of people with CFIDS experience grand mal seizures. The generalized electrical discharge characteristic of the grand mal seizure generates both motor disturbances and loss of consciousness. A person who experiences a grand mal seizure may experience a warning sign or feeling (aura)—a bad smell, a peculiar physical sensation, or a strong emotion such as fear. It is essential for anyone who has experienced a grand mal seizure to consult a neurologist.

TREATMENT TIPS

Two medications sometimes prescribed to treat symptoms of CFIDS, Klonopin and Diamox, have an effect on partial seizures involving myoclonus.

Nutritional supplements that aid in controlling seizures include manganese, which helps to correct the biochemical imbalance that results from seizures; taurine, an amino acid that helps slow nerve impulses; vitamin B_6, important for nervous system regulation; and zinc, magnesium, and GABA in small amounts.

People who have warnings of impending seizures or seizure-like episodes, either in the form of a rapidly escalating sense of urgency, surges of strange sensations, intense fear or rage, "spaciness," or any kind of sudden perceptual disturbance (such as a strong disagreeable smell), can sometimes prevent their full manifestation by immediately withdrawing from all sources of stimulation and entering into a relaxed state through meditation, relaxation exercises, or self-hypnosis techniques. This has the effect of changing the brain wave frequency to alpha waves. Once the electrical frequency of the brain waves has shifted, the seizure often is prevented (seizures occur during beta or theta wave frequencies). This technique is effective for seizures with obvious triggers (flickering lights, television, emotional upsets, and excess stimulation of any kind).

Avoiding stressors is essential for people with any kind of seizure. People who have experienced seizures must also be meticulous about avoiding the neurotoxins found in pesticides and other chemical products because of their potential seizure-inducing capacity. Prescription drug package inserts should also be examined for side effects and cautions. Wellbutrin, a medication sometimes prescribed to treat symptoms of CFIDS, is contraindicated in people who experience seizure activity.

FURTHER READING

Hyde, Byron M, and Jain, Anil. Clinical Observations of Central Nervous System Dysfunction in Post-Infectious, Acute Onset ME/CFS. In Hyde, Byron M, ed. The Clinical and Scientific Basis of ME/CFS. Ottawa, Ontario: Nightingale Research Foundation, 1992.

SEE

• Chapter 4: Antidepressant Drugs, Benzodiazepines (Klonopin), Diamox.
• Chapter 5: Amino Acids (taurine), Butyric Acid, Minerals, Vitamins.
• Chapter 6: Biofeedback, Meditation.
• Chapter 7.

SHINGLES

A number of people with CFIDS suffer from recurring shingles. Shingles is an infection from the herpesvirus, varicella zoster, the same virus responsible for chickenpox. After a person has chickenpox, the virus lies dormant and can be reactivated by another illness or immune system depression (radiation, cancer therapies, steroid treatments, immune system illnesses). The reactivated virus attacks a nerve root in the brain or spinal column and follows the course of that nerve outward to the skin, where chickenpox-like blisters erupt. The first sign of shingles can be an itching or stinging sensation on the skin, followed by intensification of pain, and finally a blistery rash. The rash can appear on any part of the body and is characteristically one-sided (left or right). The effects of shingles can be minimized if treated within the first 72 hours. A person who feels pain, itching, or tingling in a specific area that is followed by a one-sided blistery rash should see a doctor immediately.

TREATMENT TIPS

The treatment of choice for shingles is acyclovir (Zovirax), which, if taken early enough, can alleviate the worst symptoms. Famvir is used for the same purpose. If the pain persists after the initial infection (longer than a month), the resulting condition is known as postherpetic neuralgia. The sharp electric pain caused by postherpetic neuralgia is difficult to treat, but in some cases responds to antidepressant drugs. Zostrix, which can be purchased over the counter in cream form, is also now available for postherpetic neuralgia. Antihistamines may relieve itching. For numbness, Thomas Thomsen, author of *Shingles,* recommends a vibrator. This advice has a sound basis in fact because the sense of touch operates largely through vibration. To heal blisters, oatmeal, baking soda, corn starch, or cold compresses can be used. Tea tree oil can help prevent infection of healing blisters. Other treatments include Kutapressin, which can curtail outbreaks of shingles; lysine, an amino acid that halts herpesvirus replication; and colloidal silver, a natural antibiotic agent.

SINUSITIS

The sinuses are air-filled cavities located behind and around the nose and eyes. Each sinus is connected to the nasal passage by a thin duct. These ducts can be easily blocked, making drainage difficult and eventually leading to irritation, inflammation, and infection. Air pollution, cigarette smoke, dry or cold air, dental problems, bacteria, and viruses can all contribute to sinus problems. It is noteworthy that sinus problems were rated the most common chronic disease in the United States in 1981 by the National Center of Health Statistics—perhaps a testimony to growing environmental pollution.

Inflamed or infected sinuses can cause a wide range of symptoms, including headache, congestion, stuffiness, dizziness, nausea, tender cervical lymph nodes, sore throat, a feeling of facial pressure, "heavy head," and fatigue. Sinus pain can also mimic dental pain. Of these symptoms, the most frequently addressed is sinus headache. The sinus headache differs from the pressure or vascular headache in that it is felt mainly around the face and eyes. It can last for hours or even days. Sinus headaches become sharply worse with sudden increases in pressure to the region; the simple motion of bending over, air travel, a long car trip, or a change in barometric pressure can all spark intense face and head pain. The extraordinary fatigue associated with sinus problems ("nasal fatigue") has been well documented over the course of the century, receiving mention from a number of physicians from the late 1800s to the present.

Patients with CFIDS seem to be particularly vulnerable to sinus problems. The large proportion (some say as high as 75%) of allergy-related problems alone in this population seem to implicate the sinuses as a major source of trouble for CFIDS patients. Even those who do not show overt signs of allergy can have multiple sinus-related problems (headaches, increased chemical sensitivities). Some of these problems may be related to impaired immune system function, which for many is the defining feature of CFIDS. Indeed, as Dr. Alexander Chester of Georgetown Medical Center has pointed out, sinusitis may be a precipitating factor in some cases of CFIDS. Dr. Chester has proposed that, as in a similar case in which an apparent outbreak of multiple sclerosis followed sinusitis, viral diseases may be activated by a nasal mechanism. He suggests that in cases for which there are obvious signs of nasal involvement (acute onset following an upper respiratory tract infection, allergies, fluctuation of symptoms with weather changes), treating a possible underlying nasal disorder may produce substantial relief of headache, sleep disorder, mood swings, and fatigue.

TREATMENT TIPS

Although many cases of sinusitis are not bacterial in origin, and can be resolved with home treatments, sinusitis caused by bacterial infections can have serious consequences. Yellow or dark nasal discharge, severe sinus pain, or fever require a visit to the doctor. Bacterial infections are treated with antibiotic drugs. When taking antibiotics, remember to supplement with acidophilus or some other probiotic (see Chapter 5) to minimize potential side effects (the most problematic of which is Candida overgrowth). For chronic or persistent nonbacterial sinusitis, the following tips and suggestions may be useful:

- Saline nasal sprays are helpful in keeping nasal passages moist. They wash out mucus, dust, viruses, bacteria, and other sinus irritants and help reduce swelling. (Dry nasal passages are much more susceptible to infections, irritation, and subsequent inflammation.) Small, inexpensive bottles of premixed solution (Ayr, SalineX, Ocean Spray) are available in any pharmacy. Spraying may be repeated as often as needed throughout the day.

- Nasal irrigation is helpful for more severe cases and, unlike some other treatments, has the benefit of being both inexpensive and completely without side effects. To make the irrigating solution, add 1/4 to 1/2 teaspoon of salt and a tiny pinch of baking soda to 1 cup of lukewarm water. Completely fill a large all-rubber ear syringe (available in most pharmacies). Leaning forward over the sink, pinch one nostril closed, insert the syringe into the open nostril, and gently squeeze the bulb, swishing the solution around the inside of the nose. Repeat the procedure for each nostril until you have used the entire cup of solution. (The solution may run out of both nostrils or the mouth. Although this may be a bit messy, the relief provided by irrigation is well worth it.)

- Moist, warm air often alleviates sinusitis. Even standing in a shower for 5 minutes or breathing steam from a pot of boiling water can be helpful. Vaporizers and steam inhalers can also be purchased. The CFIDS and Fibromyalgia Health Resource (800-366-6056) sells a relatively inexpensive compact steam inhaler that is convenient for use in the home or when traveling. A contoured face mask allows direct flow of temperature-controlled steam. Eucalyptus, peppermint, or clove essential oil (one drop is sufficient) can be added to the water to help clear sinuses. These oils (available at most health food stores) can also be rubbed around the nostrils.

- Proper hydration is important so remember to drink lots of pure water.

- Avoid alcohol and milk, as these tend to aggravate sinus problems. Milk thickens mucous discharge, making it more difficult to keep the nasal passages clear.

- Supplements and herbs normally recommended for sinus problems include garlic (to help fight Candida and bacterial infection), vitamin A (to help repair mucous membranes), vitamin C and zinc (immune system stimulants), echinacea (an herb that acts as an immune system stimulant), and goldenseal root (available as a powder to be applied topically. Mix 1/2 teaspoonful with a drop or two of water to form a paste, spread lightly over the sinus area before bed, and wash off in the morning. Place a cloth over your pillow to prevent staining.

Apply for up to three nights.) Goldenseal is a powerful antimicrobial agent and should not be taken internally, even though it is common practice, because of potential harmful effects on the central nervous system.

- Sinusan, a homeopathic remedy that has been helpful for many people, can be purchased at most health food stores.
- Nonsteroidal anti-inflammatory drugs (NSAIDs) (aspirin and others), as opposed to simple analgesics (such as Tylenol), can be useful to reduce inflammation and pain.
- Patients with allergies usually benefit from prescription nasal sprays (Nasalcrom, Nasalcort). Although these contain cortisone, the fact that they are applied topically lowers the risk of immune system suppression normally associated with extended use of cortisone treatments.
- People with and without allergies should be careful to avoid potential sinus irritants and allergy triggers (air contaminants, sprays, fumes, dust, molds, pollen, dander). An air filter for the bedroom can be a worthwhile investment if sinus problems are severe.
- Air travel is especially problematic for people with sinus problems. Most doctors, in fact, recommend against air travel if an acute infection is present. For short-term relief, a decongestant spray such as Afrin may be useful. These sprays help open nasal passages, but should not be used for more than a day or two because they can become addictive. Excessive drying of the nasal passages also leads to greater risk of infection. Saline sprays can also mitigate some of the effects of poor air quality and airplane cabin pressure changes.

FURTHER READING

Chester, Alexander. Chronic Fatigue of Nasal Origin: Possible Confusion With Chronic Fatigue Syndrome. In Hyde, Byron M, ed. The Clinical and Scientific Basis of ME/CFS. Ottawa, Ontario: Nightingale Research Foundation, 1992.

Ivker, Robert S. Sinus Survival: The Holistic Medical Treatment for Allergies, Asthma, Bronchitis, Colds, and Sinusitis. New York: Putnam Publishing Group, 1995.

SEE

- Allergies, Candida, Secondary Infections.
- Chapter 4: Antihistamines.
- Chapter 5: Herbs, Probiotics, Vitamins.
- Chapter 6: Aroma Therapy, Homeopathy.

SKIN, HAIR, AND NAIL PROBLEMS

Skin

Skin problems are fairly common in CFIDS. Most are benign and self-limiting. Often patients don't even mention them to their doctors.

PALLOR. Pallor, although one of the few objective physical signs of CFIDS, is the symptom least observed by patients themselves. People with CFIDS are ghostly pale during the initial phase and during relapses. The whiteness of the skin is striking and can be perceived by anyone. Pallor is due to slowed blood flow.

RASHES. The rash most typical of CFIDS is lace-like and covers the face and chest. Some doctors have observed that it resembles the rash characteristic of lupus. Rashes are often experienced by those who are prone to allergies and can represent an allergic reaction to any substance consumed (urticaria or "hives") or touched (contact dermatitis). Some likely sources of contact dermatitis include acid foods (oranges, tomatoes), plant oils, permanent press bedding (treated with formaldehyde), and synthetic clothes (chemical sensitivity). Rashes can also appear after ingestion of certain medications. In his book, *Chronic Fatigue Syndrome: A Victim's Guide to Understanding, Treating, and Coping With This Debilitating Illness,* Gregg Fisher describes breaking out into hives after taking penicillin (which he explains is a classic reaction in people with infectious mononucleosis) and abdominal welts after taking acyclovir. Most skin rashes can be resolved by avoiding irritants and allergens.

DRY, PEELING SKIN. Dry skin results from loss of moisture in the outer layers of the skin. Dryness can be caused by dry air, harsh soaps, sun, fuzzy or woolen clothing, irritants (such as detergents not rinsed completely from clothes and sheets), and systemic conditions. Dry skin may also result from low thyroid function, which is not unusual in CFIDS. Paradoxically, a number of people say they have simultaneously dry and oily skin. However, as dry skin is not due to oil loss but to lack of water in the skin, it is quite possible to have an overproduction of oil due to hormonal changes while experiencing dryness due to malfunction in dermal moisture regulation. When people with CFIDS experience endocrine swings (irregular hormonal output), alternation between dry and oily skin results. Some people also notice that their skin peels (especially on the face) as though they have sunburn, even though they are spending all of their time indoors. Peeling skin can be a sign of zinc or vitamin B$_6$ deficiency, both of which are common in CFIDS. If low thyroid production is determined through appropriate endocrine tests, dry skin will improve with thyroid support. If nutritional deficiencies are suspected, skin will improve with appropriate dietary supplements, particularly vitamin B, zinc, and vitamin A. Topical treatments such as commercial lotions and creams are best avoided in patients who are prone to acne or hives because they can clog pores and may cause allergic reactions. The best remedies are to avoid harsh soaps, such as soaps with deodorants, and use a pure bath oil to aid the skin in retaining moisture. Pure soaps and bath oils that do not contain a lot of chemical additives can be found in health food stores. Dry brushing of the skin with a soft, natural bristle brush, reputed to invigorate the skin, has helped some people with CFIDS.

ACNE. Women with CFIDS are particularly prone to acne (especially around the hairline, back of the neck, and chin) before menstruation. These pimples usually disappear with the onset of menstruation. Endocrine fluctuations resulting from hypothalamus disregulation are most likely the cause of these periodic breakouts. Acne can also be exacerbated by stress because stress hormones stimulate the production of male-type sex hormones, which in turn leads to overproduction of skin oil. Certain medications, including low-dose birth control pills, cortisone, antiepilepsy medications, and vitamin B$_{12}$, can exacerbate acne as well. Good diet, vitamin supplementation, thorough cleaning with mild, easily rinsed cleansers, avoidance of creams, makeup, and skin irritants, and adequate intake of water all help reduce acne. Medication is seldom needed because acne tends to be transient.

HYPERSENSITIVITY. Many people report that they cannot stand to be touched in some places or that certain textures, types of clothing, or temperatures bother them. Like all the other senses, touch becomes hyperacute in CFIDS. Even slight pressure can be quite uncomfortable. Sensitivity to heat and cold also increases with CFIDS. People with allergic responses will be hypersensitive because of the effects of histamine (histamine sensitizes nerve endings). Antihistamines may help reduce skin sensitivity in these cases.

SPONTANEOUS BRUISING. Some people wake up in the morning to discover they have one or more dark bruises unrelated to previous injury. Sometimes bruising is related to potassium depletion, especially if the bruises appear after exposure to hot weather or periods of adrenal stress. In CFIDS it could be related to a number of factors, including altered red blood cell morphology, potassium depletion, and vitamin deficiencies. The possibility of dehydration should also be considered. If present, liquids should be increased. Water or juices can be blended with a little salt, sugar, and baking soda to increase retention.

PARESTHESIAS. Tingling, numbness, itching, prickling, crawling, and stinging sensations on the skin are common throughout CFIDS. Some paresthesias are related to nervous system activity, others are not. Spontaneous hyperventilation, which sometimes occurs in the acute stage, produces tingling in the neck and around the face. Itching can be the result of an allergic reaction. Dr. Felix Sulman has observed that stinging sensations (as though from an insect) and prickling can be produced by serotonin, an irritant that can produce skin responses similar to those of histamine. Although there is no treatment for most of these sensations, paresthesia associated with allergic reactions improves with antihistamines.

LOSS OF FINGERPRINTS. The flattening of fingertip ridges is part of the normal process of aging, usually occurring in the seventh decade. In people with CFIDS, however, this process seems to be accelerated. Dr. Philip Nelson, of Sarasota, Florida, studied a group of 165 CFIDS patients in whom he observed that a flattening of ridges occurred as early as the fifth decade. Fingerprint loss seems to predominate on the left hand and usually begins with the smallest finger. Flattening of the ridges is generally thought to reflect depletion of collagen in the skin. Fingerprint loss has been observed only in protracted cases.

Hair

The chief hair problem in CFIDS is hair loss. Normally, 50 to 120 hairs are lost each day. More than that (more than a tablespoon of hair removed from your hairbrush) is considered hair loss. Hair loss can be patchy (alopecia areata) or can be manifested as general thinning. Sometimes hair loss is slight and can go relatively unnoticed. Hair loss in CFIDS is often due to endocrine changes (such as hypothyroidism) and is usually not permanent. However, sudden loss of hair may be related to medications (notably Tagamet). Consuming excessive amounts of vitamin A also can lead to hair loss. People who are losing hair should use only mild shampoos and discuss thyroid tests with their doctor. Vitamin B and supplements that help increase circulation to the scalp such as CoQ10 or gingko may also be helpful.

Nails

Nail problems in CFIDS are usually not as dramatic as skin and hair problems. The most common are increased brittleness, bluish nail beds, and vertical ridges. Nails are made up of a soft protein called keratin, a substance composed largely of sulfur (which keeps nails hard). Nails become brittle and break or chip easily as a result of keratin deficiency or when the water content of the nail is decreased. Both causes are implicated in CFIDS. Longitudinal ridges have also been noted in many people with CFIDS. Ridges running up the length of the nail are often related to anemia, but are also associated with vitamin A deficiency and flu. A bluish nail bed is a sign that too little blood is being delivered to the nail. The nail depends on blood supplied by capillaries in the nail bed that give the nail its pinkish color. When the blood supply is diminished, nails turn blue and fail to grow. Dr. Alexander Gilliam noted in the 1934 CFIDS outbreak in Los Angeles that both bluish nails and slow nail growth (usually on one hand) were common. The best treatment for nails is to avoid contact with cleaners and other chemicals, keep them trimmed (soak them first to avoid chipping), and make sure nutrition is adequate. Calcium supplements will not help nails to become stronger because the nail plate contains very little calcium.

SLEEP DISORDERS

Sleep disturbances are so common in CFIDS that some doctors will not even make the diagnosis if a patient reports having normal, restful sleep. Nearly every CFIDS patient reports some trouble sleeping. Usually problems vary between insomnia and excessive nonrestful sleep. Some sleep patterns are fairly consistent. One person cannot fall asleep before 3:00 AM "no matter what." Another can't fall asleep for a few days, then sleeps too much for a few days, then wakes up repeatedly during the night. Every once in a while a person may be surprised by what feels like a normal night's sleep, only to have the insomnia return with a vengeance the following night. Although the disturbances can take many forms, the outcome is always the same—waking up tired. Nonrestorative sleep is a hallmark of CFIDS and is a condition that acts as a catalyst for other symptoms. Because poor sleep exacerbates other symptoms (pain, emotional swings, flu-like symptoms, fatigue), it is a focal point for treatment for most CFIDS doctors.

Any chronic alteration in normal sleep patterns is referred to as a sleep disorder. Common sleep disorders include insomnia (inability to fall or stay asleep), malsomnia (excessive light sleep or broken sleep), hypersomnia (excessive sleep), excessive rapid eye movement (REM) sleep (prolonged or hypnogogic sleep), and nightmares. Although most people experience sleep disturbances at one time or another, whether due to illness, pregnancy, emotional upset, or injury, relatively few have long-term alterations of sleep patterns. When they do, underlying physiologic causes should always be suspected. Normal sleep occurs in four stages, each of which is characterized by a distinct brain wave pattern. The first stage of sleep is light sleep, which is characterized by a reduction in the alpha waves characteristic of the waking state and an increase in theta waves (4 to 7 Hz). In the second and third stages, wave forms gradually slow and deepen until, by the fourth stage, the sleeper is producing more than 50% delta waves (3 Hz or less). In a normal sleeping adult, all four stages of sleep occur within approximately 90 minutes, followed by REM sleep, or dreaming. The entire cycle is repeated three or four times during the night. Each time, stage four sleep shortens and REM sleep lengthens, which is why the deepest sleep is at the start of the night and the most vivid dreams occur before awaking.

Most researchers agree that the sleep disturbance in CFIDS is caused by an alteration in the normal brain wave patterns required for deep, restful sleep. Dr. Russell Poland has proposed that in CFIDS the normal pattern of sleep phases is interrupted by alpha wave spikes (around 10 Hz); that is, when you should be in deep, restoring stage four sleep, your brain waves are acting as though you are awake (*CFIDS Chronicle*, Summer 1993). This is why so many people with CFIDS do not feel refreshed no matter how much they sleep and why others wake so often. Another CFIDS anomaly is the presence of excess theta waves, which cause the sleeper to remain in a light sleep state. Dr. Jay Goldstein has theorized that the brain wave disturbances are the result of alterations in hypothalamic function, the thumb-sized sector of the brain that regulates sleep (*CFIDS Chronicle*, Fall 1991). The cause of the disregulation may be attributable to the action of excess cytokines such as alpha interferon. Additional sources of sleep problems include pain, drops in blood pressure dips, irregular heart beat, and sinus congestion. Decreased blood sugar levels can also cause insomnia. As blood sugar levels drop during the night, the adrenal glands release cortisol, the "fight-or-flight" hormone. The startle reaction produced by the sudden spurt of adrenal hormone awakens the sleeper and prevents a return to sleep until the blood sugar level is raised again.

Insomnia or Difficulty Initiating and Maintaining Sleep

In the initial or acute stages of CFIDS and during severe relapse, most people have great difficulty falling asleep. Typically it takes several hours to fall asleep, although some people may not sleep until close to dawn or not at all. People may find themselves either awaking several times during the night or waking once and not being able to go back to sleep. Common wake-up times are between 11:00 PM and 12:00 midnight, 3:00 and 4:00 AM, and early dawn. A combination of tricyclic antidepressants and benzodiazepines often is recommended for people who wake frequently in the night. People who regularly cannot fall asleep until dawn may benefit from melatonin, a pituitary hormone that regulates diurnal cycles.

Hypersomnia

Excessive sleep or the inability to stay awake commonly occurs during the acute stage and may diminish as the illness progresses. Hypersomnia is generally more common in children than in adults. The hypersomniac may awaken briefly but will fall asleep shortly thereafter, sometimes at the table or wherever he or she has been recently engaged in activity. Hypersomnia is most often caused by a dysfunction in the posterior hypothalamus and upper part of the mid-brain. Prozac and other mild stimulants are often prescribed to people who have hypersomnia.

Light Sleep

Sleep that is too light or unrefreshing is typical of CFIDS and is probably due to the interference of alpha waves during deep sleep (perhaps stemming from acetylcholine deficiency). Alpha waves cause the sleeper to be too alert during sleep and may cause waking by allowing too much sensory information to be processed by the brain. Sometimes sleep may be combined with a state of wakefulness to produce a kind of half-sleep. The feeling of being neither asleep nor awake can be extremely uncomfortable.

Dysania

Dysania refers to a period lasting between 1 and 3 hours after awakening in which a person is too exhausted to get out of bed. These hours of "morning fog" are typical of CFIDS and are common in all stages of the illness.

Myoclonus

Some people are wakened by strong involuntary jerks (myoclonus) of the arms, legs (restless leg syndrome), or entire body. These in turn can trigger a startle reaction (pounding heart), making return to sleep difficult.

Dreams and Early Waking States

Nightmares are common in people with CFIDS, as are vivid, disturbing, thematic dreams. These dreams often awake the sleeper, leaving a persistent feeling of discomfort that may last well into the day. Conversely, many people also experience a complete lack of dreams or a sense that their dreams are vague and disjointed. This state of dreamlessness may last for months. Sometimes a person may awaken feeling disoriented or feel semiawake for a period of time after waking. Some people also experience a frightening inability to move any part of their body for a few minutes after waking, even after becoming fully conscious.

TREATMENT TIPS

A lot can be done to improve sleep. Pharmaceutical recommendations include low doses of Klonopin, a benzodiazepine, and Sinequan, an antidepressant, taken together. Klonopin is rapid-acting and helps induce sleep and Sinequan helps maintain sleep. Many people with CFIDS-related insomnia have found this combination helpful (although people who are sensitive to antidepressants might want to try other treatments first). Ambien, a sedative-hypnotic, is a new medication for insomnia that does not affect sleep cycles, as do benzodiazepines and antidepressants. Tylenol PM also can help induce drowsiness, especially if fibromyalgia-type symptoms are present. Antihistamines such as Benadryl may induce sleep (although antihistamines can also produce the opposite effect in some people, making them feel jittery). As always, start with a very small amount of the drug at first to check for sensitivity.

Supplements that may be helpful include magnesium, calcium, vitamin B complex, and melatonin. Patients have reported that magnesium taken before bedtime acts as a muscle relaxant, which helps them sleep. Calcium appears to have a similar effect. Vitamin B complex also can help induce sleep, especially if there is a deficiency, although it should be noted that those vitamins produced from brewer's yeast can have the opposite effect in people sensitive to yeast products. Inositol can also be taken separately to help induce sleep, although in some people with severe insomnia it may produce a rather light, unrefreshing sleep. People with sleep cycle problems (falling asleep at dawn or sleeping only during the day) have found that melatonin, a pineal gland hormone, works well. Recent research also suggests that galanthamine, a selective acetylcholinesterase inhibitor, may correct sleep disturbance by increasing the amount of acetylcholine in the brain. Because royal jelly contains natural acetylcholine, this nutritional product may be helpful for some people.

Herbs that effectively induce sleep include valerian (can be upsetting to the stomach and should be taken with a little milk), hops, passion flower, chamomile (not for those sensitive to ragweed), and skullcap. All can be blended in a tea or taken singly.

Aroma therapy works well for some people. A drop of clary sage or jasmine essential oil on a handkerchief next to the bed produces a sedative effect.

Those who wake up because of a decrease in blood sugar levels should eat something (milk or tea with a little honey or cereal). They probably can get back to sleep when the blood sugar level returns to normal. Grandma's cure for insomnia—a glass of warm milk at bedtime—also may help some people fall asleep. Warm milk contains high amounts of serotonin, which is why nursing babies often doze off before they're done feeding. Carbohydrates, such as bread or crackers, also increase the amount of serotonin in the brain. Salt sometimes helps restore sleep in people who experience insomnia as a result of low blood pressure.

Night sweats are typical of the initial or acute stages of CFIDS or relapse and as part of premenstrual syndrome (PMS). Night sweats can be drenching or can involve only the upper torso and neck. Keeping a change of nightclothes nearby can help minimize the disruption caused by having to change clothes during the night. Using light layers of bedclothes, which can be easily thrown off, is also helpful.

Last, but not least, stress must be reduced. Although CFIDS insomnia is not caused by stress, it is certainly aggravated by it. Worrisome or exciting projects should not be undertaken after dinner. A relaxing bath about an hour before bedtime or some light fiction are helpful for creating a restful state. The warm bath signals the body to cool down, which helps the person fall asleep. The rhythmic eye movements needed to read help signal the mind to produce slower brain waves. Watching television should be avoided if someone is sensitive to the effects of overstimulation. (The rapid frame changes, which force the eyes to refocus every few seconds, are arousing and may inhibit sleep onset.) If reading is not an option, listening to a tape may help induce sleep (this also works for night wakings). The act of listening changes neurotransmitter activity to induce a restful state (as anyone who has dozed through a boring lecture can attest). A tape recorder by the bed with a tape of soothing music or someone telling a calming story might help someone who wakes up in the night to try to stay calm. The more aroused and upset a person gets, the harder it will be to fall back asleep.

Be aware that skipping a night of rest to force the body into sleep is not a good idea. The person simply becomes even more exhausted and finds it harder to sleep the second night. Remember, the CFIDS sleep disorder is not caused by bad habits. It is caused by brain disturbances. Rest is permissible whenever the body allows it. Also, be aware that the long-term use of tranquilizers can be disruptive of normal sleep cycles. These drugs should be used judiciously and under the careful supervision of your doctor. CFIDS patients may need smaller doses than normally prescribed.

FURTHER READING

Orr, William C, Altshuler, Kenneth Z, and Stahl, Monte L. Managing Sleep Complaints. Chicago: Year Book Medical Publishers, 1982.

SEE

• Chapter 4: Antidepressant Drugs, Antihistamines, Benzodiazepines, Central Nervous System Stimulants, Pain Relievers.
• Chapter 5: Amino Acids, Herbs, Melatonin, Minerals (calcium, magnesium), Royal Jelly, Vitamins.
• Chapter 6: Acupuncture, Aroma Therapy, Biofeedback, Hypnosis, Meditation.
• Chapter 7.

URINARY TRACT PROBLEMS

Bladder problems are not uncommon in CFIDS. Dr. Jay Goldstein reports that some 20% of his patients experience pain on urination. Problems may include the need to go to the bathroom frequently (polyuria), difficulties urinating (dysuria), and the painful, aching, or burning sensation that are typical symptoms of inflammation of the urinary tract (cystitis). Although both men and women can experience urinary difficulties, the origins of the problems can be somewhat different. Because of anatomical differences in urinary tract structure, cystitis is more infrequent in men than in women. However, men may experience urologic problems due to inflammation and infection of the prostate gland (prostatitis).

Cystitis

Cystitis, although usually referred to as a bladder or urinary tract infection, is not limited to bacterial causes. It also can be related to an allergic response, chemical poisoning, congenital defects, or hormonal fluctuations. The distinction between the common urinary tract infection caused by overgrowth of bacteria (often *Escherichia coli*) in the urinary tract and the noninfectious bladder disorder known as interstitial cystitis is especially important because treatments for each of these disorders differ radically. In *You Don't Have to Live With Cystitis!*, Dr. Larrian Gillespie attributes interstitial cystitis to loss of the protective lining (glycosaminoglycans, or GAG layer) that normally insulates the bladder tissue from its contents. When the GAG layer is eroded (which Dr. Gillespie claims may be caused by excessive or inappropriate use of antibiotics, radiation, or chemical exposure), painful, burning urination results. Once the GAG layer has been compromised, the bladder may become repeatedly irritated by the release of certain neurotransmitters (notably serotonin) that keep the bladder in its raw, painful state. The symptoms of interstitial cystitis can be so severe that a person can qualify for disability on this basis alone.

People who have frequent symptoms of cystitis but have negative urine cultures may have interstitial cystitis and should follow the suggestions below.

TREATMENT TIPS

Treatment for bladder problems varies according to type. Medical treatments for interstitial cystitis require a diagnosis. Securing a diagnosis for interstitial cystitis, however, is not simple. It may be necessary to undergo cystoscopy or biopsy, painful procedures that involve threading a small tube through the urethra to examine or take tissue samples from the bladder wall. Because most tests for interstitial cystitis are invasive and uncomfortable, Dr. Gillespie makes some simple recommendations for short-term relief of symptoms.

In the case of interstitial cystitis acidity worsens the condition. (Dr. Gillespie likens drinking cranberry juice for cystitis to throwing gasoline on a fire.) Baking soda acts to make the urine more alkaline, which relieves burning pain. Dr. Gillespie recommends drinking a teaspoon of baking soda in water when symptoms are first noticed. In a few hours, repeat using half a teaspoon of trisodium compound (Tri-Salts), which are released more slowly into the system.

To dilute the urine, at least 10 glasses of water should be drunk during the day. If herbs can be tolerated, horsetail or corn silk tea helps flush the bladder.

Acid foods and foods high in the amino acids which eventually form serotonin and norepinephrine can irritate the bladder lining. The following foods should be avoided:

Acid Foods

Alcoholic beverages	Coffee	Pineapple
Apples	Cranberries	Plums
Cantaloupes	Grapes	Strawberries
Carbonated drinks	Guava	Tea
Chilies, spicy foods	Lemons	Tomatoes
Citrus	Peaches	Vinegar

Foods High in Tyrosine, Tyramine, Tryptophan, and Aspartate

Avocados	Cranberries	Prunes
Aged cheeses	Fava beans	Raisins
Bananas	Lima beans	Rye bread
Beer	Mayonnaise	Saccharine
Brewer's yeast	NutraSweet	Sour cream
Canned figs	Nuts	Soy sauce
Champagne	Onions	Vitamins buffered with aspartate
Chicken livers	Pickled herring	Wine
Chocolate	Pineapple	Yogurt

Not everyone notices complete relief of all symptoms by avoiding these foods; however, a substantial number of Dr. Gillespie's patients have obtained partial or significant relief. It may not be necessary to avoid all of these foods; perhaps only the very acidic foods such as citrus will trigger symptoms. Trial and error, along with keeping a food and symptoms diary, can help determine which of these foods to avoid. In addition, some dyes, additives, and chemical agents commonly found in food products can trigger symptoms. These include tartrazine (yellow dye No. 5), monosodium glutamate (MSG), sodium benzoate, and benzyl alcohol. Carefully read labels on foods and medications. Acid-free coffee and teas are available for tea and coffee lovers who can tolerate caffeine (call 800-TEA-LEAF).

Vitamin B_6, if tolerated, helps heal the bladder. It helps prevent tryptophan metabolites in urine from converting to free radicals and can convert other amino acids into free radical scavengers, thus lessening damage to the lining of the bladder. This may be the only B vitamin the more sensitive patients with interstitial cystitis can tolerate (the fermenting process used to formulate other B vitamins can cause bladder irritation in some patients). P5P is a well-tolerated form of vitamin B_6. Dosage should not exceed 50 to 100 mg/day to avoid creating dietary deficiency of vitamin B complex.

Dimethylsulfoxide (DMSO) is an industrial solvent derived from wood. Its only use approved by the Food and Drug Administration (FDA) is for treatment of interstitial cystitis. DMSO is instilled into the bladder through a catheter. Heparin, bicarbonate of soda, or a steroid (such as Kenalog) may be added to DMSO to enhance its anti-inflammatory properties. DMSO, alone or in combination, is believed to stabilize the bladder lining and provide a medium for the cells to begin self-repair. This treatment must be done in a urologist's office because the procedure requires sterile conditions. The drugs used also require a prescription. People who are highly allergic should approach DMSO with caution because it causes the release of histamine.

Elmiron has recently been approved by the FDA for general use. This drug reportedly has been quite successful in treating interstitial cystitis.

Treatments for bacterial infections of the urinary tract include Macrodantin, a urinary antiseptic, and antibiotic drugs. In all cases, bubble baths, bathing in contaminated water, synthetic underwear, and tight pants should be avoided. Pyridium can be taken for acute pain.

Caution: Patients with a diagnosis of cystitis should always request a urine culture. "Routine" antibiotic therapy without a confirmed bacterial infection may substantially worsen interstitial cystitis and, in any case, will not help treat it.

MORE INFORMATION

Interstitial Cystitis Association of America
PO Box 1553
Madison Square Station
New York, NY 10159
800-HELP-ICA (800-435-7422) (toll-free telephone)
212-979-6057 (local telephone)
212-677-6139 (fax)
www.ichelp.com (website)
> The association can help you find a doctor in your area who will treat interstitial cystitis; they also publish a newsletter that contains useful treatment information and resource materials.

FURTHER READING

Chalker, Rebecca, and Whitmore, Kristene. Overcoming Bladder Disorders. New York: Harper & Row, 1990 (available from Interstitial Cystitis Association of America, $14.00).

Gillespie, Larrian. You Don't Have to Live With Cystitis! New York: Avon Books, 1986 (to order direct, call 800-238-0658).

SEE

- Chapter 4: Antidepressant Drugs (Elavil), Antihistamines (Atarax and Vistaril).
- Chapter 5: Herbs.

Prostatitis

The prostate is a small gland, roughly the size of a large chestnut, that surrounds the neck of the bladder and the urethra. Although the principal function of the prostate gland is to produce the fluid that comprises most of the semen, its location ensures that problems that arise in this gland will cause bladder symptoms. Pressure from inflammation of the prostate, whether from bacterial or viral infection, excessive heat, radiation, or chemicals, causes pain and difficulty initiating or stopping urine flow. Infections of the prostate (and urinary tract) also produce a slight watery discharge (usually observed in the morning), an itching feeling inside the penis and discomfort while urinating, and pain in the perineal area. Acute bacterial prostatitis also can cause fever and lower back pain.

Dr. Byron Hyde, in his observations of CFIDS outbreaks, has noted that early in the illness pseudoprostatitis was observed, often in quite young men (*The Clinical and Scientific Basis of ME/CFS*, 1992). This implies that many of the urinary problems that beset men with CFIDS are not due to specific infection. However, any of the symptoms associated with prostatitis require consultation with a urologist. One male patient mentioned that, in his case, a prostate infection seemed to have triggered CFIDS. Given the increased susceptibility to infections experienced by many people who contract CFIDS and the fact that inflammation is a common problem throughout the course of the illness, problems in this area always should be thoroughly investigated by a competent physician.

TREATMENT TIPS

Because infection and inflammation of the prostate gland produce similar symptoms, doctors sometimes have difficulty making a differential diagnosis based on symptoms alone. Bacterial and viral infections of the prostate, however, can be detected by means of urinalysis or examination of prostatic fluid. Nonspecific bacterial prostatitis usually is treated with tetracycline. Chronic bacterial prostatitis is treated with a combination of antibiotics. (Nonbacterial prostatitis is not treated with antibiotics.) Sometimes muscle relaxants are used to relieve spasms in the muscles of the pelvic floor. Hot sitz baths and the occasional use of tranquilizers are also recommended. Rarely, in cases where the pain seems to be related to inflammation in the pubic bone, nonsteroidal anti-inflammatory drugs (NSAIDs) have been prescribed. Nutritional recommendations for prostate support include zinc (deficiency has been linked to some forms of prostatitis), essential fatty acids (important in prostate function), magnesium and calcium, vitamin A and vitamin E, and prostate glandular extracts, which can be found in health food stores.

FURTHER READING

Rous, Stephen. The Prostate Book: Sound Advice on Symptoms and Treatment. New York: W.W. Norton & Co., 1988.

VISION AND EYE PROBLEMS

Vision and eye problems in CFIDS cover a broad range. About 75% of people with CFIDS experience some difficulty with vision. Light sensitivity is nearly universal, at least at some stage in the illness. Because the optic nerve is so long (it traverses the entire length of the brain to process visual information), vision problems can originate in a number of areas of the brain. Most researchers agree that in CFIDS the problems probably stem from the area at the top of the brain stem (the midbrain) or in the hypothalamus (which controls pupil dilation). Eye problems in CFIDS can be both neurologic (focus problems) or mechanical (dryness, tearing), although most are probably related to nervous system disregulation. Eye problems in CFIDS tend to be transient and, although irritating, benign.

Photophobia

Many people experience extreme sensitivity to light, especially in the acute or initial stages of CFIDS. The cause of this sensitivity is a contradictory dilation of the pupil (usually on only one side), rather than the usual narrowing, when subjected to a light source. The excessive influx of light causes pain and a spontaneous impulse to shield the eyes from damage. Wearing dark sunglasses and keeping curtains drawn over windows helps ameliorate light sensitivity.

Floaters and Spots

Specks or dots that seem to float across the field of vision are common in acute phases of CFIDS. They are most noticeable against a light background and tend to follow movement of the eye. Floaters are caused by the normal condensation of collagen within the eye and are harmless, requiring no treatment. Floaters or spots accompanied by light flashes or loss of peripheral vision need to be investigated, however, because they may be indicative of inflammation or damage to the retina.

Tearing and Dry Eye

People with CFIDS report both excessive tearing and dry, irritated eyes, frequently in alternation. The periodic dry, burning eyes (keratitis sicca) common in CFIDS can lead to conjunctivitis (pink eye), in which the eye turns pink and releases a sticky discharge. It should be noted that the conjunctivitis experienced by many people with CFIDS is rarely the result of bacterial infection. In most cases, conjunctivitis results from excessive dryness, airborne allergies, or rubbing (due to itching). People who are prone to dry, burning, itchy eyes, or conjunctivitis, can benefit from artificial tears. Persistent dry eye can also be an indication of Sjögren's syndrome, an autoimmune disease that causes all mucous membranes to dry (see discussion of Sjögren's syndrome). In about half of all diagnosed cases, Sjögren's syndrome accompanies other connective tissue disorders; thus it may be worth requesting an antinuclear antibody test if symptoms are unusually persistent.

Sluggish Focus and Double and Blurred Vision

Seeing double (diplopia) can be disconcerting. Fortunately, it is usually transitory, as is blurred vision. People with CFIDS also notice that it takes longer to focus the eyes, particularly when changing focus from near to far objects. All of these difficulties are most likely caused by nervous system or muscle coordination problems, in which the normally fine-tuned response between the small muscles controlling the lens and the brain is not synchronized. The result is that when the lens of the eye overreacts to stimuli, the normal corrective mechanisms that act to straighten the eye fail to operate as quickly as they should. An alteration in brain signals also can lead to uncoordinated eye tracking (one pupil dilates or contracts at a different rate from the other). The outcome is short-term blurring, double vision, and slow focus. All of these problems are exacerbated by tiredness and improve with rest.

Tunnel Vision

Sometimes people with CFIDS experience loss of peripheral vision so severe that it appears as though they are looking through a tunnel. Tunnel vision may occur concurrently with loss of peripheral vision, making tasks such as driving risky.

Night Blindness

Night blindness is common in people who also have other visual disturbances. Night vision can decrease to the extent that a person cannot manage a trip to the bathroom at night. Leaving a night light on can remedy this problem.

Depth-of-Field Loss

People with vision problems commonly experience difficulties in tasks that require relocating objects because they have lost the ability to judge distance. As a consequence, they may mean to place a glass on a counter but miss it by an inch, walk into doorjambs, stumble on uneven sidewalks, have difficulty calculating the distance between stairs (which leads to a lot of anxiety about falling), and have problems judging the speed of oncoming traffic. Depth-of-field loss also causes visual confusion when looking at repeating objects such as stairs (particularly if they are moving, as on an escalator), oriental rug patterns, and other dense, repetitive designs. When depth-of-field loss is severe, objects can appear two-dimensional.

Nystagmus

Dr. Alfredo Sadun, a neuro-ophthalmologist at the University of Southern California, has observed nystagmus (small, rapid eye movements) in one fourth of patients with CFIDS. Nystagmus is rare (5%) in the general population and usually indicates an underlying neurologic problem. Dr. Sadun has inferred from this and other vision problems common to CFIDS that people with nystagmus may have a brain stem inflammation in the midbrain, which would cause dysfunction of the brain cells associated with vision.

Sjögren's Syndrome

Sjögren's syndrome is an autoimmune disorder that affects some 2 to 4 million patients in the United States, 90% of whom are women. In Sjögren's syndrome, the moisture-producing glands in the body, particularly those in the eyes and mouth, are attacked by the immune system. Typical symptoms include dry eyes and mouth, leading to blurred vision, eye discomfort, photophobia, hoarseness, and difficulty swallowing.

Primary Sjögren's syndrome is diagnosed in the absence of other autoimmune or connective tissue disorders. Secondary Sjögren's, the type patients with CFIDS are likely to contract, is accompanied by other illnesses that affect connective tissue (for example, rheumatoid arthritis). About 50% of patients with Sjögren's syndrome have the secondary type. Diagnosis of Sjögren's syndrome is made on the basis of blood tests that detect autoantibodies, reduced tear production in the eyes, and taking a detailed history of symptoms.

TREATMENT TIPS

A combination of vision and eye problems can make highly visual tasks such as reading or driving virtually impossible. Watching television, with its rapid shifts of scene and pulsating light effects, becomes particularly excruciating with vision problems. Dr. Alfredo Sadun recommends that people with focus problems (double vision, slow focus, poor depth perception, uneven tracking) avoid the use of bifocal eyeglasses because they make inordinate demands on the musculature of the eyes. He recommends separate glasses for near and far sight. People who have never worn glasses may find that purchasing glasses to alleviate focus problems does not help. Because most eye symptoms are transient, a person may have severe problems one month and rush to buy glasses, only to find that vision has become completely normal the next month. Symptoms that persist or worsen over time, however, should be investigated by an ophthalmologist.

Dr. David Browning, an ophthalmologist who practices in Charlotte, North Carolina, has pointed out that many vision problems can be exacerbated with use of psychoactive drugs (such as Sinequan and Xanax). Because these drugs are commonly prescribed for many individuals with CFIDS, people should be aware of potential visual side effects and exercise caution when driving or performing other demanding or dangerous tasks. It should be noted, however, that some people with CFIDS experience improvement in vision problems while taking Klonopin. Vision problems in CFIDS are rarely due to vitamin A deficiency, yet some people report improved eye function after taking beta carotene (either in supplement form or as carrot juice). Eyebright capsules and bilberry, available at health food stores, are two other common herbal remedies for eye problems.

Treatments for Sjögren's syndrome include moisture replacement therapies, nonsteroidal anti-inflammatory drugs (NSAIDs), and steroids (to downregulate immune system activity). Many patients recommend Bion Tears, an artificial tear solution that contains no preservatives or dyes and is available over the counter at most drugstores.

MORE INFORMATION

Sjögren's Syndrome Foundation, Inc.
333 N. Broadway, Suite 2000
Jericho, NY 11753
800-475-6473 (toll-free telephone)
516-933-6365 (local telephone)
516-933-6368 (fax)
http://www.sjogrens.com (website)
> Publishes a newsletter and markets *The Sjögren's Syndrome Handbook,* a guidebook for diagnosis and treatment. Annual membership: $25 in U.S., $30 in Canada, $35 overseas. Handbook: nonmembers, $29.95 plus $2.50 for shipping; members, $19.95.

FURTHER READING

Hyde, Byron M. The Clinical and Scientific Basis of ME/CFS. Ottawa, Ontario: The Nightingale Research Foundation, 1992.

WEATHER SENSITIVITY

It is common knowledge among people with CFIDS that weather changes produce a general worsening of symptoms. People in the same geographic area often exchange empathetic phone calls just before storms, cold fronts, and other climate changes. In situations where more than one member of a family is ill, the response to weather may be particularly dramatic because all ill members experience an exacerbation of symptoms simultaneously.

Fully one third of the general population may be sensitive to weather changes, according to studies performed at Hebrew University in Jerusalem. The weather sensitive commonly experience symptoms such as muscle pain, aching joints, insomnia, irritability, and the "blahs" a day or two before the weather changes. The worst weather for the sensitive individual is characterized by a falling barometer and high humidity. The reasons for the mysterious clairvoyance of those who seem to know when the weather is going to change may have to do with neurochemical changes stimulated by radiowaves sent out by advancing fronts.

Studies directed by Dr. Felix Sulman, head of the Bioclimatology Unit at Hebrew University, demonstrated that people who reported sensitivity to weather changes had unusually high amounts of serotonin and histamine in their urine a day or two before a weather change. Histamine is an inflammatory agent released during allergic reactions. Serotonin, a neurotransmitter and vasoconstrictor, is also an irritant and can be released in the body during emotional stress. According to Dr. Sulman, excessive amounts of serotonin, like histamine, can produce agitation, insomnia, irritability, runny or stuffy nose, inflammation of the eyeballs and lids, shortness of breath, sore throat, edema (in hands and feet), migraine headache, nausea, dizziness, palpitations, flushes accompanied by sweating or shivering, diarrhea, and the constant urge to urinate. Dr. Sulman maintains that the "sferics," or radiowaves, released as a consequence of the increased electrical activity preceding a front, produce positive ions that in turn act to stimulate the release of serotonin and histamine. He also speculates that weather sensitivity may be genetically adaptive because increased moodiness might have served as a warning to get back to shelter as quickly as possible. Animals may be subject to the same mechanisms. It has often been observed that their uncanny foreknowledge of coming storms leads them to seek shelter before the weather changes.

People who are weather sensitive may also react to changes in temperature. Dr. Sulman's group found that, in addition to increased histamine levels, hot weather produced decreased excretion of adrenal hormones (cortisol) signaling adrenal exhaustion. This reaction is perhaps prompted by stimulation of the hypothalamus, which is sensitive to heat. With prolonged hot weather, the symptoms of adrenal exhaustion become evident: low blood pressure, fatigue, listlessness, depression, confusion, difficulty performing mental tasks, and hypoglycemia. In some individuals the period of exhaustion may be preceded by transient hyperarousal of the thyroid (particularly at the onset of hot, dry weather), causing overactivity, insomnia, irritability, restlessness, palpitations, sweating, and diarrhea. Cold weather can produce similar effects.

Many people with CFIDS and fibromyalgia note a definite worsening of symptoms, including anxiety, myalgia, headache, inflammation, and insomnia just before storms and the passing of weather fronts, particularly during conditions of high positive ions (low barometer and high humidity). Many also note a worsening of symptoms during hot weather. We are not aware of anyone with CFIDS who has been tested for serotonin, histamine, or adrenal hormone levels in the urine before a storm or during hot or cold weather so it cannot be certain that altered hormone levels cause the weather sensitivity experienced by people with CFIDS. However, many of Dr. Sulman's findings corroborate what is known about hormonal irregularities caused by CFIDS.

Dr. Sulman has noted that prolonged hot weather stimulates the hypothalamus, a brain structure that seems to act as a focal point for many CFIDS-related problems and can eventually lead to adrenal exhaustion. The adrenal irregularities common in CFIDS (as noted by Dr. Mark Demitrack and colleagues) may be responsible for unusually rapid depletion of adrenal hormones and ensuing malaise brought about by heat. Increased histamine levels also have profound implications for the substantial number of people with CFIDS, who may also experience oversensitivity to histamine itself (*CFIDS Chronicle*, Summer 1993). Dr. Sulman's findings also predict higher reactivity to weather changes in women, who produce far fewer adaptive stress hormones than men and more histamine and serotonin in response to weather stress.

A number of people with CFIDS report worsening of depression during the winter. Seasonal affective disorder (SAD) is a medically recognized condition in which the decreased amount of light during the winter months triggers mood changes. Some patients have found that SAD treatments (exposure to full-spectrum light from full-spectrum lightbulbs, lightboxes, and spending time outdoors) may help alleviate symptoms.

TREATMENT TIPS

To minimize the effects of impending storms, Dr. Sulman recommends avoiding sources of positive ionization (forced-air heating and cooling, friction between synthetic fabrics, air pollution) as much as possible. Exposure to negative ions is also helpful, although this solution is difficult to implement. Negative-ion machines, because they produce ozone and nitrous oxide, are not recommended. Some people have observed that their symptoms improve during a stay by the ocean, where negative ionization is high, but this is not a practical solution for most. Some essential oils reputed to increase the effectiveness of negative ions are cypress, lemon, orange, bergamot, pine, bois de rose, cedarwood, grapefruit, pettigraine, patchouli, and sandlewood. For people with SAD, full-spectrum lightbulbs and lightboxes can be purchased from the CFIDS and Fibromyalgia Health Resource (800-366-6056).

Other suggestions that Dr. Sulman makes to increase adrenal hormones and minimize the effects of heat and impending weather changes include low levels of monoamine oxidase inhibitors (MAOIs) and serotonin blockers. In CFIDS, however, these drugs should be used with caution because they entail risks that may outweigh their potential value.

For people sensitive to humidity, it may be worthwhile to purchase a dehumidifier for the bedroom. Air-conditioning systems also reduce the amount of humidity inside the house. Although Dr. Sulman cautions against forced-air cooling, sometimes the relief brought by the decrease in humidity offsets any negative effects of the machinery. For all types of weather sensitivity, it is important to be aware of impending storms and fronts. Listen to weather forecasts and keep a log of symptoms before weather changes to see which ones produce the most severe effects. Plan to take it easy on those days.

FURTHER READING

Sulman, Felix G. *Short- and Long-Term Changes in Climate.* Boca Raton, Fla.: CRC Press, 1982.

WEIGHT LOSS OR GAIN

Weight fluctuations are common in CFIDS. These changes can be dramatic, with a sudden gain or loss of 10 pounds or more in less than a week. In long-term cases, weight problems may be demonstrated as a tendency to gain weight easily.

There are many competing theories to explain weight fluctuation in people with CFIDS. Increases and decreases in weight can occur as the result of faulty cell metabolism, immune system overactivation, hypothyroidism or hypoadrenalism, loss of appetite due to excess catecholamine production (adrenaline), gastrointestinal upset, and carnitine deficiency. Hypothalamic disregulation is another prime reason for weight problems. The hypothalamus controls thyroid and adrenal function. It is a potent regulator of the immune system and also regulates appetite. Studies performed in rats some 50 years ago demonstrated that damage to the ventromedial hypothalamus resulted in obesity, whereas electrical stimulation to the same region produced anorexia. More recent research has proposed that alterations in neurotransmitter activity in the hypothalamus, specifically norepinephrine, are ultimately responsible for appetite. Since hypothalamic dysfunction is central in mediating other CFIDS symptoms, there is good reason to suspect its involvement in appetite disorder and weight problems associated with the illness.

Weight Loss

The sudden weight loss common to the acute stages of CFIDS can be dramatic. First, surface fat reserves, then muscle seem to disappear daily. The reasons for the weight loss are multiple. Some symptoms common in the acute stage (loss of appetite, gastrointestinal upset, changes in taste perception, exhaustion, difficulty swallowing, nausea, vomiting) result in serious reduction in caloric intake. Lowered intake reduces the supply of available vitamin B complex, which in turn diminishes appetite. As intake is further reduced, deficiencies become established, leading to continuation of the vicious cycle. Lack of food intake is not the only reason people lose weight in this stage. Immune system overactivity, in particular the expression of tumor necrosis factor (TNF), a cytokine released by activated T cells, causes severe weight loss. Dr. Nancy Klimas has found increased expression of tumor necrosis factor in patients with CFIDS (*Journal of Chronic Fatigue Syndrome,* 1995). In theory, the acute stage of the illness, when the immune system is overactive, may produce sudden weight loss due to the increased production of tumor necrosis factor. This is true even for patients who eat copious amounts of food.

TREATMENT TIPS

Treatments that have been helpful in acute-stage weight loss include alpha ketoglutarate (a citric acid metabolite that halts wasting syndrome), L-carnitine, vitamin B complex, and general nutritional supplementation. Ensure, protein powders, and shakes are also effective in increasing weight. Antidepressants, mild tranquilizers (benzodiazepines), stress-reduction techniques (hypnosis, meditation) may all help increase appetite.

Weight Gain

A number of theories have been proposed for the weight gain typical of many people with CFIDS. One is that in some people thyroid function is reduced, leading to generally slower metabolism, constipation, drowsiness, and a tendency to gain weight. Another theory is that along with altered cell metabolism comes an inability to utilize fat and carbohydrates. The well-known L-carnitine deficiencies observed in CFIDS seem to bear this theory out. The inability to utilize carbohydrates could feasibly lead to their storage as fat in the body. Reduced levels of glucose resulting from insufficient carbohydrate metabolism can produce carbohydrate craving. The late-afternoon sugar and starch cravings experienced by so many people with CFIDS can lead to overeating and the consequent storage of underutilized carbohydrates as fat (although not all those who experience cravings gain weight). A third theory proposes that the weight gain in CFIDS is largely due to edema, that is, water weight. According to this theory, water weight buildup is due to adrenal insufficiency, with adrenal hormones the agents responsible for regulating water retention. Because secondary adrenal insufficiency has been noted in CFIDS, this theory also seems relevant.

One of the biggest problems associated with weight gain is loss of self-esteem. Patients who, in addition to their illness, have to cope with a change in appearance may feel unattractive. Sometimes it helps to remember that the increase in weight is not due to poor eating habits or laziness but is a symptom of an illness. As the illness recedes and other symptoms wane, weight tends to return to normal.

TREATMENT TIPS

The weight loss drugs, fenfluramine plus phentermine (Fen-phen) and dexfenfluramine (Redux) have recently been banned by the Food and Drug Administration (FDA). These drugs decrease carbohydrate and sugar cravings by altering levels of serotonin and dopamine, two neurotransmitters that affect appetite. Weight loss medications do not increase metabolic rate, nor do they "melt fat off your body." In addition, they can be dangerous. Patients with CFIDS should avoid weight loss drugs because side effects can be severe. Side effects include pulmonary hypertension, dry mouth, diarrhea, weakness, sleepiness, dizziness, and gastrointestinal pain. Ephedrine, an herb currently being marketed as "herbal Fen-phen," can produce similar side effects (see Chapter 5: Herbs).

Some central nervous system stimulants such as Ionamin can also help in weight reduction. Ionamin activates dopamine in the brain, which may produce unpleasant side effects such as insomnia, agitation, and restlessness. Prozac, an antidepressant sometimes prescribed for people with CFIDS, depresses the appetite and can indirectly cause weight loss. Maintaining good dietary habits is essential. Pay careful attention to eating a wholesome, nutritious diet, even within the confines of food restrictions (see Chapter 9). Some clinicians recommend taking the supplement L-carnitine for weight loss. L-Carnitine helps convert fat into muscle, which is beneficial for people who gain a lot of weight while ill. However, it should also be noted that a few patients with CFIDS, particularly those with low-weight problems, have gained weight while taking L-carnitine supplements. It is possible that L-carnitine acts to normalize weight. The mineral chromium may help curb sugar cravings, as can the amino acid L-glutamine.

People who are taking antidepressants should note that a number of these drugs, including monoamine oxidase inhibitors (MAOIs) and tricyclic drugs, can cause weight gain. Sudden weight gain after taking these medications should be reported to your physician. People with persistent weight gain should undergo tests for thyroid hormone insufficiency.

FURTHER READING

Wurtman, Judith J. The Serotonin Solution. New York: Fawcett Columbine, 1996 (provides an interesting and informative discussion of the role of serotonin in carbohydrate cravings; several chapters outline diet recommendations for specific problems).

III

TREATMENT OPTIONS

The following chapters summarize the treatments currently used for CFIDS and its major symptoms. For the sake of convenience, they are divided into three categories.

1. Pharmaceutical agents (Chapter 4) include all prescription and over-the-counter drugs currently recommended by CFIDS clinicians. All of these treatments must be supervised by a physician, regardless of whether a prescription is required. The information in this chapter can be used to make preliminary investigations of medications referred to in the CFIDS literature, to increase knowledge of medications suggested by physicians, or to inform physicians about currently used CFIDS medications. The *Directory of Prescription Drug* patient assistance program lists companies that participate in providing prescription drugs for patients who cannot afford them (800-762-4636).

2. Nutritional supplements and botanical agents (Chapter 5) can be purchased without a prescription from health food stores, mail-order vitamin suppliers, and some drugstores and supermarkets. The information in this chapter can be used to plan any treatment protocol designed with a nutritionist, chiropractor, osteopath, neuropath, herbalist, or physician.

3. Alternative and complementary medical and supportive therapies (Chapter 6) are often useful in treating CFIDS. Many, such as acupuncture, require the services of trained practitioners. This chapter also presents information about many of the supportive therapies that have been used successfully to alleviate symptoms of CFIDS.

The fact that these treatments are presented in separate chapters does not mean they must be kept separate in practice. Most CFIDS clinicians use an eclectic approach, freely combining nutritional supplements, complementary and alternative medical practices, and traditional drug-oriented medicine. Most patients with CFIDS use the same strategy, changing back and forth from prescription drugs to supportive therapies to home remedies. With the plethora of symptoms and the ever-changing nature of CFIDS, flexibility is the best policy.

TREATMENT TIPS

- *Start small.* People with CFIDS tend to be sensitive to many medications. By starting with small doses, the risk of negative reactions is minimized. A patient can always build up to a larger dose. CFIDS clinicians nearly always start patients on a much lower than normal dosage for prescription medications.

- *Go slow.* Try one treatment at a time. Otherwise it will be impossible to identify which treatment was effective and which was not. Remember, many treatments, especially nonpharmaceutical treatments, may require several weeks to have an effect.
- *Recycle.* Throughout the different stages of the illness, treatment strategies need to change. What was not effective at an earlier stage in the illness may be helpful at a later one. Don't throw away supplements or pharmaceutical agents. Store them in the refrigerator, but remember to check the expiration dates before using them.

We hope that somewhere among these pages will be a remedy that alleviates your worst symptom, or that helps you progress so that you can see the light at the end of the tunnel. Remember, keep trying. In the world of CFIDS treatments, persistence pays.

Pharmaceuticals and Prescription Drugs

AMPLIGEN

DEFINITION. Ampligen (poly I:poly C12U) is a mismatched double-stranded RNA (ribonucleic acid) with immodulatory and antiviral properties. Because Ampligen has not yet been approved by the Food and Drug Administration (FDA), its use to date has been experimental.

BACKGROUND. In the early 1980s a molecule called Poly(I)-Poly(C) was discovered to inhibit tumor growth and stimulate interferon production. As a result, it was used in a number of cancer trials. However, it was found that the substance was toxic and made patients quite ill with serious side effects. While Poly(I)-Poly(C), the parent of Ampligen, is extremely toxic, the toxicity decreases significantly when the structure of the RNA is altered. Fortunately, the effectiveness of the new substance remains intact despite the change in structure.

In 1987 Ampligen was used experimentally in a small group of patients with AIDS (acquired immunodeficiency syndrome). The positive results of this trial seemed to confirm the claim that Ampligen is believed to augment natural killer cell function and influence 2-5A synthetase pathway. This pathway is vital in the defense against viral infections. According to Dr. Robert Suhadolnick of Temple University in Philadelphia, there are defects in key components in the antiviral system in some CFIDS patients, the most notable of which are low latent 2-5A synthetase and upregulated RNase (ribonuclease) L activity (*Journal of Interferon and Cytokine Research*, 1997). Ampligen is thought to help correct both of these defects.

USES IN CFIDS. In August 1988, Dr. Daniel Peterson, a pioneer in CFIDS treatment, was the first physician to use Ampligen in an extremely ill patient with CFIDS. Because of the severity of the patient's illness, Dr. Peterson was able to obtain permission from the FDA to use Ampligen under compassionate care status. The results were impressive and encouraging. One year into therapy the patient had recovered near-normal function in some areas and demonstrated a 46-point increase in IQ. This justified the next pilot study by Dr. Peterson, as well as several other formal studies conducted independently.

At the 1990 CFIDS Conference in Charlotte, North Carolina, and at the Cambridge Symposium, Dr. Peterson reported positive results after treating 15 patients with Ampligen. At the end of 24 weeks, most of the patients demonstrated increased performance status (Karnofsky scores) and exercise tolerance (as measured by treadmill testing). Cognitive improvement was demonstrated by improved memory and increased IQ scores. No significant toxicity was reported. Ampligen's antiviral properties were confirmed by evidence that human herpesvirus 6 reactivation was absent after treatment and abnormal components of the 2-5A pathway returned to normal range. It is of interest that of the two or three patients who did not respond to Ampligen therapy, the only significant pretreatment difference was measurable differences in 2-5A synthetase pathways.

The encouraging results of the small study by Dr. Peterson paved the way for a larger FDA-approved double-blind study in 1991 involving 92 patients in four U.S. cities. Again the results were encouraging. Many of the participants had been severely disabled before treatment and required assistance for simple daily activities. More than half of those in the study who received Ampligen demonstrated improvement and many were able to carry out daily activities with minimal assistance.

A study in Brussels, Belgium, presented at the 1996 American Association for Chronic Fatigue Syndrome (AACFS) Conference, to evaluate the safety and efficacy of intravenously administered Ampligen also showed encouraging results. Eleven patients with myalgic encephalomyelitis (ME) (as CFIDS is called in Belgium) were given intravenous Ampligen twice a week for 24 weeks. The Belgian physicians reported that at the end of 24 weeks, all 11 experienced some improvement. In addition, no adverse effects to treatment were noted. These positive results paved the way for expanded trials currently being conducted in Belgium.

PROTOCOL. Because this drug is in the experimental phase, treatment protocols are still evolving. Ampligen is quite fragile, which makes administration difficult (it must be given intravenously). Two intravenous injections a week are given over a 9- to 16-month period. Longer courses of treatment seem to produce longer lasting results.

PROS AND CONS. The CFIDS community is watching the evolving status of Ampligen with great interest. As one of the few drugs that has been held out as a possible cure for CFIDS, Ampligen may hold great promise for the future. Its rate of success, at least in clinical trials, is to date unequalled by any other treatment. Dr. Kenny DeMeirleir claims that close to 80% of his patients reported "complete clinical recovery" after taking an extended course of treatment. Patients report improvement in overall function, energy levels, cognitive performance, and some have been able to return to work.

Although test results are encouraging, it is important to note that Ampligen is not a surefire cure. The percentage of patients who demonstrate substantial improvement with the drug has yet to be determined. Side effects are not uncommon. Patients who have taken the drug report that they felt worse initially and that it took some time before the side effects (dizziness, nausea) were no longer felt. Dr. Peterson reported at the 1990 CFIDS Conference that some patients experienced an interferon-like reaction, with headaches, myalgias, and rarely, hair loss. A puzzling effect noted by Dr. Paul Cheney was that although patients report overall lessening of symptoms, particularly cognitive symptoms, they do not necessarily equate this lessening of severity to "feeling good" (*CFIDS Chronicle,* Physicians Forum, 1991).

AVAILABILITY AND COST. Currently, Ampligen is available in the United States on an experimental basis only to a limited number of patients. Dr. Patricia Salvato, Dr. Daniel Peterson, and Dr. Charles Lapp are among a select number of physicians in the United States who have completed the necessary paperwork to begin treating patients meeting specific age and severity of illness criteria. As the program gets underway, more patients may gain access to the drug. Meanwhile, physicians interested in treating patients with Ampligen can apply to HemispherX Biopharma (formerly HEM). Canadian physicians can request Ampligen for their patients using the Emergency Drug Release Program. In Belgium, Ampligen is being administered to patients with CFIDS by Dr. DeMeirleir at the University of Brussels.

At present, Ampligen is quite expensive. A single infusion costs $140. At this rate, 1 year of treatment will cost over $14,500. Patients must pay for the cost of the treatment because Ampligen is available on a cost recovery basis only. If Ampligen is approved by the FDA after additional double-blind studies are completed, the cost may be covered by insurance.

MORE INFORMATION

http://www.helixbio.com
http://www.cais.net/cfs-news/ampligen.htm

> These websites provide up-to-date information about the current status of Ampligen and other related compounds such as Oragen.

ANTIDEPRESSANT DRUGS

DEFINITION. Antidepressant drugs are a class of pharmaceutical products used to alleviate or prevent symptoms of depression by influencing neurochemistry.

BACKGROUND. It is estimated that one in four women and one in ten men can expect to experience at least one episode of mood disorder in the course of a lifetime. The prevalence of mood disorders has prompted a boom in research and, as a result, several new drugs have been approved in recent years that provide relief from depression.

In the late 1950s, the first antidepressants, monoamine oxidase inhibitors (MAOIs), were developed to treat depression and severe panic disorder. They operate by inhibiting the action of monoamine oxidase, the enzyme that breaks down epinephrine (adrenaline), norepinephrine (noradrenaline), serotonin, and other monoamines. In the late 1960s, a new type of drug, the tricyclic antidepressant, was introduced. The tricyclics increased amounts of serotonin and norepinephrine in the brain. In 1987, Prozac (fluoxetine), a new neurochemical modulator, was approved by the Food and Drug Administration (FDA). Prozac is one of the family of drugs known as selective serotonin reuptake inhibitors (SSRIs). These act directly on a brain cell's ability to reabsorb serotonin, a neurotransmitter involved in many neurologic functions, including sleep, digestion, blood flow, and, of importance, mood elevation.

Although antidepressants were developed to treat mood disorders such as anxiety and depression, clinicians have found that the symptoms of many chronic illnesses seem to respond to antidepressant therapy. Antidepressants have been used to treat chronic pain syndromes, migraine headaches, bladder and urinary problems, and bulimia.

USES IN CFIDS. Patients with CFIDS often are dismayed and concerned when their physicians suggest an antidepressant. It appears they are being diagnosed with depression, which, although sometimes a symptom of CFIDS, is clearly not the underlying cause. Antidepressants do have a place in the treatment of a number of CFIDS symptoms. They have proven helpful in improving sleep, energy levels, and cognitive impairment, as well as alleviating pain and perhaps even enhancing immune function.

Although there are various antidepressants to choose from, not all patients with CFIDS respond to these medications. Often CFIDS patients with sensitivities to medications cannot tolerate any antidepressant, even in the smallest doses. In a survey of patients with chemical sensitivities conducted by a DePaul University research team, more than 50% of respondents reported negative effects of antidepressants. Dr. Fred Friedberg, author of *Coping With Chronic Fatigue Syndrome: Nine Things You Can Do*, also found that a substantial proportion (about one third) of 249 patients with CFIDS reacted negatively to antidepressants. It is important for physicians and patients to remember that CFIDS patients usually require much lower doses of these medications than other patients, and therefore the dose prescribed should be one tenth or less (depending on the sensitivity of the patient) of the standard dose. In his book, *The Doctor's Guide to Chronic Fatigue Syndrome,* Dr. David Bell, pediatric CFIDS specialist, states that giving patients with CFIDS a standard dose of antidepressants can virtually serve as a diagnostic test for the illness; most patients are immobilized by it. Antidepressants can provide some degree of symptomatic relief to many patients. It is important, however, to be attentive to side effects, which frequently mimic the symptoms of the disease itself. Excessive fatigue and drowsiness, headaches, nausea, diminished libido, insomnia, and agitation can either be due to the effects of the drug or to the illness itself so it is important to be observant and increase the dosage cautiously.

TRICYCLIC ANTIDEPRESSANTS

NOTE: Tricyclic antidepressants increase the amount of norepinephrine in the brain. They cannot be given in conjunction with MAOIs because of the risk of producing dangerously high blood pressure.

Sinequan

Sinequan (doxepin), one of the most commonly used medications in the treatment of CFIDS, is of major benefit in treating sleep disturbance. It is believed that Sinequan may help correct the slow-wave sleep defect found in CFIDS and fibromyalgia. Improvement in the sleep disturbance often brings an increase in energy levels. Reduction in the pain associated with CFIDS and fibromyalgia is also noted after treatment with Sinequan. Many patients with CFIDS also report improvement in allergies as a result of Sinequan's histamine-blocking properties. Because general improvement has been noted in immune function, it has been speculated that Sinequan at low doses may function as an immune modulator.

PROTOCOL. Low doses (2 to 10 mg) of Sinequan, taken 1 to 2 hours before bedtime, are usually prescribed to treat CFIDS symptoms. Liquid formulations allow for even smaller doses.

PROS AND CONS. Side effects include weight gain, constipation, and dry mouth. Many patients with CFIDS report excessive sedation or a drugged feeling and therefore cannot tolerate treatment. Paradoxically, some feel depressed after taking the drug (but not before). However, most people report improved quality of sleep, better endurance, and energy. While some patients experience daytime sedation during the first few days, this problem usually resolves rapidly. Benefits are often noted fairly quickly, within a few days to weeks.

AVAILABILITY AND COST. Sinequan is inexpensive ($5 to $30 per month, depending on the dose) and is available by prescription in generic and brand-name formulations.

Elavil

Elavil (amitriptyline) is beneficial in treating pain, sleep disturbance, headaches, and gastrointestinal problems and may be recommended if Sinequan produces excessive sedation. In addition, Elavil is often helpful in treating interstitial cystitis, a disorder that affects many women with CFIDS. Some interstitial cystitis symptoms that may respond to Elavil are frequent urination and bladder and pelvic pain. Dr. Alan Wein, a urologist who specializes in treating interstitial cystitis, has noted that Elavil is effective in nearly 50% of his patients, probably because of its antihistamine properties.

PROTOCOL. Dosage varies, but generally 10 mg or less nightly is prescribed to minimize side effects.

PROS AND CONS. The side effects of Elavil are similar to those of Sinequan, although exacerbation of muscle weakness in CFIDS seems to be more common with Elavil than with other antidepressants. Benefits are noted quickly. On the negative side, some patients have had to discontinue the drug because of weight gain, dry mouth, or palpitations.

AVAILABILITY AND COST. Elavil is available by prescription and is inexpensive. The generic drug costs about $7 for a 30-day supply, compared with about $14 for the brand-name drug.

Pamelor, Norpramin, and Tofranil

Pamelor (nortriptyline), Norpramin (desipramine), and Tofranil (imipramine) are sometimes used in patients with CFIDS. They are helpful in treating fatigue, pain, sleep disturbance, and anxiety. Their main side effects are similar to those of other tricyclic antidepressants.

SELECTIVE SEROTONIN REUPTAKE INHIBITORS

NOTE: SSRIs must not be taken within 14 days of discontinuing MAOIs.

Prozac

The first SSRI to be approved in the late 1980s, Prozac (fluoxetine) differs from earlier antidepressants in that its mode of action is more specific. It works directly on altering the level and action of serotonin only (the tricyclic antidepressants inhibit uptake of norepinephrine as well). The SSRIs, also referred to as second-generation antidepressants, are often prescribed in place of tricyclic antidepressants because they have fewer side effects. Unlike other antidepressants, SSRIs do not cause sedation. In fact, Prozac can often act as a stimulant to increase energy. Nor do they cause the dry mouth, palpitations, and dry cough that are common with use of the tricyclic drugs.

USES IN CFIDS. Dr. Nancy Klimas, CFIDS specialist and immunologist at the University of Miami, has studied the effect of SSRIs on the immune system. At the 1990 CFIDS conference in Charlotte, North Carolina, Dr. Klimas reported that more than half of 25 CFIDS patients given Prozac for 3 months showed moderate to marked improvement. Improvements in the number of natural killer cells seem to indicate that Prozac (and other serotonin-influencing drugs) may have a modulating effect on the immune system.

PROTOCOL. When used in CFIDS, Prozac is generally given in considerably smaller dosage (2 to 10 mg, taken in the morning) than the standard dose used to treat depression.

PROS AND CONS. Prozac is effective in treating the fatigue of CFIDS, the hallmark symptom of the syndrome. Other symptoms that may respond to treatment are pain, cognitive dysfunction, and sometimes excessive sleep. The drug is also helpful in treating the physiologic depression that may accompany CFIDS as a result of metabolic changes, as well as the secondary depression that stems from the devastating experience of having a chronic, debilitating illness. An additional benefit is that, unlike the tricyclic antidepressants, Prozac does not cause weight gain. Some people have reported substantial improvement with Prozac. One patient reported that within a few weeks he was much better and has since been looking for part-time work. Another woman claimed she would have had to leave her job without Prozac. Others find it gives them an all-around boost and helps control mood swings. However, an equal number of people are unable to tolerate the side effects of Prozac and have stressed emphatically that they will never try it again. Reports of anxiety, agitation, and even excessive sedation (a paradoxical reaction not uncommon in CFIDS patients) are common. One woman said her fatigue while taking Prozac was so profound, it seemed she could not remember her own name. People who have difficulty sleeping almost universally report worsening of insomnia. In addition, many clinicians advise their patients who have been taking MAOIs to allow a longer than usual interval (up to 5 weeks) before taking Prozac. This drug's long half-life may also require a longer interval after discontinuation before starting new antidepressant treatments.

It is worth noting that Prozac has received more than its share of publicity—good and bad—in recent years. It has been praised as a miracle drug by some and labeled a danger to society by others, capable of inciting homicidal and suicidal rages. Although Prozac may have settled into its rightful place in medicine—as a new and sometimes effective weapon against depression, anxiety, obsessive-compulsive disorder, and bulimia— its effectiveness in CFIDS is still open to debate. A recent double-blind study conducted by Dr. J.H. Vercoulen of the University Hospital of Nijmegen in The Netherlands concluded that fluoxetine (20 mg/day) had no beneficial effect on fatigue or any other symptoms of CFIDS (*Lancet,* 1996). Despite conflicting reports, Prozac is still one of the more frequently prescribed antidepressants.

AVAILABILITY AND COST. Prozac is available in liquid to allow smaller doses. There is no generic formulation. The cost can range from $10 to $100 per month, depending on the dose prescribed. Insurance usually covers the cost.

FURTHER READING

Kramer, Peter. Listening to Prozac. New York: Penguin Group, 1993 (a best-selling nonfiction book).

Zoloft and Paxil

Zoloft (sertraline) and Paxil (paroxetine) are two newer drugs that are similar to Prozac, but because they are associated with fewer side effects, they may be more easily tolerated. Both drugs have a shorter half-life than Prozac does. Both have been used to treat CFIDS and have demonstrated effectiveness in treating symptoms such as fatigue, cognitive dysfunction, mood swings, pain, sleep disorders, and immune dysfunction. One patient reported that after taking Paxil for 3 months she felt stronger and was sleeping better than she had for years. Another patient believed Zoloft enabled her to recover enough to seek part-time work. Along with Prozac, Zoloft is effective in treating the depression that may accompany CFIDS. A few patients have mentioned that they felt as bad while taking these drugs as they did with other antidepressants, reminding us that many patients cannot tolerate any of these drugs. For these patients, alternative treatments have been suggested, including vitamins, amino acids, herbs, and other complementary therapies.

MONOAMINE OXIDASE INHIBITORS
Nardil and Parnate

MAOIs are used much less frequently than other antidepressants to treat CFIDS. The side effects associated with Nardil (phenalzine) and Parnate (tranylcypromine) can be severe. An additional drawback is the dietary restrictions that accompany MAOI use. Foods that contain the amino acid tyramine (aged cheese, yogurt, wine, avocado, among many others) must be avoided to prevent severe hypertensive crisis. Because these foods are so common, patients may find compliance difficult. Some patients with CFIDS have found MAOIs effective. Others have reported ill effects. One patient believed an MAOI may have contributed to a prolonged relapse, producing even greater neurologic and cognitive problems than she had experienced before.

OTHER ANTIDEPRESSANTS
Wellbutrin

Not a tricyclic antidepressant, SSRI, or MAOI, Wellbutrin (bupropion) frequently is used to treat the fatigue associated with CFIDS. Many physicians who specialize in the treatment of CFIDS have prescribed Wellbutrin when Prozac or Zoloft failed, and find it of great benefit in improving energy and controlling mood. In some patients, Wellbutrin does not produce the side effects noted with other antidepressants. The drug may be taken alone or with other tricyclic antidepressants to improve sleep. Because Wellbutrin is a nonsedating antidepressant, side effects can be similar to those of Prozac (jitters, anxiety, insomnia). The biggest drawback to the use of Wellbutrin is the risk of seizures.

PROTOCOL. The standard initial prescribed dose is 75 mg daily. CFIDS patients may wish to start with a lower dose to check for tolerance.

AVAILABILITY AND COST. A 1-month supply costs about $24. Wellbutrin is not yet available in a generic formulation.

Desyrel

Among the most sedating antidepressants, Desyrel (trazodone) is often used to treat insomnia. It is not, however, as helpful as many of the other antidepressants in treating anxiety and depression in CFIDS. Some patients report improved sleep with a low dose of Desyrel, but experience severe orthostatic hypotension with higher doses. Side effects include dizziness, nervousness, tremors, weakness, tinnitus, nausea, dry mouth, constipation, sexual dysfunction, and sweating.

PROTOCOL. The prescribed dose in CFIDS is generally 25 to 50 mg at bedtime.

AVAILABILITY AND COST. A 30-day supply of the generic drug (50 mg) costs about $17.

Effexor

When approved for commercial use, Effexor (venlafaxine) received a remarkable amount of publicity and was touted as a newer and better Prozac. Effexor is chemically unrelated to the other antidepressants and has a unique mode of action, blocking serotonin, norepinephrine, and dopamine reuptake. However, effects of the drug in CFIDS have been less than dramatic. No patient in our survey noted any substantial improvement or benefit. One patient felt more anxious and jittery. Another complained of recurring cold sores, which disappeared when the drug was discontinued. Dr. Jay Goldstein commented that, while Effexor may have been marketed as "the best thing since sliced bread," his experience was to view it as another alternative treatment rather than the most effective antidepressant (*CFIDS Chronicle,* Physicians Forum, Fall 1993). Dr. Goldstein reports nausea and hypertension as possible side effects. As more CFIDS specialists experiment with this drug, reports may be more favorable.

ANTIFUNGAL AGENTS

DEFINITION. Antifungal drugs are used to treat *Candida albicans* infection and other fungal infections.

Nystatin

In the 1940s two scientists found a mold in soil that could inhibit the growth of other molds (including *Candida albicans*). They named the substance nystatin, after New York State, where it was discovered. The drug was patented in the 1950s and for the next 20 years nystatin was primarily used in suppositories to treat vaginitis. It was popularized in the early 1980s when studies by several clinicians chronicled the successful treatment of chronic candidiasis (systemic yeast infection) with nystatin.

Candidiasis produces extreme fatigue, depression, muscle pain, and concentration problems, among other symptoms (see Chapter 3: Candida).

USES IN CFIDS. When many cases of what was then called chronic Epstein-Barr virus infection (now CFIDS) appeared in the 1980s, patients began searching for any effective treatment for the symptoms that plagued them. The alternate diagnosis of Candida infection, whether considered as the cause or an effect of CFIDS, led many patients to experiment with antifungal regimens. Although some physicians consider Candida treatments controversial and without scientific basis, many CFIDS clinicians use nystatin and other antifungal agents to treat CFIDS. Dr. Murray Susser and Dr. Michael Rosenbaum, among other physicians, use antifungal medications when symptoms of Candida infection are present along with a medical history of antibiotic or steroid use that may have contributed to Candida overgrowth. As an additional aid to determining whether an antifungal regimen might be helpful, a number of physicians use blood tests to measure Candida antibodies in the blood stream.

PROTOCOL. Many CFIDS physicians suggest using the powdered form of nystatin, citing that it works better than the pill form and is more pure (free of dyes or additives). The usual dose is 500,000 to 1,000,000 units, four times a day. Lower doses may be used initially to prevent die-off reactions. In *Chronic Fatigue Syndrome and the Yeast Connection,* Dr. William Crook notes that flush, fever, and agitation may indicate that the dose is too high. Indications that the dose is too small include excessive fatigue, cold, and achiness.

PROS AND CONS. Nystatin is considered safe, with few side effects. A surprisingly large number of the patients surveyed reported that nystatin (in combination with dietary changes and nutritional supplements as part of Candida control) has helped improve symptoms of CFIDS. Patients often report increased energy, improved immune function, and better overall health after taking nystatin. Some symptoms (thrush, gastrointestinal complaints) respond quickly to treatment, but it can take weeks or months before overall improvement is observed.

While a number of patients note steady improvement over time, others experience no benefit after long trials of nystatin, and still others are not able to tolerate the drug at all. One patient reported an extreme allergic reaction to nystatin. Those who have a negative reaction, however, can often tolerate other antifungal medications. It is important to note that with antifungal medications the phenomenon of "die-off" may create problems; that is, as the antifungal medications kills the yeasts, they secrete toxins into the body and symptoms may worsen initially. Symptoms of die-off include increased fatigue, muscle aches, and headaches. It can be difficult to differentiate between symptoms that could be due to die-off, intolerance for the drug, or perhaps a "bad CFIDS day."

AVAILABILITY AND COST. Nystatin is available over the counter in suppository form to treat vaginitis and is widely available in creams for topical use. It is available in pill form by prescription at most pharmacies, but the powdered form is difficult to find. Pharmacies that carry the powdered form are Apothecary (800-869-9160) and Willner Chemists (800-633-1106). Pills or powder may cost $30 to $50 a month. Insurance coverage varies.

Diflucan

Diflucan (fluconazole), an antifungal introduced in the United States in 1990, is extremely valuable in treating the life-threatening Candida infections that sometimes occur in immunocompromised patients, such as those with AIDS (acquired immunodeficiency syndrome) or advanced cancer.

Diflucan differs from nystatin in that it is absorbed through the intestinal wall and traverses the blood stream, thereby penetrating anywhere excessive yeast colonization is found. Therefore, in theory at least, Diflucan may be more beneficial than nystatin to treat systemic or pervasive yeast infections.

USES IN CFIDS. Many clinicians have found Diflucan beneficial for treating CFIDS symptoms. A respected CFIDS specialist, Dr. Carol Jessop, a one-time skeptic of Candida as a symptom of CFIDS, has used antifungal therapies when patients have symptoms suggestive of Candida overgrowth. She has stated that, although other agents may be of benefit, Diflucan was her treatment of choice. Dr. Jessop found that because Diflucan penetrates the central nervous system, her patients experienced improvement in cognitive problems. This was not the case with nystatin or Nizoral. Dr. Jay Goldstein, on the other hand, has reported only limited success with Diflucan. He prescribes it chiefly to treat gastric disturbances (*CFIDS Chronicle*, Physician's Forum, Spring 1991).

PROTOCOL. Some physicians prescribe 200 mg for 1 week, followed by 100 mg for 3 to 6 weeks. A reevaluation is recommended after that time.

PROS AND CONS. Diflucan is usually well tolerated. The principal side effects are nausea and other gastrointestinal complaints. It works very quickly and patients will usually see improvement within a few days to weeks. Diflucan is extremely expensive, thereby prohibitive for some patients.

AVAILABILITY AND COST. Diflucan is available by prescription. The cost may range from $250 to $600 a month, depending on the dosage. Insurance plans usually cover the cost (if your insurance does not include Diflucan to treat CFIDS, you may qualify for a compassionate free supply; contact Pfizer, Inc., Roerig Division; 800-869-9979).

Nizoral

Nizoral (ketoconazole) is somewhat similar to Diflucan but is used less frequently because of its serious side effects, including liver toxicity and endocrine system disturbances. Although the drug is effective and inexpensive, many physicians are cautious about prescribing it. Patients taking Nizoral generally undergo blood tests, including liver profile, every 30 days. Nizoral is available by prescription. A 30-day supply generally costs about $30.

Sporanox

Sporanox (itraconazole), the newest antifungal drug to be approved by the FDA, is rapidly gaining popularity as an effective antifungal agent. Like Diflucan and Nizoral, Sporanox is used to treat systemic Candida overgrowth. It is slightly less expensive than Diflucan and, because it is less toxic to the liver, is safer than Nizoral. Sporanox also is used to treat infections that are resistant to other therapies. Some patients who have found little benefit from Diflucan have noted improvement with Sporanox. The drug is generally well tolerated. The most common side effects are transient nausea and headache. Doses range from 100 to 200 mg/day. The cost is $135 to $200 a month, depending on the prescribed dosage. Because the capsules contain chemical dyes, patients with chemical sensitivities can place the Sporanox in a dye-free capsule.

ANTIHISTAMINES

DEFINITION. Antihistamines are a class of drugs that appear to compete with histamine for cell receptor sites on effector cells, thereby blocking the effects of histamine.

BACKGROUND. Antihistamines have been used for many years to treat allergies and allergic reactions. Some antihistamines are also used to treat motion sickness and mild Parkinson's disease.

USES IN CFIDS. Because many patients with CFIDS have allergies (usually preceding but sometimes developing after the onset of CFIDS), antihistamines are often prescribed for relief of seasonal and general symptoms. Antihistamines are also of benefit in treating many other symptoms of CFIDS, including insomnia, bladder problems (interstitial cystitis), anxiety, and muscle pain. Benefits are noted rapidly, usually within 24 hours to a few weeks. The side effects produced by antihistamines are generally minor, although some patients with CFIDS report heart palpitations.

Claritin and Hismanal

Claritin (loratadine) and Hismanal (astemizole) are useful in the treatment of the symptoms of seasonal allergies, such as runny nose, sneezing, itching, and watery eyes. They have the distinction of being nonsedating, which may be of value in some patients with CFIDS. Some patients have reported that, although they are usually sensitive to medications, Claritin has brought great relief from hay fever symptoms, without adverse effects.

AVAILABILITY AND COST. Claritin and Hismanal are available by prescription, and generally cost about $60 to $65 for a 30-day supply. Claritin (10 mg) is one of the most expensive antihistamines, at about $70 for a 30-day supply. Insurance plans usually cover prescription antihistamines.

Benadryl

Benadryl (diphenhydramine) is useful for treating hives, seasonal allergies, upper airway congestion, and severe allergic reactions (anaphylactic shock). The drug is very sedating and can be used as a sleep aid for CFIDS-related insomnia if taken at bedtime. Like the other antihistamines, Benadryl is not addictive, and thus may offer a good alternative to habit-forming sleeping pills. However, as Dr. David Bell points out in *The Doctor's Guide to Chronic Fatigue Syndrome*, Benadryl can lose effectiveness with continuous use for longer than a few weeks and therefore may be better used only occasionally. One woman noted that, although Benadryl ensures a good night's sleep, she rotates it with a benzodiazepine so that she does not develop a tolerance to either drug (see Benzodiazepines). Although Benadryl is generally well tolerated, adverse reactions (notably agitation and tachycardia) have been reported. It is important to check with a physician before trying it, especially if you are prone to heart beat irregularities.

Benadryl is inexpensive, costing less than $10 per bottle or package. It is also available as a dye-free pill and in liquid form, which may be of benefit to CFIDS patients with chemical sensitivities. Benadryl can be purchased without a prescription.

Chlor-Trimeton

A patient with long-term CFIDS wrote of her positive experience using Chlor-Trimeton (chlorpheniramine maleate) (*CFIDS Chronicle,* Winter 1994). She reported that a dose of 2 mg improved her sleep and she felt "less miserable in the day. There was less aching, less fatigue, a little more mental clarity." After the drug effect reached a plateau, she increased the dose and noticed that all her symptoms improved, not just sleep disturbances. Other patients have also reported similar benefits. Chlor-Trimeton is available over the counter.

Atarax and Vistaril

Atarax and Vistaril (hydroxyzine) have a wide range of uses in treating CFIDS symptoms. Dr. Paul Cheney prescribes Vistaril to treat muscle pain (*CFIDS Chronicle,* Spring 1995). Two physicians who specialize in treating interstitial cystitis, Dr. Grannum Sant and Dr. Theoharis Theoharides of Tufts University, have published several papers detailing the effectiveness of Atarax and Vistaril. Dr. Theoharides noted that several patients given hydroxyzine experienced improvement in urinary frequency and bladder pain. He theorizes that this drug may inhibit secretion of mast cells, a type of cell involved in allergic reactions that may be responsible for many symptoms in interstitial cystitis. Dr. Theoharides states that other antihistamines do not seem to be effective in treating interstitial cystitis (*Seminars in Urology,* 1991). The initial dosage is 25 mg a day, which can be slowly increased to 100 mg. Daytime sedation, the most common side effect, generally disappears in a few days. Because Atarax and Vistaril are not a cure for interstitial cystitis, symptoms often recur after discontinuation of the drug. However, the success rate is high and the risks low, compared with many other invasive therapies for interstitial cystitis. Several of our survey respondents have used Atarax to treat bladder problems, with good results. One patient, however, could not tolerate the sedative effect and another reported that she developed an intolerance to Atarax after a few months. Another patient reported that the drug simply stopped working after several months.

AVAILABILITY AND COST. Atarax and Vistaril are available by prescription, in brand-name or generic formulations. These drugs are inexpensive. Thirty tablets of the lowest strength (10 mg) generic drug costs about $6.

Antivert

Antivert (meclizine) is used to treat vertigo, dizziness, and motion sickness. In CFIDS, it is frequently prescribed to treat vertigo associated with CFIDS as well as balance problems, nausea, motion sickness, and Meniere's disease. Antivert is safe to use. The most common side effect is excessive sedation. Brand-name or generic formulations are available by prescription. The usual dosage is 25 mg one to three times a day. The cost, about $10 a month, is covered by most health insurance plans.

ANTIVIRAL AGENTS

DEFINITION. Antiviral agents are a group of drugs used to inhibit the replication of viruses.

Acyclovir

In the early 1980s, acyclovir (Zovirax) was hailed as one of the first drugs proven effective against genital herpes. Although later shown to be not as universally helpful as researchers first thought, acyclovir does relieve the severity, duration, and frequency of outbreaks for many patients with genital herpes. Acyclovir is not a cure for the infection because it does not kill the virus but merely inhibits its ability to replicate. In addition to treating herpesvirus, which causes genital herpes, acyclovir has been used with some success to treat other types of herpesvirus infections, such as chickenpox (varicella zoster virus), shingles (herpes zoster), cytomegalovirus (CMV), and infectious mononucleosis (Epstein-Barr virus), among others.

USES IN CFIDS. In the mid-1980s, Epstein-Barr virus was thought to be the cause of the illness now known as CFIDS. Because Epstein-Barr virus is one of the herpesviruses, it was logical for acyclovir to be used to treat cases of what was then called chronic Epstein-Barr virus or chronic mononucleosis. At that time, physicians using acyclovir noted symptomatic improvement in many of their patients. However, the first formal study was not completed until 1988, when Dr. Steven Straus of the National Institutes of Health (NIH) headed a double-blind, placebo-controlled study to determine the effectiveness of acyclovir against CFIDS. Dr. Straus' results revealed no difference between the placebo group and patients given acyclovir (*New England Journal of Medicine,* 1988). Notwithstanding these inconclusive results, many physicians familiar with CFIDS continue to prescribe acyclovir, citing both their success rate and the flawed methods of Dr. Straus' study as justifications. Dr. Charles Lapp, for example, reported "remarkable results with this medication." Other physicians also recommend acyclovir, especially in the presence of high titers of herpesvirus, recurrent shingles, or other clinical evidence of viral infection (*CFIDS Chronicle,* Spring 1991).

PROTOCOL. The oral form is most commonly recommended because intravenous injections carry some risk of toxicity. Daily doses range from 800 to 4000 mg divided throughout the day. Topical creams or ointment can be applied directly to the skin to treat surface blisters and other lesions. Despite the associated risks, patients with acute infections may require intravenous administration. Because resistance can develop, 30- to 60-day intervals between courses of therapy are recommended to ensure continued effectiveness.

PROS AND CONS. Acyclovir, while not a cure for CFIDS, may lessen the viral load in patients with CFIDS who demonstrate a lot of viral activity (high titers of herpesvirus, recurrent flu-like symptoms, shingles). A number of patients with CFIDS have reported success with acyclovir in controlling shingles and eliminating chronic sore throat. In their book, *CFIDS, An Owner's Manual,* Barbara Brooks and Nancy Smith reported success with acyclovir, claiming it to be the most important component of their respective treatments. Positive results are far from universal, however. An equal number of patients with CFIDS report little or no benefit, even after months of trial. For those who do receive some benefit, the results are generally short-lived. Many patients must take the drug daily to see any result at all. Acyclovir, although usually well tolerated, produces some common side effects, notably lightheadedness, nausea, and headache. Patients with kidney disease should not take acyclovir.

AVAILABILITY AND COST. Oral acyclovir is available by prescription. Because a generic formulation is not available, the drug is quite costly. Depending on the prescribed dose, a month's supply may cost upward of $200 or $300. Insurance plans sometimes cover the cost (Burroughs-Wellcome, the manufacturers of Zovirax, have a program for patients without insurance or with other financial hardship; call 800-722-9294 for information).

Famvir

Famvir (famcyclovir) is a newly approved medication with antiviral activity against herpesviruses, particularly herpesviruses 6 and 7, two viruses that play an important role in CFIDS. Technically, Famvir is a prodrug; that is, a substance that is converted into an active drug once in the body. Famvir functions the same as Zovirax, but with fewer side effects. There is some indication that it may be more effective, as well. Currently, only a few CFIDS clinicians prescribe Famvir so not much information is available as to its effectiveness in treating CFIDS. Famvir is available by prescription. This drug is expensive. A 1-month supply can cost as much as $500, depending on the dosage.

Amantadine

Amantadine (Symmetrel) is prescribed for viral infections (type A influenza virus) and Parkinson's disease. It acts by blocking the penetration of cell membranes by the infectious material from viruses. As an antiviral agent, it is of no benefit unless administered at the onset of infection. In patients with CFIDS who cannot tolerate flu shots, amantadine might be a good alternative, especially for those patients susceptible to frequent episodes of influenza. In CFIDS, its most common use is not as an antiviral agent but as a stimulant. It is used to treat fatigue and lethargy in mild cases. Common side effects include insomnia, confusion, headaches, and dizziness. Amantadine interacts with antidepressants and antihistamines. Some patients with CFIDS cannot tolerate this drug so the initial dose should be small. Amantadine is available by prescription. A 1-month supply of the generic amantadine costs approximately $12.

BENZODIAZEPINES

DEFINITION. Benzodiazepines are central nervous system depressants.

BACKGROUND. The benzodiazepines are a group of drugs used to treat anxiety, skeletal muscle spasm, insomnia, and panic. Their calming effect is produced by a general slowing of the central nervous system. Within a decade of their introduction on the market, they had become one of the most frequently prescribed medications in the United States and, by the late 1980s, more than 10% of the U.S. population had taken some form of tranquilizer.

Although the benzodiazepines do not pose as many problems as the major tranquilizers, they too produce tolerance and dependence if used over a long period of time. Benzodiazepines can be classified into two main groups, depending on their half-life (how long it takes to clear half the drug from the body). In general, the shorter acting benzodiazepines (with a half-life of 4 to 20 hours) are more habit forming than those with a longer half-life (24 to 72 hours). In cases where dependence develops, doses should be tapered off *slowly* to avert withdrawal symptoms (anxiety, jitters, insomnia, confusion, sweating, heart palpitations, and depression).

USES IN CFIDS. The benzodiazepines are frequently prescribed, often in combination with a small dose of antidepressant, to treat insomnia. The logic behind prescribing both drugs is that one gets you to sleep and the other keeps you asleep. The majority of CFIDS physicians also recommend some form of benzodiazepine for patients with panic disorder or agitation due to upregulation of the sympathetic nervous system. It is important to note that benzodiazepines are usually prescribed in small doses to treat CFIDS. Normal doses of these drugs can produce paradoxical reactions, creating the very symptoms the drug is supposed to control. Even tiny doses can produce adverse reactions in patients hypersensitive to chemicals and drugs. It may be worthwhile to do a toothpick test (crush the pill and take only what clings to the end of a moistened toothpick) before embarking on a full program.

Klonopin

Klonopin (in Canada, Rivotril) (clonazepam) acts directly on the limbic system, thalamus, and hypothalamus to produce anticonvulsant effects. It has been used since the late 1970s to control seizures. Klonopin is easily absorbed through the digestive tract and has a half-life of 24 to 72 hours. Effects are noticeable within 20 minutes and can last for 12 hours.

USES IN CFIDS. Klonopin is the most widely recommended benzodiazepine for patients with CFIDS. It is usually taken in conjunction with Sinequan to control insomnia. A number of patients have reported that Klonopin helps improve cognitive symptoms, particularly poor concentration and "brain fog." Some patients also report that Klonopin helps alleviate flu-like achiness.

PROTOCOL. The dose recommended to treat CFIDS-related insomnia is low, generally 0.5 to 1 mg taken before bedtime.

PROS AND CONS. The side effects of Klonopin are mild, especially compared to those of some of the other benzodiazepines. Some patients with CFIDS, however, experience sedation, excessive thirst, depression, and gastrointestinal upset even with small doses. If taken for longer than a month, Klonopin should not be discontinued suddenly. On the positive side, Klonopin appears to be well tolerated by many patients with CFIDS.

AVAILABILITY AND COST. Klonopin is available by prescription. A 30-day supply of the generic drug (clonazepam, 0.5 mg) costs about $24. The cost is usually covered by insurance (but check for time limitations).

Valium

Valium (diazepam), an antianxiety drug, was introduced in the United States in 1963. It acts by depressing the area of the central nervous system that controls the emotions (limbic system). It is also used as an anticonvulsant in patients with epileptic seizures and to relieve skeletal muscle spasms. Side effects from long-term use can include depression, drowsiness, lethargy, fainting, slurred speech, tremor, blurred or double vision, gastrointestinal disorders, nausea, and respiratory depression. It has a half-life of 20 to 50 hours. Onset occurs within 30 minutes to an hour, with peak action in 1 to 2 hours.

USES IN CFIDS. Valium is less frequently recommended than Klonopin, nevertheless some people have found it to be very effective. In most cases, Valium is used for insomnia. It is taken just before bed. As with Klonopin, it should be taken at the lowest possible dose. If side effects or tolerance develop, Valium should be eliminated by slowly tapering off the dose.

AVAILABILITY AND COST. Valium is available by prescription. A 1-month supply (30 tablets) of the generic drug at the lowest dose (2 mg) costs about $11.

Xanax

Xanax (alprazolam) was introduced in 1982 to treat anxiety, muscle spasms, and insomnia. It is also widely prescribed to treat panic attacks, agitated depression, and phobias. Xanax is more rapidly metabolized and eliminated than other benzodiazepines and causes less "hangover." It has a half-life of 12 to 15 hours, rapid onset (about 15 minutes), and its peak action occurs within 1 to 2 hours.

USES IN CFIDS. Because Xanax acts so quickly, it is usually recommended to treat panic and anxiety attacks. It is not often prescribed for persistent insomnia, although it may be recommended on a short-term basis. As with other benzodiazepines, Xanax should be taken at the lowest possible dose. It is not recommended as a daily medication, but only as needed to alleviate the effects of panic or anxiety due to overactive nervous system responses.

AVAILABILITY AND COST. Xanax is available by prescription. It is inexpensive; a supply of 30 tablets of the generic drug at the lowest dose (0.25 mg) costs about $7.

BETA BLOCKERS

DEFINITION. Beta blockers slow heart activity by interfering with adrenal hormones.

BACKGROUND. Beta blockers are used primarily to treat angina and high blood pressure and to control irregular heart beat in damaged hearts. They can also be used to prevent migraine headaches, control ocular fluid pressure, and reduce anxiety. Beta blockers work by occupying the specific receptors in the heart, airways, and blood vessels (beta$_1$ and beta$_2$ adrenergic receptors) designed to receive the stimulating neurohormone, norepinephrine. By preventing the action of norepinephrine, beta blockers reduce the force and rate of heart beats and prevent dilation of blood vessels surrounding the brain and of the airways leading to the lungs. The action of most beta blockers makes them useful for treating neurally mediated hypotension (NMH), an abnormal reflex interaction between the heart and brain. Patients with NMH experience sudden drops in blood pressure, leaving them feeling faint and weak. Beta blockers are used to help maintain constant blood pressure in NMH.

USES IN CFIDS. Beta blockers have been prescribed to treat idiosyncratic heart problems (palpitations, mitral valve prolapse, and rapid or irregular heartbeat) and, in some circumstances, anxiety and headaches. Beta blockers are also used to treat low blood pressure common in CFIDS because researchers at Johns Hopkins University have published findings that seem to demonstrate a link between CFIDS and NMH. Although NMH does not cause CFIDS, treating it may help to alleviate some of the more troubling symptoms of CFIDS.

PROTOCOL. The beta blockers recommended in NMH are propranolol and atenolol (Tenormin). These are normally prescribed as part of a program that includes increased intake of dietary salt and Florinef (fludrocortisone), a steroid drug (see Florinef). Beta blockers should not be taken with any food, drug, or other medication that contains caffeine or alcohol because the combination may increase heart rate or blood pressure.

PROS AND CONS. Recently, a Johns Hopkins University study has created quite a stir in the CFIDS community (*Journal of the American Medical Association,* 1995). Of the 22 patients with CFIDS and NMH treated in this study, nine reported full recovery and seven noted some improvement. (However, not all of these patients received beta blockers; some were given only Florinef.) These initial results were encouraging. However, symptoms of CFIDS do not always respond favorably to beta blockers. Some patients report little or no effect and others observe that symptoms have actually worsened. Moreover, long-term and severe cases have not shown substantial improvement using this regimen.

Beta blockers can cause orthostatic hypotension (the feeling of fainting on standing), fatigue, dizziness, lightheadedness, depression, and headaches. In at least one patient with CFIDS, the beta blocker Sectral (acebutolol) caused NMH to progress to postural orthostatic tachycardia syndrome (POTS), a much more serious disorder, which left him bedridden for months. An additional consideration for those who have taken beta blockers for a long period of time is that the drug should not be discontinued suddenly but should be tapered off gradually over several weeks to avert irregularities in heart rate. People with poor circulation in the arms and legs, a frequent problem in CFIDS, are also cautioned not to take beta blockers because these drugs make the problem worse.

AVAILABILITY AND COST. Beta blockers are available by prescription. The cost ranges from $10 to $30 a month and usually is covered by insurance.

CALCIUM CHANNEL BLOCKERS
(Nicardipene, Nimodipine, Nifedipine, Verapamil)

DEFINITION. Calcium channel blockers inhibit the transmembrane influx of calcium ions into cardiac and smooth muscle.

BACKGROUND. Calcium channel blockers work by preventing calcium ions from entering smooth muscle cells. Calcium is especially important for the functioning of these cells and specialized cells in the heart. When calcium levels are lowered, the result is a relaxation of blood vessels, allowing an increased supply of blood and oxygen to the heart while decreasing its work load. As a consequence of their effect on blood vessels, calcium channel blockers are useful in treating cardiovascular disorders, such as angina (chest pain) and coronary artery disease, and to lower blood pressure. These drugs also may improve exercise capacity and subsequently reduce the need for surgery in patients with cardiac problems.

USES IN CFIDS. At the 1990 CFIDS conference in Los Angeles, Dr. Ismael Mena presented evidence of cerebral dysfunction in patients with CFIDS. Using neurologic spectroscopic scanning techniques, Dr. Mena reported that 71% of CFIDS patients have low blood flow (hypoperfusion) in the temporal lobe of the brain. He further reported that after treatment with calcium channel blockers, some of these patients exhibited clinically improved cerebral blood flow (*CFIDS Chronicle,* Spring/Summer 1990).

A number of CFIDS clinicians have noted improvement in cognitive function in patients given calcium channel blockers. Cardene also is helpful in treating migraine-type headaches. Dr. Jay Goldstein also observed improvements in cognitive function and energy level in patients given calcium channel blockers. He has also noted increased exercise tolerance, decreased tender point sensitivity, and alleviation of panic disorder with nimodipine. In October 1994, Dr. Robert Keller, Medical Director of the Center for Special Immunology in Miami, reported improvement of symptoms in 25 patients with CFIDS after treatment with the calcium channel blocker verapamil. Within 1 month of finding the optimal dose of verapamil, patients reported improvement in fatigue, memory, and myalgia. Dr. Keller also reported a decrease in the number of activated T cells, demonstrating that calcium channel blockers may have some immunomodulatory properties.

PROTOCOL. The most commonly prescribed calcium channel blockers in patients with CFIDS are nimodipine, nicardipene, and verapamil. Doses must be individualized for each patient, but generally are quite low:

Nimodipine	30 mg, 2 or 3 times daily
Nicardipene	20 mg, 2 or 3 times daily
Verapamil	120 to 240 mg, taken nightly

PROS AND CONS. Symptomatic relief can be obtained quickly with calcium channel blockers; therefore a trial is often worthwhile in many cases, even in the absence of a single-photon emission computed tomography (SPECT) scan. Improved cognitive function, fewer headaches, increased energy, and decreased muscle spasms have all been reported with use of these drugs. Although calcium channel blockers can be effective for some of the more problematic CFIDS symptoms (cognitive dysfunction), side effects can be a problem. The most common are lowered blood pressure (which can be serious if blood pressure is already low), severe pressure headaches, dizziness, gastrointestinal problems (diarrhea, constipation), and weakness. In addition, hypertensive effects can be exaggerated by concomitant use of other drugs that affect blood pressure, such as beta blockers. Tagamet (cimetidine) also increases the effects of calcium channel blockers. The use of calcium channel blockers requires close supervision by a physician.

AVAILABILITY AND COST. Calcium channel blockers are available by prescription. Nimodipine is expensive, costing almost $5 per pill, or more than $300 a month. Nicardipene and verapamil are much less expensive, about $30 a month.

CENTRAL NERVOUS SYSTEM STIMULANTS
(Cylert, Ritalin, Dexedrine, Ionamin)

DEFINITION. Central nervous system (CNS) stimulants are a class of drugs that, much like the amphetamines, speed CNS responses by releasing stored norepinephrine from nerve terminals in the brain.

BACKGROUND. Prescription CNS stimulants were first promoted in the 1950s as a treatment for hyperactivity, attention deficit disorder (ADD), and narcolepsy. They also gained popularity as weight-loss drugs. Although routinely prescribed for children with ADD, the use of CNS stimulants in children has been the focus of much controversy since the 1980s, when they received a great deal of adverse publicity.

USES IN CFIDS. CNS stimulants are generally used to increase energy and cognitive function in CFIDS. The drugs most commonly recommended for CFIDS patients are Cylert (pemoline) and Ritalin (methylphenidate), although Dexedrine (dextroamphetamine) is also sometimes prescribed. Ionamin (phentermine), a mild CNS stimulant that activates dopamine in the brain, is sometimes recommended in CFIDS patients with hypersomnia or significant cognitive impairment. The mild stimulation induced by a low dose of any of these drugs can often dispel feelings of lethargy and "brain fog" and, because effects are so immediate, they can act as a "quick fix" in an emergency. While there is great appeal in seeing immediate improvement in energy levels and cognitive function, most CFIDS clinicians prescribe these drugs with caution. A number of CFIDS clinicians believe that the disabling fatigue of CFIDS may be a protective mechanism. Therefore, creating energy artificially may in the long run cause relapse and may even exacerbate the disease process.

PROTOCOL. Dosage varies according to the individual needs of the patient, as determined by a physician. Patients with CFIDS, however, are advised to start with the smallest dosage to avert the negative effects of overstimulation. Dexedrine, for example, is prescribed at the lower than usual dose of 5 to 10 mg. Ionamin dosage varies between 15 and 30 mg (taken in the morning).

PROS AND CONS. Stimulants, while appearing to provide more energy, tax the system. As a consequence, they are beneficial only if the system is strong to begin with. Whereas CNS stimulants have been effective in some patients, they are of modest to little benefit for others. Some patients even report feeling much worse. It appears that the less ill the patient the better the response. The boost received from these drugs may enable patients with mild symptoms to work full-time or part-time. One patient surveyed, in fact, believed Cylert had been the only medication he had tried in 3 years that had had any beneficial effect. Most people use Cylert and Ritalin only "as needed" to provide extra energy on particularly long or important days. The most common side effects are anxiety, excitation, insomnia, gastrointestinal problems, dizziness, headache, palpitations, dry throat, appetite loss, and hypertension. As with other medications that affect the CNS, some patients experience a paradoxical reaction of extreme fatigue and weakness. Drug interactions are numerous, including antidepressants (especially MAOIs), anticonvulsants, and caffeine. As with MAOIs, foods high in tyramine should be avoided (see Chapter 3: Urinary Tract Problems, Cystitis). CNS stimulants are contraindicated in patients with cardiovascular disease or hyperthyroidism.

AVAILABILITY AND COST. CNS stimulants are available by prescription, either as brand-name or generic drug. Most are inexpensive. Cylert and Ritalin, for example, cost $20 to 50 per month. Insurance usually reimburses the cost.

CYTOTEC

DEFINITION. Cytotec (misoprostol) is a synthetic prostaglandin E_1 analogue that replaces depleted gastric prostaglandins.

BACKGROUND. Cytotec is routinely used to prevent gastric ulcers in elderly or debilitated patients who are receiving nonsteroidal anti-inflammatory drug (NSAID) therapy. In these patients, the action of natural prostaglandins (hormone-like substances that regulate inflammation, blood vessel dilation, and a host of other physiologic responses) are blocked.

USES IN CFIDS. Cytotec is primarily recommended for patients suffering from leaky gut. It is believed the drug actually helps "patch" the damaged lining of the small intestine, thereby reducing symptoms associated with food sensitivities.

PROTOCOL. Physicians recommend taking four 100 µg tablets a day (one with each of three meals and one before bedtime). When reducing dosage, the bedtime dose should be the last tablet eliminated.

PROS AND CONS. Cytotec has relatively few side effects. Many patients who have tried Cytotec report an increase in the number of foods they can tolerate and a decrease in related gastrointestinal symptoms. One patient with severe food intolerance noted sustained improvement even after eventually discontinuing Cytotec. The most common side effects are diarrhea, flatulence, nausea, headache, and, rarely, vaginal bleeding. If side effects last longer than a week or are severe, the dosage should be lowered. Cytotec is contraindicated in pregnant women because it may induce miscarriage.

AVAILABILITY AND COST. At the highest recommended dosage (four per day), a month's course of Cytotec costs about $108. Cytotec is available by prescription and the cost is covered by most insurance plans. Uninsured patients may meet the manufacturer's criteria for its "Patients in Need" program and qualify for a free supply (contact Searle, 5200 Old Orchard Rd., Skokie, IL 60077; 800-542-2526).

DIAMOX

DEFINITION. Diamox (acetazolamide) is a diuretic drug.

BACKGROUND. Diamox was introduced in 1953 as a diuretic. Because it reduces intraocular pressure, it is used to treat glaucoma and can also be used to treat edema, high-altitude sickness, and as an anticonvulsant. Diamox blocks the action of carbonic anhydrase, an enzyme that helps form hydrogen and bicarbonate ions from carbon dioxide and water. It promotes excretion of sodium, potassium, water, and bicarbonate. By blocking carbonic anhydrase in the central nervous system and increasing carbon dioxide tension, Diamox also helps decrease abnormal neuronal discharge that may lead to convulsions.

USES IN CFIDS. Because it increases cerebral blood flow, Diamox is used to treat cognitive dysfunction, as well as pressure headaches and balance problems. Patients taking Diamox often report increased energy.

PROTOCOL. Diamox usually is prescribed at 250 mg to be taken two or three times a day. As with other medications, however, physicians sometimes wish to begin with a lower dose. Because Diamox is a diuretic, potassium supplementation or potassium-rich foods (bananas and apricots) may be necessary. Diamox can be taken with food to lessen the chance of nausea or stomach irritation.

PROS AND CONS. For severe, hard-to-treat cognitive problems, Diamox can be a real boon. Diamox acts quickly; therefore, a long trial is not necessary. On the negative side, it can create metabolic acidosis, weakness, skin tingling, loss of appetite, and near-sightedness; may cause allergic reactions in persons allergic to sulfa drugs; and may activate gout or cause syndromes similar to lupus if taken for extended periods. Diamox can potentiate the effects of tricyclic antidepressants.

AVAILABILITY AND COST. Diamox is available by prescription only. It is inexpensive. A 1-month supply costs $11 (generic drug) and $35 (brand-name drug).

FLEXERIL

DEFINITION. Flexeril (cyclobenzaprine) is a muscle relaxant used to treat pain and skeletal muscle spasms.

BACKGROUND. Flexeril is closely related to the tricyclic antidepressants such as Elavil and Tofranil. It blocks nervous system impulses from the spinal cord to skeletal muscle.

USES IN CFIDS. Flexeril is a commonly prescribed medication that can be extremely beneficial in treating the fibromyalgia component of CFIDS. It may also help treat insomnia because it is sedating.

PROTOCOL. For muscle pain, 10 mg one to three times a day is recommended. To treat insomnia, take 5 to 10 mg at bedtime.

PROS AND CONS. Flexeril is an older drug with a good safety record and minimal side effects. The most common side effects are excess sedation and dry mouth. Flexeril is most useful during episodes of muscle or back pain. In addition, it may relieve insomnia in persons unable to tolerate other sleep medications. Flexeril is not addictive, as is the case with many sleeping pills, but it may lose its effectiveness over time. Flexeril is contraindicated in patients who have taken an MAOI within 14 days, have a history of heart arrhythmias, or are taking anticholinergic drugs because of its adverse anticholinergic effects.

AVAILABILITY AND COST. Flexeril is available by prescription, in generic or brand-name formulations. The drug is inexpensive. A 1-month supply is $20 and is covered by most insurance policies.

FLORINEF

DEFINITION. Florinef (fludrocortisone) is the acetate salt of a synthetic steroid with a mineralocorticoid activity.

BACKGROUND. Florinef was developed to help the body retain salt, which otherwise would be passed in the urine. Because it has mineralocorticoid activity, its effects are limited to regulation of electrolyte and water balance. It has none of the anti-inflammatory effects of prednisone and no effect on blood sugar levels, as does cortisone.

USES IN CFIDS. Florinef has received considerable attention as a CFIDS medication as a direct result of the highly publicized Johns Hopkins study of neurally mediated hypotension (NMH). In NMH, sudden decrease in blood pressure leads to fainting (syncope), lightheadedness, trouble concentrating, and dizziness. As nearly all of the CFIDS patients in the Johns Hopkins study tested positive for NMH, researchers have been hopeful about treatments that would address this particular symptom. Florinef, because of its ability to increase sodium retention, helps to raise blood pressure. In so doing, many symptoms associated with decreased blood pressure can be relieved.

PROTOCOL. A full dose of Florinef is one 0.1 mg tablet taken nightly. Most physicians currently working with CFIDS patients recommend starting at a low dose (one fourth tablet for four consecutive nights) to avert any possible drug reactions. The dose can be increased incrementally to a half tablet for 4 days, three fourths of a tablet for 4 days, and finally a full tablet. One patient noted that Florinef must be taken exactly every 24 hours or symptoms return; thus a rigid schedule is advised once the medication is started.

A potassium supplement is advised because Florinef causes the body to excrete more than the usual amount of potassium. In addition, plenty of fluids should be consumed while taking this medication. The side effects of headache or stomachache can be lessened when Florinef is taken with a full glass of water. The small amount of lactose in Florinef may cause some discomfort to those who are lactose intolerant or allergic to milk protein.

PROS AND CONS. Although Florinef has been highly touted as a broad-spectrum CFIDS treatment, CFIDS specialists have pointed out that the overall success rate is not high with this drug.

Florinef can produce serious side effects, the most common of which are high blood pressure and depression. Some patients experience such severe side effects that treatment with Florinef becomes untenable. Midodrine (Amatine), a newly approved drug, has proved effective in treating orthostatic hypotension. However, patients in a double-blind study also experienced significant numbers of adverse effects (*Journal of the American Medical Association,* 1997). Although midodrine is not widely used in the CFIDS community, a few patients have reported no benefit. Some patients have turned to alternative treatments such as licorice (which can mimic the action of steroids).

Before embarking on a course of treatment with Florinef or its substitutes, patients are advised to undergo thorough testing to confirm NMH. Because these drugs affect blood pressure, treatment must be closely supervised by a physician.

AVAILABILITY AND COST. Florinef is available by prescription. A 30-day supply of 0.1 mg tablets costs about $14.

SEE
• Chapter 5: Herbs (licorice).

GAMMA GLOBULIN

DEFINITION. Gamma globulin is a fraction of human blood that contains pooled antibodies.

BACKGROUND. Gamma globulin, or immunoglobulin, is a blood product pooled from many donors and processed so that it contains a high concentration of immunoglobulin G (IgG) and other antibodies that mitigate against and prevent certain diseases. Gamma globulin has been in use for more than 40 years to prevent hepatitis, particularly in health care workers, as a prophylactic during epidemics of measles and rubella, and as an immune modulator in Kawasaki syndrome and in myasthenia gravis (a disease that affects the muscles).

USES IN CFIDS. Gamma globulin is one of the earliest CFIDS treatments. The rationale behind the use of gamma globulin is twofold. First, it was thought that if CFIDS were caused by a virus, particularly a common virus that most of the general public had been exposed to (such as Epstein-

Barr virus), gamma globulin would contain certain antibodies to fight the virus. Second, certain patients with CFIDS had demonstrated deficiency of IgG subclasses and it was proposed that gamma globulin could correct this deficiency. While gamma globulin has sometimes been helpful in treating CFIDS, it is not easy to determine why. There is no proof of a specific causative virus as of yet and it seems that patients who demonstrate IgG deficiency do not always respond better to gamma globulin therapy than do those without IgG deficiency. Several studies, both controlled and open, have been completed in the United States and other countries with inconclusive results.

- In 1986, Dr. James Oleske and colleagues from the New Jersey School of Medicine in Newark conducted an open trial of 12 patients with chronic Epstein-Barr virus infection (CFIDS) with IgG or IgG subclass deficiency. These patients underwent intravenous gamma globulin therapy for 1 year. Symptoms improved in eight and showed no improvement in four, but did not worsen in any patients.
- Also in 1986, Dr. Richard DuBois of Atlanta, Georgia, reported the results of a double-blind controlled study of patients with chronic mononucleosis syndrome (CFIDS) treated with intramuscular gamma globulin. Symptoms in 52% of the patients who received gamma globulin improved after treatment.
- In 1988, Dr. Phillip Peterson of the University of Minnesota headed a double-blind controlled trial of intravenous gamma globulin in 30 patients with CFIDS. Patients received an infusion of gamma globulin every month for 6 months. Of these 30 patients, 12 (40%) had low IgG concentrations and 29 (9%) had a viral onset. Given the immunologic deficiencies, a presumed viral component, and a severely affected group of patients, the results fell short of expectations. No significant difference was demonstrated between the placebo and drug responses.
- In 1991, Dr. Denis Wakefield of Sydney, Australia, concluded a study of 49 patients with CFIDS enrolled in a double-blind placebo-controlled study of intravenous gamma globulin. Twenty-three patients received gamma globulin infusions over 90 days, with encouraging results. Symptoms in 10 patients improved. In addition, several immune parameters tested showed improvement after treatment. Some side effects were reported, but they may have been due to the high dose of gamma globulin. Dr. Wakefield and his colleagues reported interest in undertaking a larger trial with a lower dose of gamma globulin.

- In 1997, Australian pediatrician Dr. K.S. Rowe published the results of a study of 70 adolescents (ages 12 to 18 years) with chronic fatigue syndrome who received intravenous gamma globulin therapy. After 3 months of treatment, significant improvement was noted, but there were some side effects.

PROTOCOL. Intravenous gamma globulin may be infused once a month for 6 months or longer. Intramuscular gamma globulin can be injected once or twice a week for 6 weeks, after which the patient is reassessed.

PROS AND CONS. Many leading clinicians continue to use gamma globulin therapy, with varying degrees of success. Gamma globulin is not usually a first-line treatment and is often used after other therapies have been attempted. Dr. Paul Cheney uses both intramuscular and intravenous gamma globulin, with different rates of success. He has stated that intravenous gamma globulin may be more effective than intramuscular gamma globulin (*CFIDS Chronicle,* Spring 1995). However, he found intramuscular gamma globulin, which is much less costly than intravenous gamma globulin, particularly useful in helping reduce the frequency of upper respiratory tract infections in some patients. Dr. Murray Susser and Dr. Michael Rosenbaum, authors of *Solving the Puzzle of Chronic Fatigue Syndrome,* state that, although CFIDS is a complex disease that requires an integrative approach, if they had to choose the single most effective treatment, it would be gamma globulin.

Only a few of our survey respondents found some relief from gamma globulin therapy. The more severely ill patients noted improvement of almost all symptoms (cognition, energy, and mood). They were not cured, but were able to increase their level of activity. Several patients noted little or no benefit. No side effects were reported in our survey, but headaches, dizziness, and nausea are mentioned in the CFIDS literature, particularly if the dose is high or the rate of infusion is too fast.

A number of patients with CFIDS have expressed concern about the safety of gamma globulin, inasmuch as it is a blood product. Most physicians believe it is safe because, to date, there is no record of anyone contracting human immunodeficiency virus (HIV) from gamma globulin therapy. However, in early 1994 there were reports in newspapers concerning batches of gamma globulin overseas that were contaminated with hepatitis C virus. In May 1994, however, a new manufacturing process for intravenous gamma globulin was developed that inactivates any viral contaminants. Gamma globulin therapy is now considered safe. Nevertheless, it is important to carefully discuss the risks and benefits with a physician.

AVAILABILITY AND COST. Gamma globulin is obtained through a physician and is usually administered in the office. Intravenous infusions are costly and can be as much as $1000 per infusion. Some insurance companies reimburse the cost if the claim carefully documents specific immune dysfunction such as IgG subclass deficiency or hypogamma globulinemia. Intramuscular gamma globulin is much less costly, generally less than $100 per injection.

GUAIFENESIN

DEFINITION. Guaifenesin is an expectorant that helps clear mucus from congested passageways by increasing production of respiratory tract fluids.

USES IN CFIDS. Guaifenesin, an expectorant that is the primary active ingredient in many cough syrups, may seem an unlikely candidate as a CFIDS treatment. However, some years ago Dr. Paul St. Armand at the University of California at Los Angeles observed that this medication helped his patients with fibromyalgia. From his observations, Dr. St. Armand speculated that patients with fibromyalgia and CFIDS might have an inherited metabolic defect that causes faulty excretion of phosphates. According to Dr. St. Armand, if phosphate accumulates in the mitochondria of cells, then adenosine triphosphate (ATP) and energy production are impaired. The accumulation of phosphates also leads to increased calcium within the cells, possibly creating the tender points so commonly seen in fibromyalgia. It appeared to Dr. St. Armand that this defect in phosphate excretion could account for the symptoms of fibromyalgia and CFIDS. In support of his theory, Dr. St. Armand observed that gout medications, which increase excretion of both uric acid and phosphate, also produced positive results, although they were not as well tolerated or as effective as guaifenesin.

PROTOCOL. For people with CFIDS, guaifenesin LA (long acting) is usually prescribed. It can be purchased in pill form, without added antihistamines or decongestants. Dr. St. Armand recommends an initial dosage of 300 mg of pure guaifenesin twice a day. If that proves ineffective, the dosage is increased to 600 mg twice a day. About 30% of his patients may require higher doses. Dr. St. Armand has observed that 2 months of treatment reverses a year of illness, which should provide a baseline for calculating how long the medication may be needed (a person who has been ill for 4 years will need 8 months of treatment). Dr. St. Armand cautions that, for guaifenesin to be effective, salicylate must not be used (salicylate or salicylic acid ingredients are in Pepto-Bismol, Ben-Gay, Myoflex Creme, aspirin, Alka-Seltzer, cosmetics, plant-containing shampoos and conditioners, plant-derived vitamins, and herbal remedies). Dr. St. Armand also recommends that patients take a calcium and magnesium supplement with meals to block absorption of phosphates in food.

PROS AND CONS. Few controlled studies have been performed to confirm or disprove the effectiveness of guaifenesin in treating symptoms of CFIDS so commentaries on this drug are anecdotal. One patient with long-term CFIDS reported dramatic symptomatic improvement with guaifenesin (*Mass CFIDS Update,* Summer 1996). She began taking guaifenesin in 1994 to treat a stubborn bout of bronchitis and was surprised to note a number of other symptoms began improving. After several months she noticed she was beginning to have clusters of "good days" and that her pain was "almost nonexistent." She also noted improvements in cognitive function, energy, and vision.

Although few side effects are directly attributable to guaifenesin, CFIDS symptoms may initially worsen. Often a patient may feel much worse for the first 2 to 4 months of treatment. Dr. St. Armand warns that this treatment "takes confidence and strength" because results may not be seen for several months. He also warns that patients with both fibromyalgia and hypoglycemia will not notice any improvement with guaifenesin treatment unless the hypoglycemia is corrected (see Chapter 3: Hypoglycemia for dietary and other recommendations). Although Dr. St. Armand believes the long-term benefits are worthwhile for patients with fibromyalgia, many patients with CFIDS may be wary of risking relapse.

Patients interested in trying guaifenesin should also note that, although Dr. St. Armand claims significant improvement among his patients, studies have not replicated his results. A double-blind controlled study conducted at the Oregon Health Sciences University by Dr. Robert M. Bennett and Dr. Sharon Clark found no difference between the guaifenesin and placebo groups after a year of treatment. Neither did they find an increase in urinary excretion of phosphates, which seems to undercut the basis for guaifenesin's (theoretical) mode of action. In light of these findings, it is apparent that guaifenesin's role in the treatment of fibromyalgia and CFIDS is yet to be determined.

AVAILABILITY AND COST. Guaifenesin is available by prescription. Although it is also found in many over-the-counter cough syrups, these may contain other active ingredients, as well as alcohol, dyes, and flavoring. A month's supply costs about $26 (generic drug) and $36 (brand-name drug) and is usually covered by insurance.

MORE INFORMATION

Paul St. Armand, M.D.
4560 Admiralty Way, Suite 355
Marina del Rey, CA 90292

> Copies of papers on fibromyalgia: "One Disease–Two Names," "Hypoglycemia," and "The Use of Uricosuric Agents in Fibromyalgia" for clinicians.

HYDROCORTISONE

DEFINITION. Hydrocortisone is a glucocorticoid hormone excreted by the adrenal cortex in response to stress, inflammation, and low blood sugar levels.

BACKGROUND. Cortisone and hydrocortisone are two adrenal hormones that have numerous effects on body functions, including reduction of inflammation and maintenance of sodium and potassium balance and blood sugar. They have profound effects on protein and carbohydrate metabolism. Cortisone is used medically to treat inflammatory conditions such as rheumatoid arthritis, lupus, and allergies.

USES IN CFIDS. Whether cortisone or hydrocortisone should be used to treat CFIDS is a topic of much debate among CFIDS clinicians. Recent studies performed by Dr. Mark Demitrack and colleagues showing endocrine system deficiency along the hypothalamic-pituitary-adrenal axis (HPA axis) seem to indicate chronic adrenal insufficiency in patients with CFIDS (*Journal of Clinical Endocrinology and Metabolism,* 1991). The low levels of cortisol found in some CFIDS patients, combined with increased or new inflammatory responses (allergies, irritable bowel syndrome, and rheumatic conditions), also seem to point to the use of cortisol as a potentially effective treatment. However, not all clinicians agree that treatment with hydrocortisone is beneficial. Cortisone is an immune system suppressant and, in cases in which the immune system is already compromised, its effects could be disastrous. Clinicians who are critical of cortisone's usefulness as a CFIDS treatment point out that glucocorticoids are best used as a short-term treatment for severe allergic reactions. Long-term use may exacerbate the disease process.

PROTOCOL. Hydrocortisone (cortisone, cortisol) may be given as a single injection of 100 mg or less to treat severe allergic response or in acute cases of CFIDS when immediate intervention is required. It may also be administered in low doses (5 to 20 mg) on a daily basis.

PROS AND CONS. Cortisone is a naturally occurring chemical. However, its use, especially on a long-term basis, carries significant risk. When the body registers the presence of cortisone, the adrenal glands decrease production. Over a long period of time, the adrenal glands may fail to produce glucocorticoids altogether, making the patient entirely dependent on a drug source for this essential hormone. In addition to the risk of dependency and adrenal failure, the dosage must not be excessive, or Cushing's syndrome may eventually develop, with tendencies for obesity, hypertension, osteoporosis, and mental disturbances. Side effects of even small doses of cortisol may include headache, gastrointestinal disturbances, insomnia, and weakness. On the positive side, single ("pulse") administrations of cortisol can be lifesaving for patients with severe allergic reactions or acute-onset CFIDS. To date there are not enough data regarding small, regularly administered doses to draw any conclusion. Hydrocortisone is contraindicated in systemic fungal infections.

AVAILABILITY AND COST. Cortisone is available by prescription, in generic and brand-name formulations. The cost ranges from $15 to $30 a month, depending on the dosage.

KUTAPRESSIN

DEFINITION. Kutapressin is a peptide and amino acid solution derived from porcine (pig) liver.

BACKGROUND. In the late 1920s, it was discovered that liver helped patients with acne vulgaris. As a result of this observation, attempts were made to isolate the active factor from liver. Not until the 1940s was activity demonstrated in a specially purified liver fraction. Subsequent refinements in isolation of the active material led to the introduction of Kutapressin. Since then, Kutapressin has been used to treat poison ivy, hives, eczema, severe sunburn, herpes zoster, and other dermatologic conditions. According to Dr. Thomas Steinbach, Kutapressin was used decades ago to treat neurasthenia, a condition that bore a remarkable resemblance to CFIDS. Dr. Steinbach observes that Kutapressin's antiviral and anti-inflammatory properties make it an effective treatment for infectious mononucleosis.

USES IN CFIDS. Kutapressin's value as a CFIDS treatment did not become generally known until Dr. Thomas Steinbach and Dr. William Hermann used Kutapressin successfully in the early 1980s to treat shingles and what was then referred to as Epstein-Barr virus reactivation (*CFIDS Chronicle,* Summer 1990). Because of Kutapressin's excellent safety record and the positive results in treating Epstein-Barr virus infection, they conducted an informal unblinded study of some 270 patients with CFIDS. The results were impressive. Of the study participants, 75% showed improvement, and in some cases marked improvement, after only 40 injections of Kutapressin. Even more promising was that many of these patients had been ill with CFIDS for more than 5 years. The study riveted the attention of CFIDS clinicians because no drug treatment to date had produced such impressive results. A second study published by Dr. Steinbach and Dr. Hermann demonstrated the same impressive results (as presented at the International CFIDS Conference, Albany, N.Y., 1992). Of the 130 patients who participated in the second study, 85% reported notable or marked reduction of symptoms while receiving Kutapressin injections. Of 111 patients who reported significant reductions in symptoms, 103 noted results within 6 months of treatment. As a result of these studies, many CFIDS clinicians began to incorporate Kutapressin in their treatment plans, particularly when there is evidence of viral activity (high titers of human herpesvirus 6 and high interferon levels).

Because the underlying cause of CFIDS remains unknown, it is difficult to determine why Kutapressin has such dramatic effect. Some researchers have theorized that Kutapressin must have both antiviral and immunomodulatory properties to simultaneously curtail viral reactivation and the characteristic immune system overreaction typical in CFIDS. Kutapressin's role in suppressing viral activity is fairly well documented. A study published by Dr. D.V. Ablashi and colleagues proved that Kutapressin is a potent inhibitor of herpesvirus 6 in vitro without causing cell damage (*In Vivo*, 1994). A later study conducted in 1996 by Dr. E. Rosenfeld and colleagues found that Kutapressin was also effective against Epstein-Barr virus (*In Vivo*, 1996). However, its role in immunomodulation remains speculative. Dr. Steinbach and Dr. Hermann postulated that Kutapressin may act to mediate the action of lymphokines, the immune system chemicals that are thought responsible for many of the symptoms characteristic of CFIDS.

PROTOCOL. The original protocol developed by Dr. Steinbach and Dr. Hermann consists of a daily intramuscular injection of 2 ml of Kutapressin for 25 days followed by 2 ml injections every other day for 25 days, followed by 2 ml injections three times a week for several months.

Currently, Dr. Steinbach is prescribing daily injections of 2 ml of Kutapressin, tapering off after a 6-month period to one injection a week, using natural killer cell function as a treatment guideline.

A 23-gauge 1-inch-long needle is recommended for deep intramuscular injection. Dr. Steinbach also administers vitamin B_{12} shots as an important therapeutic adjunct. He prefers that the first few injections be given in the office, after which the patient is instructed in how to administer the injections at home. Follow-up is on a monthly basis.

PROS AND CONS. Kutapressin, although quite effective for some patients, is not universally helpful. Not everyone has achieved the remarkable success rate reported by Dr. Steinbach and Dr. Hermann. Kutapressin can involve a lot of time and money, with little gain. To that end, many patients do not continue with it for 6 months if they have noted no results after 3 or 4 months. Most patients who have benefited from it note an immediate cessation of sore throats, a reduction in flu-like feelings, pain, and fatigue, and improvement in energy level. One patient who had been bedridden became self-sufficient after treatment with Kutapressin. Many others have reported decreased duration and severity of episodes of flu, increased energy and stamina, and a feeling of overall improvement with Kutapressin. Gregg Fisher, in his book *Chronic Fatigue Syndrome: A Comprehensive Guide to Symptoms, Treatments, and Solving the Practical Problems of CFS,* states that he and his wife, both CFIDS patients, experienced notable improvement with Kutapressin. He further adds that it was the first medication that genuinely helped them both. Although Kutapressin is considered safe, it does produce a few minor side effects initially, but which usually pass quickly after the first few injections are given. In most patients, side effects subside within the first 20 days of treatment. A small number of patients, however, may feel worse. People with allergies to pork and women who are pregnant should not take Kutapressin.

AVAILABILITY AND COST. Kutapressin is available by prescription only. It costs between $90 and $140 per 20 ml vial (10 injections). A full 6-month course of treatment costs between $700 and $900. Many insurance companies cover the cost; however, some companies consider Kutapressin an experimental drug and do not cover the cost.

NALTREXONE

DEFINITION. Naltrexone (Trexan or ReVia) is an opioid antagonist.

BACKGROUND. Because naltrexone binds to opioid receptors in the nervous system, it is used to block the effects of narcotics. As a consequence, it has been useful for treating drug dependency. Naltrexone (ReVia) has recently been approved by the FDA to help treat alcohol addiction as well. Naltrexone is also useful in a number of medical conditions, including Alzheimer's disease, bulimia, and multiple sclerosis.

USES IN CFIDS. CFIDS clinicians have expressed interest in naltrexone, especially in light of findings regarding naltrexone's effect on T and B cells as well as natural killer cells. Dr. Susan Levine, a well-known CFIDS expert affiliated with Mt. Sinai Hospital, New York, explains the rationale for the use and success of naltrexone. "Naltrexone can act to counteract some of the negative effects of excess stimulation by endorphins, such as diminished immune function, and may help to improve cognition and listlessness" (*CFIDS Chronicle*, January/February 1989). (Endorphins are naturally occurring substances present in high concentrations during various illnesses, including viral and autoimmune disease.) One study by Dr. Levine provided encouraging results. Cognitive symptoms improved in six of ten CFIDS patients treated with 5 mg naltrexone. No clinically important side effects were observed. Other physicians continue to prescribe naltrexone to treat cognitive disorders.

PROTOCOL. Dosage ranges from 5 to 50 mg. Lower doses usually are most effective.

PROS AND CONS. A few people have found naltrexone of minimal or modest benefit. One patient believed naltrexone improved memory; another felt less fatigue and less body achiness. However, side effects typically include anxiety, insomnia, and headache.

AVAILABILITY AND COST. Naltrexone is available by prescription. The cost is approximately $150 for a 30-day supply of 50 mg tablets and less for lower doses. Insurance coverage may vary; check with your carrier.

NITROGLYCERIN

DEFINITION. Nitroglycerin is a nitrate commonly used to relieve angina.

BACKGROUND. Nitroglycerin is one of the oldest drugs in continual use, having been used for more than 100 years to treat angina. It is a vasodilator; that is, it causes relaxation of the blood vessels. This in turn increases the supply of blood and oxygen to meet the needs of the heart.

USES IN CFIDS. Nitroglycerin has been used primarily to treat fibromyalgia-type pain in people with CFIDS, although it has other uses as well. At the 1992 CFIDS conference in Albany, New York, Dr. Jay Goldstein reported that nitroglycerin not only relieved pain but often helped alleviate many other symptoms associated with low blood flow (hypoperfusion) in the brain. After initiating nitroglycerin treatment, Dr. Goldstein's patients reported a decrease in headaches, sore throat, irritable bowel–type symptoms, anxiety, and depression. They also noted increased energy and improved cognition. A point of great interest regarding nitroglycerin as a CFIDS treatment is that some patients with concurrent multiple chemical sensitivities report improvement in symptoms.

PROTOCOL. Because nitroglycerin affects the heart, it is best to determine a specific dose with your physician (individual requirements vary). Dr. Goldstein prescribes sublingual nitroglycerin, generally 0.04 mg (more information on Dr. Goldstein's protocol can be obtained from *CFIDS Chronicle,* which provides a transcript on nitroglycerin, or by reading Dr. Goldstein's book, *Chronic Fatigue Syndrome: The Limbic Hypothesis*).

PROS AND CONS. In marked contrast to other CFIDS medications, nitroglycerin acts very quickly. Improvement in symptoms can be noted within minutes, making them easy to evaluate. Benefits can be global; energy, pain, cognitive function, and mood may improve significantly. However, side effects are common. The most frequent problems are reduced blood pressure, fainting, dizziness, and headache. For this reason, nitroglycerin is usually administered while the patient is sitting. Patients with migraine headaches should not take this drug because it will worsen the condition. An additional drawback to nitroglycerin is that it loses its effectiveness over time. Dr. Goldstein states, "The most vexing problem in my use of nitroglycerin has been the development of tolerance, which is sometimes extremely rapid, occurring even after the first dose" (*CFIDS Chronicle,* Summer 1993). Concurrent use of any drug that lowers blood pressure or alcohol will exaggerate the hypotensive effect of nitroglycerin.

AVAILABILITY AND COST. Nitroglycerin is available by prescription, in pill or patch formulation. It can be purchased as a generic drug or any of more than two dozen brand-name drugs. Nitroglycerin is inexpensive; 100 pills cost less than $10. Insurance usually covers the cost.

OXYTOCIN

DEFINITION. Oxytocin is a hormone produced in the posterior lobe of the pituitary gland.

BACKGROUND. Oxytocin is a pituitary hormone that stimulates uterine muscle contraction and sensitizes nerves. It also controls microcirculation in the brain. Oxytocin is naturally produced in large quantities during childbirth, lactation, in response to certain stressors (hypoglycemia, exercise, hypothermia), and during sexual intercourse. Its most common medical use has been as an aid in stimulating contractions during labor.

Oxytocin is also used to control postpartum uterine bleeding. The neurotransmitter dopamine stimulates oxytocin production.

USES IN CFIDS. CFIDS clinician, Dr. Jorge Flechas, suggests that patients with CFIDS might well have a deficiency in oxytocin (*CFIDS Chronicle,* Spring 1995). Dr. Flechas bases his theory on the fact that CFIDS patients have lower levels of two other hormones, corticotropin-releasing hormone (CRH) and arginine vasopressin (AVP), which are coexpressed with oxytocin in the same region of the brain. He points out that many of the symptoms of CFIDS (pain, loss of libido, sleep disturbances, low exercise tolerance, circulatory problems, and metabolic disorders) could be generated by oxytocin deficiency. Several CFIDS clinicians, including Dr. Flechas and Dr. Jay Goldstein, use oxytocin to treat CFIDS symptoms. They have reported increased stamina, decreased pain, and improved cognitive function in those patients who have used it. In his book, *Betrayal by the Brain,* Dr. Goldstein has also noted a decrease in fibromyalgia pain, anxiety, depression, and perhaps even food allergies.

PROTOCOL. Oxytocin may be administered orally, sublingually, or as an intramuscular injection.

PROS AND CONS. Because use of oxytocin to treat CFIDS symptoms is new, little information is available as to its efficacy. Side effects, most commonly associated with the injectable forms of oxytocin, can be serious, and include nausea, irregular heart beat, changes in blood pressure, convulsions, headache, weight gain, dizziness, difficulty breathing, and mental disturbances. Any side effects should be reported to your physician. Pregnant women should not take oxytocin.

AVAILABILITY. Oral oxytocin (Pitocin, Syntocinon) is available by prescription only.

PAIN RELIEVERS

NOTE: Most analgesics are available over the counter, but it is still important to discuss dosage and side effects with your physician, especially if any of these medications are taken regularly.

DEFINITION. Analgesics are agents that diminish pain.

BACKGROUND. Pain killers work by blocking the body's production of hormones that send pain messages to the brain (prostaglandins) or by occupying the sites that receive those messages. The two general types of analgesics are nonnarcotics, which block chemical production, and narcotics, which block reception in the brain. Nonnarcotic pain killers include aspirin and other salicylates, acetaminophen (Tylenol), and nonsteroidal anti-inflammatory drugs (NSAIDs) such as ibuprofen (Advil, Motrin). Narcotic pain killers include the opiates and opioids, such as codeine, Darvon or Wygesic (propoxyphene), Demerol (meperidine), and morphine. Because narcotics are habit-forming, they are used on a short-term basis only. A number of prescription analgesics contain a combination of nonnarcotic and narcotic pain killers. The most common combinations contain codeine and acetaminophen or aspirin. These drugs are used when pain persists or is not relieved by other nonnarcotic or narcotic drugs.

Aspirin

Aspirin is classified as a nonsteroidal anti-inflammatory drug (NSAID) because it reduces inflammation. It blocks pain by inhibiting the enzyme cyclooxygenase, which helps the body produce inflammation-causing prostaglandins. The main active ingredient in aspirin is acetylsalicylic acid, a chemical that was first derived from willow bark.

USES IN CFIDS. Aspirin is recommended for those CFIDS patients with continual or severe joint and muscle pain. In his book, *The Doctor's Guide to Chronic Fatigue Syndrome,* Dr. David Bell notes that aspirin is beneficial for CFIDS patients with "prominent joint and muscle pain, headache, lymph node pain and general aching, and is less effective in patients with prominent fatigue, nausea, and neurologic symptoms."

PROTOCOL. Aspirin can be taken as needed to prevent or treat pain. Dr. Bell suggests that some patients with intractable pain may benefit from daily use of aspirin. To avoid stomach upset, aspirin should be taken with food or in buffered form. As with other drugs, it is best to begin with a small dose to assess tolerance.

PROS AND CONS. Although aspirin is generally regarded as safe, frequent use can lead to a number of side effects, including tinnitus (ringing in the ears), nausea, and heartburn. If aspirin is taken on a regular basis, an antiulcer medication (such as Zantac or Tagamet) may also be recommended to protect the lining of the stomach. Patients with a history of ulcers, gastroesophageal reflux, or other gastrointestinal problems should avoid aspirin. Aspirin should not be given to children because it can cause Reye's syndrome.

AVAILABILITY AND COST. Aspirin is available over the counter at any pharmacy and most supermarkets. It is inexpensive. Check the label carefully because some aspirin brands contain other potentially irritating ingredients, such as caffeine.

NSAIDs

Nonsteroidal anti-inflammatory drugs (NSAIDs) act by inhibiting prostaglandin production. Like aspirin, they reduce inflammation, pain, and fever. Unlike aspirin, which is cleared from the body quickly, NSAIDs have a long half-life and thus require less frequent administration. Their lower dosage leads to fewer side effects.

USES IN CFIDS. NSAIDs are recommended to treat recurring pain in muscles and joints. Many patients with CFIDS who have chronic acute pain prefer ibuprofen (Advil, Motrin) over other pain medications.

PROTOCOL. NSAIDs are generally taken as needed. Patients should start with a small dose to assess tolerance.

PROS AND CONS. Because all NSAIDs can produce gastrointestinal problems, caution must be exercised. Buffered or enteric-coated drugs help protect the stomach lining. The medication should always be taken with food. Finally, patients should be alert for signs of gastrointestinal distress (heartburn, reflux, pain).

AVAILABILITY AND COST. NSAIDs are available over the counter. The most common is ibuprofen (Advil, Motrin). Prescription NSAIDs include Clinoril, Feldene, and Tolectin. Intramuscular Toradol may be prescribed for severe pain. NSAIDs are generally more expensive than aspirin or acetaminophen.

Acetaminophen

In contrast to those NSAIDs that work by inhibiting prostaglandin production, acetaminophen (Tylenol) acts in the brain, where it blocks the perception of pain. As a consequence, acetaminophen is not of particular benefit in treating joint or muscle pain due to inflammation. Its primary uses in CFIDS are to relieve headache and generalized achiness and to reduce fevers.

PROS AND CONS. Acetaminophen does not cause stomach irritation, as do aspirin and other NSAIDs. However, a number of patients with CFIDS find they can tolerate only low or infrequent doses. An additional and serious problem associated with acetaminophen is that high doses can lead to liver damage—as can any dose of this drug taken with alcohol. If signs of liver malfunction develop (jaundice or pain under the right side of the rib cage), acetaminophen should be discontinued immediately.

AVAILABILITY AND COST. Acetaminophen is available over the counter in brand-name and generic formulations.

Ultram

Ultram (tramadol) is a new, centrally acting analgesic. Its mode of action is not yet fully understood, but, much like acetaminophen, it is believed to act on pain receptors in the brain.

USES IN CFIDS. Ultram has been prescribed to treat muscle and fibromyalgia-type pain.

PROS AND CONS. Some patients report that Ultram is the most effective medication for pain and that it also helps relieve insomnia and fatigue. The drug is reputedly nonaddictive, although some patients have reported tolerance to the drug. Ultram acts quickly and does not seem to produce as many side effects as other pain medications, although some patients have reported headaches. This drug is contraindicated in patients with seizure disorders and those taking monoamine oxidase inhibitors (MAOIs).

AVAILABILITY AND COST. Ultram is available by prescription only. Dosage varies, but the manufacturer recommends a maximum of 50 mg every 4 hours. Depending on dosage and frequency, a month's supply could cost as much as $100. No generic formulation is available.

Narcotics

The subset of CFIDS patients with severe, burning, intractable pain that does not respond to other treatments may need stronger medications. In these cases, narcotics (codeine, hydrocodone, Demerol, Darvon, Tylenol with codeine) may be recommended. Although effective, narcotics are addictive and therefore should be used only when other pain treatments have failed to alleviate pain.

PROS AND CONS. Narcotics offer immediate and sometimes total relief from certain types of pain. Some CFIDS patients with fibromyalgia report that a single injection of Demerol may relieve pain for up to 6 months. The reasons for this are not clear, but for some patients breaking the cycle of pain reception in the brain seems to have decided long-term effects. Narcotics can be used only infrequently and in small doses because the risk of addiction is high. The most common side effects are drowsiness, mood changes, and constipation. Codeine also causes stomach upset.

The higher the dose, the more serious the side effects. High doses, for example, may cause breathing problems; therefore, patients with a history of respiratory problems should exercise caution or avoid narcotics entirely.

PENTOXIFYLLINE

DEFINITION. Pentoxifylline (Trental) is a hemorrheologic agent derived from xanthine.

BACKGROUND. Pentoxifylline improves capillary blood flow by increasing the flexibility of red blood cells and lowering blood viscosity. This double action enables blood cells to squeeze through tiny capillaries with greater ease. Traditionally, pentoxifylline is used to treat vascular diseases, especially those that inhibit blood flow.

USES IN CFIDS. Some clinicians have recommended pentoxifylline in CFIDS to increase blood flow to the brain. Single-photon emission computed tomography (SPECT) scans consistently reveal lowered blood flow in patients with CFIDS. In theory, pentoxifylline should resolve that problem. Pentoxifylline may also address another blood problem common to CFIDS. Dr. L.O. Simpson, a pathologist from the University of Otago Medical School in Dunedin, New Zealand, discovered that patients with CFIDS have irregularly shaped red blood cells, which makes it more difficult for blood cells to pass through capillaries. Dr. Simpson believes the decreased cerebral blood flow in CFIDS is the consequence of abnormally shaped blood cells. Many of the symptoms of inadequate blood supply such as lightheadedness, vertigo, and cognitive problems might be alleviated if blood flow is increased.

PROTOCOL. The usual recommended dose is 400 mg three times a day, with meals. Patients with CFIDS may want to begin with a lower dose to assess sensitivity.

PROS AND CONS. CFIDS patients who have benefited from pentoxifylline report dramatic improvement in cognitive function. One man who was in danger of losing his job because of problems of concentration and memory reported that pentoxifylline restored his cognitive function to normal. Pentoxifylline should not be used by those who cannot tolerate stimulants. Xanthine, from which pentoxifylline is derived, is closely related to caffeine. Pentoxifylline is contraindicated in patients with peptic ulcers and those at risk for hemorrhage.

AVAILABILITY AND COST. Pentoxifylline is available by prescription. A month's supply costs about $55.

TAGAMET AND ZANTAC

DEFINITION. Tagamet (cimetidine) and Zantac (rantidine) are histamine H_2 receptor antagonists that inhibit acid secretion in the stomach.

BACKGROUND. Before Food and Drug Administration (FDA) approval of Tagamet in 1977, the pain resulting from duodenal ulcers was nearly impossible to treat with standard medications. While not a cure, Tagamet is thought to allow ulcers to heal by blocking acid secreted by the stomach in response to histamine. Millions of patients now take Tagamet (and Zantac, approved in 1983) and a substantial number have obtained significant relief from pain. Tagamet, Zantac, and two other approved H_2 blockers, Axid (nizatidine) and Pepcid (famotidine), are also prescribed to treat heartburn and gastritis.

In the early 1980s, Dr. Jay Goldstein used Tagamet to treat infectious mononucleosis (confirmed by monospot test, enlarged spleen, and other clinical findings consistent with the diagnosis) in a college student. The symptoms resolved within 24 hours. Dr. Goldstein's rationale for treatment was based on the fact that Epstein-Barr virus, which causes mononucleosis, is a herpesvirus and, in most herpes infections, there is an increased number of T suppressor cells. It had been recently demonstrated that T suppressor cells had H_2 receptors on their surfaces, and it was thought that the cells were activated by histamine. Dr. Goldstein theorized that perhaps the T cells could be inactivated by Tagamet, an H_2 blocker. His theory appears to have validity, as Dr. Goldstein reports positive results in 90% of cases of mononucleosis treated with Tagamet. He has received positive feedback from physicians around the United States who have replicated his results (*CFIDS Chronicle,* 1988 Compendium).

USES IN CFIDS. In 1985, Dr. Goldstein began to see his first cases of what was then called chronic Epstein-Barr virus infection (now CFIDS). Using the same logic that he used to treat mononucleosis, Dr. Goldstein gave his patients Tagamet and Zantac. He has found over the course of years that at least 20% of patients with CFIDS have responded favorably to treatment with H_2 blockers. Although the cause of CFIDS remains undetermined, it is known there is activation of T suppressor cells, probably due to viral activity. It is believed that H_2 blockers have a modulatory effect on the immune system in that they probably inhibit overproduction of lymphokines responsible for some of the flu-like symptoms of CFIDS.

Several leading CFIDS clinicians, including Dr. Charles Lapp, use H_2 blockers to treat gastrointestinal symptoms as well as for immune system modulation. Dr. Murray Susser and Dr. Michael Rosenbaum use H_2 blockers to treat immune system dysfunction.

PROTOCOL. Whereas some patients take only low doses of these H_2 blockers (even a sliver of a pill can be effective, according to Dr. Goldstein) others take the standard prescribed dose for ulcers:

Tagamet   300 to 400 mg, one or more tablets per day
Zantac   75 to 300 mg/day

PROS AND CONS. H_2 blockers work rapidly and results can often be seen in less than 2 weeks, thereby making a trial worthwhile. Many patients have reported a variety of benefits. A few of our survey respondents with allergies felt much better overall after taking Zantac and several found significant relief from digestive disturbances as well. Two respondents reported that Tagamet gave them more energy and lessened the weak, achy feeling of CFIDS. Another respondent thought Zantac relieved bladder pain due to interstitial cystitis, perhaps because it blocked stomach acid. Many acidic foods cause bladder disorders (see Chapter 3: Urinary Tract Problems).

Dr. Goldstein has noted that some patients feel nervous and agitated while taking Tagamet. Other clinicians believe H_2 blockers cause depression (a less common side effect according to the *Physicians Desk Reference*). Because Tagamet may interact with and increase blood concentrations of many drugs, some of which are commonly prescribed in CFIDS (antidepressants and benzodiazepines), it is important to advise your physician of all medications you are taking. Zantac may be prescribed more frequently than Tagamet to treat symptoms of CFIDS because it is less interreactive with other medications and may pose less risk for side effects.

AVAILABILITY AND COST. Tagamet and Zantac are available by prescription. The cost may range from $40 to $100 per month, depending on the dose, and is usually covered by insurance. Pepcid AC and Zantac 75 are available over the counter. The cost of Pepcid AC is approximately $7.50 for a package of 18 tablets, 10 mg strength.

TRANSFER FACTOR

DEFINITION. Transfer factor, an extract from peripheral blood lymphocytes (white blood cells) of a healthy donor, facilitates the transfer of T cell–mediated immunity from one person to another.

BACKGROUND. Transfer factor has been used for more than 40 years to transfer immunity from a presumably healthy donor to a recipient. It has been used to treat viral, parasitic, and bacterial infections, as well as certain autoimmune diseases and cancers. Distinctive types of transfer factor may be used, depending on the condition being treated. Nonspecific transfer factor from a pool of healthy donors may be used for immune system modulation. Disease-specific transfer factor is used to treat a specific virus or infection, such as herpesviruses or human immunodeficiency virus (HIV). In addition, donor-specific or dedicated donor transfer factor can be obtained from a relative or other household member.

USES IN CFIDS. Transfer factor, at least in theory, would appear to be valuable as a primary therapy in CFIDS. Because the cause of the disease is still unknown, it has been difficult to find a universally effective treatment. Transfer factor is considered adaptogenic; that is, it can boost a deficient immune system or, conversely, can downregulate the immune system in certain autoimmune conditions. This makes it an ideal immunomodulator in CFIDS. However, as the following data reveal, reports of the efficacy of transfer factor have been conflicting.

- At the May 1994 CFS/ME conference in Dublin, Ireland, information was presented regarding a study of 20 patients with CFS treated with oral transfer factor by Dr. Giancarlo Pizza and colleagues from Bologna, Italy. Of the 20 patients, improvement was noted in 12 and remission was observed in two. There were no significant side effects. This oral form of transfer factor was specific for Epstein-Barr virus, cytomegalovirus, human herpesvirus 6, and herpes simplex virus. Despite these positive findings it is important to note that it is difficult to accept the premise that a combination of a few known viruses would help the vast majority of CFIDS patients, some of whom may not have these viruses present or may have other viruses not being addressed by this specific transfer factor.
- Dr. Perry Orens of Great Neck, New York, reported a positive experience with transfer factor (*CFIDS Chronicle,* Fall 1993). With Dr. Hugh Fudenberg, a leading international expert on transfer factor, Dr. Orens used injectable, donor-specific transfer factor to treat symptoms of CFIDS in nine patients. The results were complete remission in two patients, marked improvement in two, partial improvement in two, and no improvement in three.
- In 1991, Dr. Denis Wakefield of Australia reported the results of an extensive double-blind study of transfer factor. Of 90 patients with CFIDS, 46 received the transfer factor and 44 received a placebo. Twenty-five patients received specific transfer factor donated by a family member and 21 received transfer factor from an unrelated donor (a healthy control). Follow-up 3 months later showed no difference in quality of life, immunologic assessment, or activity levels.

It was concluded that neither specific nor nonspecific transfer factor were of benefit. It is important to note that the treatment consisted of only eight injections, given over the course of a month. It is possible that the short duration of treatment affected the outcome.

PROTOCOL. Transfer factor may be given in oral or injectable form. It may take at least 6 months before improvement is noted.

PROS AND CONS. Because transfer factor is not widely used to treat CFIDS, it is difficult to assess its efficacy. It is worth noting that when transfer factor is effective, the results are global, with significant improvement of symptoms. In *The Type 1/Type 2 Allergy Relief Program*, Dr. Alan Levin wrote of his extensive experience with transfer factor. After using it to treat severe allergic conditions in more than 300 patients, he reported a 68% success rate, with miraculous results in some patients. However, he pointed out some serious side effects, including heart or muscle malfunction, temporary or permanent brain damage, and aggravated vasculitis, and recommended that transfer factor should probably be used only in patients with incapacitating symptoms. Other physicians do not share Dr. Levin's enthusiasm or success rate, however, and a number of CFIDS patients have reported not only lack of improvement but even a worsening of allergic-type symptoms, even after lengthy treatments with transfer factor. In fact, treatment surveys conducted by De Paul University and independent researchers have shown that about a third of those who try transfer factor consider it "harmful."

In sum, there are many drawbacks to use of transfer factor: (1) it is not widely available and is considered an experimental treatment; (2) it is costly and not usually covered by insurance; (3) many patients and physicians have raised questions about its safety and side effects; and (4) because it is a blood product, the risks of disease transmission should not be ignored, although donors are extensively screened and the transfer factor undergoes a filtration process that should eliminate viruses. Side effects of treatment may vary. Dr. Pizza notes that fatigue, sore throat, fever, and headache may occur within the first few days of treatment, but these resolve quickly. These side effects might be the result of immune system activation in response to transfer factor.

AVAILABILITY AND COST. Transfer factor therapy for CFIDS is not widely available. Currently, Dr. Hugh Fudenberg of Spartanburg, South Carolina, Dr. Lewell Brenneman of San Francisco, and Dr. Giancarlo Pizza of Bologna, Italy, are using transfer factor. A CFIDS specialist should be able to refer you to other physicians who use this therapy. Currently, the cost of injections is approximately $250 per month.

5

Nutritional Supplements and Botanicals

Alpha Ketoglutarate

Amino Acids

Antioxidants

Bioflavonoids

Blue-Green Algae

Butyric Acid

CoQ10

DHEA

Entero-Hepatic Resuscitation Program

Essential Fatty Acids

Glucosamine Sulfate

Herbs

LEM

Malic Acid

Melatonin

Minerals

NADH

Probioplex

Probiotics

Pycnogenol

Royal Jelly

Sambucol

Vitamins

ALPHA KETOGLUTARATE

DEFINITION. Alpha ketoglutarate is an ionic form of alpha ketoglutarate acid, an intermediate in the tricarboxylic cycle (Krebs cycle).

BACKGROUND. Alpha ketoglutarate fulfills a vital role in the metabolism and utilization of carbohydrates, proteins, and long-chain fatty acids. Its best known function is as a component of a number of energy-producing cycles at the cellular level. The first of these, the Krebs cycle, breaks down and transforms citric acid through a series of enzyme-controlled reactions to produce adenosine triphosphate (ATP), a crucial energy source for many cell processes. Alpha ketoglutarate, as an early intermediate in the Krebs cycle, forms the basis for all further transformations. It is also required for catabolism of many amino acids, another process that generates energy. Another important function of alpha ketoglutarate involves the formation of nonessential amino acids (amino acids that are biosynthesized in the body), notably glutamate and, through its action, proline, alanine, aspartic acid, and asparagine.

USES IN CFIDS. Alpha ketoglutarate is used as a short-term energy enhancer and for Krebs cycle support in patients with CFIDS. Because of its essential role in energy production and carbohydrate metabolism, it may be useful as a general CFIDS treatment as well. Patients with low levels of alpha ketoglutarate (as confirmed by an Organic Acids Test) have noted significant improvement in energy levels with alpha ketoglutarate supplementation.

PROTOCOL. Suggested dosage of alpha ketoglutarate is one or two 300 mg capsules per day, which can be taken with meals. Because of its location in the Krebs cycle, alpha ketoglutarate is generally more effective if taken with other Krebs cycle supports such as vitamin C, B vitamins, essential fatty acids (evening primrose oil, borage oil, or fish oil), magnesium, nutritional supplements, and NAC (*N*-acetyl-L-cysteine).

PROS AND CONS. Because alpha ketoglutarate is not a stimulant but works through natural metabolic pathways, it is a relatively risk-free source of energy. People who take alpha ketoglutarate usually do not "crash" afterward. It has no reported side effects at recommended doses. Results tend to be less dramatic than those obtained with CoQ10, however, which may make this product less attractive to those who want a greater boost.

AVAILABILITY AND COST. Alpha ketoglutarate is sold in many health food stores and by mail-order vitamin suppliers. One bottle of Alpha KG+ (Metabolic Maintenance Products; 800-772-7873), a quality, hypoallergenic brand that contains no preservatives, additives, colorings, or fillers, costs about $10 and lasts 1 month at the highest recommended dosage.

AMINO ACIDS

DEFINITION. Amino acids are nitrogen-containing chemical units (amines) that, bound together, make up protein.

BACKGROUND. The amino acids, in various combinations, form the hundreds of types of proteins present in every living organism. These proteins are essential for nearly all processes that induce cell growth and repair, as well as for continued maintenance of every body tissue, organ, and structure within the body. Amino acids link together to form tens of thousands of proteins and enzymes, each of which has a specific function. They can also perform as individual units. Single amino acids can act as neurotransmitters or as precursers to neurotransmitters in the central nervous system. Therefore, not only are they responsible for providing and maintaining the very substance of which we are made, but also for the communications system that enables us to plan, dream, think, feel, and direct our every action.

There are 20 primary amino acids. About 80% are produced in the liver and the remaining 20% must be obtained from food. Whether an amino acid can be produced within the body is what distinguishes the essential from nonessential amino acids. The essential amino acids (those that must be obtained from food sources) are arginine, histidine, isoleucine, leucine, lysine, methionine, phenylalanine, threonine, tryptophan, and valine. Nonessential amino acids include alanine, glutamine, asparagine, glycine, proline, and serine. Given the countless functions that amino acids perform, a protein shortage or congenital defect in amino acid synthesis can lead to problems that involve every system in the body.

USES IN CFIDS. Specific amino acids, both essential and nonessential, have been recommended as treatments by a number of CFIDS clinicians. Their applications include mediation of hyperactive nervous system responses, repair of leaky gut and other intestinal disturbances, and regulation of the CFIDS metabolic dysfunction that results in loss of cellular energy.

In CFIDS there is an imbalance in amino acid ratios. Dr. Alexander Bralley and Dr. Richard Lord have noted that people with CFIDS commonly have deficiencies in tryptophan, phenylalanine, taurine, isoleucine, and leucine. They also have found lower than normal amounts of arginine, methionine, lysine, threonine, and valine in a smaller number of CFIDS patients. It is significant that the most common deficiencies are of phenylalanine and tryptophan because these two amino acids are precursers to the catecholamines and serotonin, neurotransmitters that are closely involved with sleep function, stress responses, and regulation of pain and mood. Dr. Scott Rigden has also noted that many of their patients with metabolic abnormalities have an imbalance in amino acid ratios. The implication is that, for these patients, amino acids may be either synthesized or utilized at a slower rate or appear in such disequilibrium that they no longer function together with full efficiency (perhaps giving a clue to the origins of the collagen formation problems and enzyme disturbances common in many patients with CFIDS).

Amino acid supplementation has recently received some attention as a specific CFIDS treatment. Using an amino acid analyzer to measure specific imbalances, Dr. Bralley and Dr. Lord tailored a supplement to correct amino acid deficiencies. In a study of 25 CFIDS patients, they found that correcting specific amino acid imbalances resulted in 50% to 100% improvement in symptoms (*Journal of Applied Nutrition,* 1994). The greatest effect was noted in energy levels. Two patients who had had CFIDS symptoms for 15 years experienced dramatic improvement. Patients also reported improvement in cognitive function and elimination of "brain fog." It should be noted that single amino acids taken as dietary supplements may not be well tolerated by patients with serious metabolic disturbances.

Carnitine

Carnitine (L-Carnitine) is a betaine, one of the methyl group donors. It is crucial for the transport of long-chain fatty acids into the mitochondria of cells, which provides energy to skeletal and heart muscle. Carnitine also aids in reducing toxic buildup of organic acids, which are a natural by-product of cell metabolism. Carnitine deficiency produces fatigue, muscle weakness, malaise, exercise intolerance, heart beat abnormalities, and tissue acidosis. Carnitine deficiency can result from congenital metabolic defects and some antibiotic therapies.

USES IN CFIDS. Japanese researchers have shown that CFIDS patients have a deficiency in intracellular levels of acylcarnitine. They found no deficiency in serum levels of free carnitine, however, indicating the deficiency is not the result of lack of carnitine in the system but of its derivative. Acylcarnitine deficiency can be expected to produce not only the fatigue and weakness characteristic of interruption in mitochondrial processes but also the malaise typical of autointoxication. Dr. Hiroko Kuratsune and colleagues discovered that in their sample group of 38 CFIDS patients, low levels of acylcarnitine covaried with the severity of the illness (*Clinical Infectious Diseases,* 1994). As symptoms improved, so did acylcarnitine levels. In a recent study comparing amantadine and carnitine, Dr. Audrius Plioplys and Dr. Sigita Plioplys found "statistically significant clinical improvement" after 8 weeks of treatment (*Neuropsychobiology,* 1997).

PROTOCOL. Carnitine can be taken in liquid or pill form as an over-the-counter nutritional supplement or as a prescription medication. As a food supplement, the general recommended dosage is 1000 mg/day taken with a meal. The prescription medication Carnitor (levocarnitine) can be taken as a tablet, liquid, or injections. The recommended oral dosage of liquid Carnitor is 50 mg/day in divided doses, taken with meals, and of tablets is 330 mg three times a day. The liquid is better tolerated than the pill form although patients with chemical sensitivities should note that the liquid drug also contains artificial flavors, colors, preservatives (methylparaben), and sucrose.

PROS AND CONS. Carnitine as a food supplement is widely available. The only side effect reported is weight change (gain or loss). Patients have reported increased muscle function, decreased weakness, and overall improved stamina and well-being after 1 to 2 months of carnitine supplementation. In some cases, the benefits remained even after finishing the course of treatment. Side effects of Carnitor include diarrhea, upset stomach, and body odor. The manufacturers recommend taking divided doses with meals to avoid stomach upset.

AVAILABILITY AND COST. A 12 oz bottle of the liquid nutritional supplement Mega L-Carnitine (made by Twin Labs) can be purchased over the counter at most vitamin and health food stores for about $20. At the recommended dosage of 1 tablespoon a day, the bottle will last for 1 month. A 1-month supply of prescription tablets (Carnitor) costs about $79.

Glutamine

Glutamine is a nonessential amino acid used to treat sugar craving, fatigue, peptic ulcers, and personality disorders. When converted to glutamic acid, it acts as an excitatory neurotransmitter in the brain. In the intestinal tract, glutamine strengthens the gut's function as an immune barrier by supporting the production of secretory immunoglobulin A (sIgA) and maintains the structure, metabolism, and function of the mucosal lining of the intestines. Glutamine can help heal injured gut mucosa after surgery and, in a high percentage (92%) of patients, completely heals ulcer damage. Glutamine is an important detoxifying agent for ammonia, a neurotoxin and one of the toxic by-products of protein metabolism.

USES IN CFIDS. Glutamine is primarily used to treat leaky gut because it is so important in gastrointestinal growth and function. Clinicians recommend 1000 mg of glutamine daily, divided into equal doses (patients with many sensitivities may want to test a very small amount of this amino acid before taking the full dose). A number of CFIDS patients have noted improvement in gut function and increased food tolerance with this treatment. Side effects from this amino acid are relatively rare; the most common are lethargy and depression. Glutamine in tablet form is fairly inexpensive. A 100-tablet bottle (500 mg) costs less than $15. The cost of the powdered form (for those who need a higher dose) is about $29 for a 280 gm jar (Cambridge Neutraceuticals; 800-265-2202).

Glutathione

Glutathione, a tripeptide composed of glycine, cysteine, and glutamic acid, is found in high concentrations in every tissue in the body. It is a powerful antioxidant and detoxification agent, protecting the body against damage from oxygen radicals such as hydrogen peroxide and superoxide. It also helps reduce injury caused by radiation, chemotherapy, heavy metals (mercury), and drugs (including cigarettes and alcohol). NAC (*N*-acetyl-L-cysteine), a precurser to glutathione, is an antidote to acetaminophen poisoning and helps deter the toxic effects of naphthalene, benzene, and anthracine.

USES IN CFIDS. Glutathione is used primarily as an antioxidant and as an aid in detoxification. Because a number of CFIDS patients have low glutathione levels, this peptide is increasingly gaining attention among CFIDS clinicians as a means to combat some of the symptoms associated with impaired detoxification processes. The important role it plays in liver function makes it particularly useful for patients with numerous sensitivities, allergy-type reactions, and autointoxication symptoms (malaise, headache, muscle pain). Dr. Paul Cheney has noted a striking improvement in patients' symptoms, especially headache, within days of initiating glutathione treatment. Because glutathione is poorly absorbed in the gut, he recommends reduced glutathione (*CFIDS Chronicle,* Spring 1995). Initial doses are high, from 150 to 425 mg three times a day. After a short time, doses can be reduced to 75 to 150 mg three times a day and maintained at those levels. Glutathione is available from health food stores and mail-order suppliers. A bottle of 60 reduced glutathione capsules (100 mg) costs about $21.50. Capsules should be taken with meals to avoid stomach upset.

Lysine

Lysine is needed for bone growth in children and to maintain nitrogen balance in adults. It also aids in the production of antibodies, hormones, and enzymes and helps in collagen formation, muscle building, and tissue repair. Lysine deficiency can result in hair loss, anemia, bloodshot eyes, loss of energy, and irritability.

USES IN CFIDS. Lysine is recommended chiefly because of its ability to inhibit reproduction of herpesviruses (herpes simplex virus, varicella zoster virus, human herpesvirus 6, and Epstein-Barr virus), which require arginine in order to reproduce. Lysine's structure is similar enough to arginine, however, that herpesviruses can be fooled into using lysine instead. Since the virus cannot use lysine for replication, once the lysine is used, the virus loses its ability to reproduce, effectively halting the spread of the infection. Some CFIDS doctors recommend lysine to treat frequent outbreaks of cold sores (herpes simplex) or shingles (herpes zoster).

PROTOCOL. Dr. Charles Lapp recommends 1 to 2 gm of lysine, taken daily with meals (*CFIDS Chronicle,* March 1991). Foods high in arginine, such as chocolate, nuts, raisins, whole wheat, cereal, and brown rice, should be avoided. Side effects of lysine can include dizziness, sweating, nausea, appetite loss, and difficulty swallowing. Lysine should be discontinued if these symptoms develop. Lysine is available in most health food stores and can be purchased inexpensively. Most brands retail for less than $10 for a 100-capsule bottle (500 mg).

Taurine

Taurine acts as a building block for all other amino acids and consequently is present in every cell in the body. It is a prime component of bile (thus aiding in fat digestion and vitamin absorption) and is found in high concentrations in heart muscle, white blood cells, and the central nervous system (CNS). Anxiety, hyperactivity, and poor brain function are related to taurine deficiency. Taurine can be synthesized in the body from cysteine, with the aid of vitamin B_6.

USES IN CFIDS. Dr. Majid Ali, author of *The Canary and Chronic Fatigue,* makes extensive use of taurine as an antioxidant and has reported excellent results in treating fatigue and chronic constipation. He recommends a dosage of 250 mg/day, along with magnesium and potassium. Taurine may also be of benefit in treating hyperactive nervous system responses. Because taurine slows CNS impulses, it may help relieve symptoms such as insomnia, anxiety, and restlessness. Taurine can be purchased in most health food and vitamin stores and costs less than $10 a bottle.

ANTIOXIDANTS

DEFINITION. Antioxidants are a group of vitamins, minerals, and enzymes that help protect cells from free radical damage.

BACKGROUND. Antioxidants have long been used as preservatives because of their ability to retard the oxidation that causes oils to become rancid. However, they have come under increasing scrutiny over the past few years for their medical value. The same process that allows them to prevent oils from becoming rancid also protects the body from damage caused by free radicals. Free radicals are atoms or groups of atoms that have lost an electron. These molecules containing unpaired electrons are highly unstable and can easily pick up other elements, causing volatile reactions. When large numbers of free radicals are formed, whether from exposure to radiation, toxic chemicals, or rancid oils, or because of prolonged illness and immune activation, significant damage can result. When dangerously high levels of free radicals are present, changes in protein structure can result. The body may identify the altered proteins as foreign elements and launch an immune system attack.

The body has its own defenses against excess free radical formation. The group of biochemicals known as antioxidants are found abundantly in nature in the form of vitamins, minerals, and enzymes. The most widely used antioxidants are vitamins A, C, and E, gamma-linoleic acid (GLA), the amino acids cysteine and glutathione, the mineral selenium, the enzyme superoxide dismutase (SOD), CoQ10, and the bioflavonoids in pycnogenol, milk thistle, and gingko (see specific discussions of these agents).

Antioxidants operate in concert to prevent free radical damage. A single antioxidant, once it has neutralized the free radical, can itself cause cell damage. The action of other antioxidants is necessary to return antioxidants to their reduced state, in which they can continue to scavenge free radicals. Therefore, antioxidants should be taken in combination rather than single forms. An article in *The New England Journal of Medicine* reports that heavy smokers in Finland who took very high doses of the antioxidant beta carotene had a *higher* rate of lung cancer than those taking a placebo (*CFIDS Chronicle*, Spring 1995). However, when beta carotene was combined with vitamin E, this was not the case.

USES IN CFIDS. Patients with CFIDS demonstrate evidence of considerable free radical formation, which means some form of antioxidant therapy should be included in any treatment program. Orthomolecular clinicians recommend a broad-spectrum approach, as opposed to single-supplement therapy. Pycnogenol is a particularly potent antioxidant, but not always well tolerated. Grape seed extract can be used as a substitute. Vitamin E, because it is the only fat-soluble antioxidant, is particularly good in combination with other antioxidants such as selenium, beta carotene, and vitamin C.

BIOFLAVONOIDS

DEFINITION. Bioflavonoids are glycosides (sugars) derived from citrus, paprika, and other plants, which serve to protect capillaries. Although formerly known as "vitamin P," bioflavonoids are not vitamins.

BACKGROUND. Bioflavonoids were first extracted from paprika in 1936 by a scientist who claimed that the substance had a greater effect than vitamin C in reducing capillary bleeding. It was later shown that the substance, or rather substances, helped maintain capillary strength by inhibiting permeability of the walls (rather than maintaining the actual structure, as does vitamin C). This may be because bioflavonoids inhibit oxidation of epinephrine (adrenaline), the hormone directly responsible for capillary wall integrity. Bioflavonoids enhance absorption of vitamin C and, when taken together, can help protect and preserve capillaries, increase circulation, prevent cataracts, and produce a mild antibacterial effect. Dietary sources include buckwheat, black currants, peppers, blue-green algae, and the white part of citrus peel. Some bioflavonoids are hesperidin, rutin, and quercetin.

USES IN CFIDS. The bioflavonoid in widest use among patients with CFIDS is quercetin. It is chiefly used to treat asthma and allergies. Quercetin has properties similar to those of antihistamines and can inhibit mast cell production, two functions that together can curb many allergic responses. Quercetin is also reported to help relieve muscle pain, particularly along the upper back and shoulders.

PROTOCOL. Bioflavonoids may be taken through indirect dietary sources such as blue-green algae or directly in pill form. Quercetin needs to be taken with bromelain, an enzyme found in pineapple, because it is so poorly absorbed. Dr. James Balch, author of *Prescription for Nutritional Healing,* recommends 1000 to 2000 mg one to three times a day to prevent or lessen the severity of asthma attacks and allergies.

PROS AND CONS. A number of allergy-prone patients with CFIDS have noted that allergy symptoms subside with quercetin. For patients with many allergies, this may provide overall improvement because allergy symptoms can cause systemic problems. The primary side effect is that high doses may cause diarrhea.

AVAILABILITY AND COST. Quercetin is available from health food stores and most vitamin catalogs. A 3-month supply may cost as little as $15. The CFIDS and Fibromyalgia Health Resource (800-366-6056) markets a 100-tablet bottle of a quercetin-bromelain combination (also contains vitamin C and magnesium) for about $30.

BLUE-GREEN ALGAE

DEFINITION. Blue-green algae *(Aphanizon flos-Aquae)* is a microorganism found in lakes and oceans and in soil.

BACKGROUND. In evolutionary terms, blue-green algae is one of the oldest plants on Earth. It is also the most self-sufficient, needing only water, sunlight, and air to flourish. Blue-green algae is considered by some to be nature's ideal food. It contains all of the essential amino acids, beta carotene, B complex vitamins (especially vitamin B_{12}), and other vitamins and minerals. Much like related "green" products that have been popular in the past (chlorella, spirulina, barley green, and green magma), blue-green algae contains high amounts of chlorophyll. However, unlike most other green supplements, blue-green algae contains choline, a precurser of the neurotransmitter acetylcholine. Blue-green algae is reputed to improve memory and concentration, enhance immune system function, and increase energy.

USES IN CFIDS. Blue-green algae has recently become popular in the CFIDS community as an energy booster. People with CFIDS have reported that blue-green algae tablets give them greater stamina, more energy, and greater resistance to stress.

PROTOCOL. The generally recommended dosage is three to six 250 mg tablets a day. Patients should start with the lowest dose and increase it incrementally. Patients with food sensitivities may want to start with a half-tablet or quarter-tablet.

PROS AND CONS. Blue-green algae seems to work quickly. A number of patients with CFIDS have reported good results within a day or two.

Some patients have noted that whereas a moderate dose (two to four tablets per day) gives them energy, the maximum dose (five or six tablets per day) keeps them up at night. Many patients also report headaches and an overall worsening of symptoms. The Food and Drug Administration (FDA) has received complaints of side effects (nausea, diarrhea, numbness, and headaches). Although the FDA is not certain that blue-green algae is the cause of these symptoms, some experts believe the algae may be contaminated with neurotoxic substances or other algae that may be toxic to the liver (*Health,* 1997). Severely ill patients may want to delay trying this product until later.

AVAILABILITY AND COST. Blue-green algae is available from health food stores, mail-order vitamin suppliers, and private distributors (who often charge more and may market impure products). The CFIDS and Fibromyalgia Health Resource (800-366-6056) markets a bottle of 120 tablets (250 mg) for $24. At a dose of four tablets a day, a bottle lasts a month. Klamath, the brand most often recommended, retails a 130-tablet bottle (500 mg) for $36. Discounts are possible through L&H Vitamins (800-221-1152).

BUTYRIC ACID

DEFINITION. Butyric acid (butanoic acid) is a short-chain saturated fatty acid found naturally in the human intestine and in butter fat.

BACKGROUND. Short-chain fatty acids (volatile fatty acids) are produced in the colon as natural by-products of the bacterial fermentation of fiber. These fatty acids provide an energy source for the mucosal cells of the lining of the colon, enabling them to check the proliferation and establishment of pathogens (such as Salmonella and Candida) and allowing greater absorption of magnesium and vitamin K. Deficiency of these fatty acids results in absorption problems, diarrhea, and, over the long term, colitis. Of the three fatty acids found in all mammals (butyrate, acetate, and proprionate), butyrate is the preferred energy substrate. It stimulates the normal proliferation of mucous cells, enabling greater efficiency of all colonic functions. Butyric acid has been used successfully to treat Candida overgrowth (yeast infection), cancer, ulcerative colitis, and nonspecific inflammatory conditions of the colon. It is one of the treatments recommended for leaky gut and for alleviating food sensitivities.

USES IN CFIDS. The use of butyric acid in CFIDS has been limited, probably because few clinicians other than nutritionists and oncologists are familiar with its potential value. Of the few patients with CFIDS who have tried butyric acid, however, none has reported side effects other than transitory queasiness. General improvement in digestion, reduction in leaky gut symptoms, and increased food tolerance have all been noted. Although butyric acid is recommended for treating digestion disorders, it may also have a positive effect on some neurologic problems associated with CFIDS. Dr. Cheney proposes that an imbalance in the actions of the neuroexcitatory chemical NMDA (*N*-methyl-D-aspartate) and the neuro-inhibitor GABA (gamma amino butyric acid) may lead to many of the troubling neurologic symptoms experienced by patients with CFIDS (insomnia, intolerance of sensory stimuli, seizure-like activity, pain) (*CFIDS Chronicle*, Spring 1995). For many patients, downregulation of the NMDA receptors, accomplished with small doses of Klonopin (clonazepam), magnesium, Nimotop (nimodipine), melatonin, or calcium channel blockers, leads to general improvement of all symptoms. Butyric acid, because it forms a component of GABA, may also rectify some of this proposed neurochemical imbalance by increasing the amount of neuroinhibitory action in the brain.

PROTOCOL. Butyric acid is usually taken orally. The suggested dose is one or two capsules with each meal.

PROS AND CONS. Butyric acid is inexpensive, safe, and does not require a prescription.

AVAILABILITY AND COST. ButyrEn capsules, marketed by Allergy Research Group (800-782-4274), are hypoallergenic, containing no yeast, wheat, corn, soy, dairy products, or artificial colors or resins. They are buffered with calcium and magnesium. They are available from nutritionists and some specialized vitamin stores. One bottle of 100 capsules costs about $17.

CoQ10

DEFINITION. CoQ10 (ubiquinone) is a fat-soluble coenzyme found in the mitochondria of most mammal cells.

BACKGROUND. CoQ was first discovered by R.A. Morton, a biochemist who gave it the name ubiquinone after its ubiquitous presence in nearly all living things. "Co" stands for coenzyme (a vitamin-like substance), "Q" for quinone (the group of organic chemicals to which CoQ belongs), and "10" for the number of isoprene units that characterize the particular CoQ found in animal cells. CoQ10 is vital in electron transport, the intracellular function that ultimately provides the energy necessary to sustain life. CoQ10 is also a powerful antioxidant and is important in immune system function. The Japanese have successfully used CoQ10 to treat gum disease, heart disease, and high blood pressure, and to enhance the effectiveness of the immune system. Research performed in Japan and elsewhere indicates that CoQ10 can be of benefit in treating allergies (owing to its ability to block the effects of histamine), asthma, candidiasis, obesity, diabetes, and mental function diseases such as Alzheimer's disease and can slow the aging process (CoQ10 levels decline with age).

USES IN CFIDS. CoQ10 is one of the most frequently recommended supplements for the treatment of CFIDS-related fatigue because of its importance in the production of adenosine triphosphate (ATP), the cellular source of energy. In addition to reducing fatigue, CoQ10 may alleviate muscle weakness and pain. It is also one of the few supplements that seems to reduce cognitive dysfunction. Its role as a free radical scavenger may lead to improvement in immune responses in patients with CFIDS. Although its effects as a natural antihistamine have not yet been specifically explored in CFIDS, patients with allergies may benefit from CoQ10.

PROTOCOL. CoQ10 can be taken in a single dose or divided into two 100 mg doses taken at different times during the day. The normal recommended dose is between 50 and 200 mg/day. Sublingual troches, reputedly more effective against cognitive dysfunction, may be taken at higher doses. Oral CoQ10, although primarily absorbed by the digestive tract and liver, is also effective for some patients. The oral dosage varies, but is usually 25 to 50 mg/day.

PROS AND CONS. CoQ10 is a supplement with few side effects. Responses to it are far from uniform, however. A significant number of patients, particularly those with fibromyalgia, find that CoQ10 increases their energy over the course of the day. Others, however, report that CoQ10, while giving them an initial energy boost, also increases insomnia and causes jitters. Some people report, paradoxically, that CoQ10 increases exhaustion, although this effect may be more common in the acutely ill than in those with stable symptoms.

AVAILABILITY AND COST. CoQ10 can be purchased at most health food stores. High-grade brands are preferred because CoQ10 deteriorates rapidly when exposed to heat and light. The CFIDS and Fibromyalgia Health Resource (800-366-6056) retails sublingual CoQ10 (50 mg) for $25.45. High-potency sublingual troches are available by prescription through specialized compounding pharmacies. These can be requested in pure form, without added flavoring or coloring. A package of 24 sublingual troches costs about $54. These have a 30-day shelf life so must be used within a month. Sun-Ray Supply (800-437-1765) markets an over-the-counter form of sublingual CoQ10 with a 2-year shelf life. (These may be more appropriate for patients who take smaller doses over a longer time.) A 30-day supply of 200 mg troches costs $43.95. CoQ10 is not usually covered by insurance because it is classified as an experimental therapy. High amounts of CoQ10 occur naturally in fatty saltwater fish, especially mackerel, salmon, and sardines.

DHEA

DEFINITION. DHEA (dehydroepiandrosterone) is a naturally occurring adrenal hormone.

BACKGROUND. DHEA, a hormone produced in the adrenal cortex, generates the sex hormones estrogen and testosterone. It is the most common hormone in the blood and is found in greatest concentrations in the brain. Perhaps because DHEA levels decrease with age, it has been called "the fountain of youth." Preliminary research has provided evidence that DHEA may help the elderly by strengthening bones and muscles, decreasing joint pain, and improving sleep and mood. In addition to influencing hormone production, DHEA has several effects on immune system function, not the least of which is the regulation of lymphokine production. A study conducted in 1993 by researchers at the University of Tennessee showed that DHEA decreases the amount of circulating interleukin-6 (a potent bone resorber) and enhances the function of natural killer cells. Because of these and other immune system–enhancing properties, DHEA has been used to treat systemic lupus and AIDS.

USES IN CFIDS. Inspired by mounting evidence of adrenal cortical hypofunction in CFIDS, clinicians have begun testing for blood levels of DHEA in CFIDS patients and have discovered lower than normal levels. Based on these results, low doses of DHEA have been administered in hopes of raising immune function and normalizing the metabolic and endocrine disturbances that commonly accompany CFIDS. It is believed that DHEA could also act as an antiviral agent because testosterone, a DHEA derivative, has demonstrable antiviral effects.

PROTOCOL. The usual dosage of DHEA is 25 to 100 mg/day, although a number of clinicians report good results with smaller doses. Dr. Majid Ali states that he frequently prescribes DHEA in doses of 50 mg taken on alternating days for up to several months. In contrast, Dr. James McCoy has found that smaller doses (10 mg or less) are equally, if not more, effective than larger doses (*CFIDS Chronicle,* Fall 1993). He recommends starting at one tenth the normal dose to minimize the chance of negative reactions. Many patients with CFIDS confirm that the smaller doses (10 mg) work well for them.

PROS AND CONS. Patients with CFIDS have reported weight loss, increased energy, improved cognitive function, and better immune system responses with DHEA. However, a number of patients have reported heart palpitations, jitters, and altered mental and emotional states. Dr. Paul Cheney points out that DHEA is often most beneficial in mild CFIDS and notes that even in cases where DHEA deficiency can be documented, administration of this hormone has caused severe relapse in some of his more severely ill patients (*CFIDS Chronicle,* Spring 1995). It is important to remember that even though DHEA is a natural substance, it is still a powerful hormone. Hormones, because they are released directly into the blood stream, produce profound metabolic effects, not all of which are intended. Like other steroid or hormone treatments, DHEA is not without some risk and must be approached with caution.

AVAILABILITY AND COST. DHEA can be synthesized from wild yam and other roots and thus is fairly easy to produce commercially. It can be purchased through mail-order catalogs and at most health food stores. Some patient-recommended brands are available from Pure Encapsulations (800-753-2277) and AMNI (800-356-4791). A single bottle generally lasts 1 to 3 months, depending on the dose taken, and costs $15 to $30.

One of the natural precursers to DHEA, pregnenolone, also seems to produce positive results in patients with CFIDS. Patients report increased energy, enhanced mental clarity, and general improvement after taking pregnenolone. The dosage is 10 mg every other day in patients younger than 50 years and 20 mg every other day in patients over 50 years old. Pregnenolone can be purchased from the CFIDS and Fibromyalgia Health Resource (800-366-6056).

ENTERO-HEPATIC RESUSCITATION PROGRAM

DEFINITION. The Entero-Hepatic Resuscitation Program is a dietary supplementation plan designed to support and increase efficient functioning of the intestines and liver.

BACKGROUND. The Entero-Hepatic Resuscitation Program is basically a modified diet plan accompanied by a powdered nutritional supplement (UltraClear) that was designed to improve liver and gastrointestinal function. The program was developed to assist patients with compromised digestion, liver detoxification system impairment, and cellular metabolic abnormalities. The main theory behind the program is that these patients have similar problems in removing toxins, whether originating from outside sources or from the metabolic waste produced naturally in the body. As these toxins build up, a number of symptoms develop (gastrointestinal problems, fatigue, skin problems, malaise, weakness, insomnia, and poor concentration), indicating that the body's natural systems of detoxification are not functioning properly. The Entero-Hepatic Resuscitation Program, in combination with an elimination diet, is designed to help rebuild or support the major organs responsible for detoxification and digestion. Once these are restored to full function, they will be able to speed the process of elimination and reduce the number of metabolic poisons that result from faulty or incomplete digestion. The program accomplishes this by providing the specific nutrients the body needs to ensure smooth functioning and repair of intestinal mucosal linings and by enhancing liver function with liver enzymes.

USES IN CFIDS. Dr. Scott Rigden has designed a program specifically for patients with CFIDS (*CFIDS Chronicle,* Spring 1995). It is based on the principle that, because of underlying metabolic abnormalities, most patients with CFIDS are unable to effectively clear toxins from their systems, resulting in what amounts to a perpetual condition of self-poisoning. Dr. Rigden attributes many CFIDS symptoms, including cognitive problems, depression, fatigue, weight gain, sleep disorders, and recurrent yeast infections, to faulty detoxification originating in the liver and intestines. He backs up his theory with study results from his own patients that show not only impaired elimination pathways but also marked improvement in those patients who have completed one of two entero-hepatic resuscitation programs. Those patients who would best benefit from entero-hepatic resuscitation are those who experience recurrent gastrointestinal problems; have food, chemical, or environmental sensitivities; demonstrate abnormal findings on liver function tests; or have chronic headache or muscle and joint pain.

PROTOCOL. The Entero-Hepatic Resuscitation Program can be adjusted to fit specific needs and symptoms. To this end, Dr. Rigden uses two programs, tailored to the degree of severity and type of symptoms of each patient. One program utilizes UltraClear Sustain, a supplement that contains Jerusalem artichoke flour; the other utilizes UltraClear, which does not. Severity of illness or gastrointestinal problems are measured by means of liver function tests, detoxification pathways, and the Metabolic Screening Questionnaire (MSQ), a self-administered questionnaire designed to rate symptom intensity and frequency duration (for a copy of the MSQ, send a self-addressed stamped envelope to The CFIDS Association of America, PO Box 220398, Charlotte, NC 28222-0398).

Dietary restrictions vary according to the severity of symptoms, but all patients are encouraged to avoid alcohol, caffeine, sugary foods, fatty foods, processed foods, and foods that may provoke allergic reactions (wheat, barley, rye, oats, and, for some patients, dairy products or meat), as well as any foods to which there are suspected sensitivities. Among those who begin the program, Dr. Rigden notes that many experience temporary worsening of gastrointestinal symptoms 2 to 3 days into the program, but this passes within 2 weeks. To avert the transient problems associated with the program, patients are advised to take the supplement with a meal and to divide it over the day in small amounts. In addition, all participants in the program are urged to drink 2 quarts of pure water daily.

PROS AND CONS. Although Dr. Rigden points to a very high success rate (80%) in the 200 patients in his study, the program may not be appropriate for many in most need of its benefits. Patients who have numerous food sensitivities, for example, may not be able to follow the dietary restrictions required by the program. Dr. Rigden also notes that patients with leaky gut may have to heal the mucosal membrane *before* embarking on entero-hepatic resuscitation. In addition, Dr. Rigden's success in patients who have either been ill for long periods of time or have significant impairment in mitochondrial function (resulting in many amino acid abnormalities) is less than encouraging. Dr. Rigden remarks that in severely ill patients (those who have urinary sulfate/creatine ratios less than 1) this program may actually make symptoms worse. Dr. Paul Cheney has also noted that patients with low glutathione levels may have a severe relapse because UltraClear acts as a liver stimulant. Stimulating the liver increases the demand for glutathione, which in patients who already have glutathione deficiency, may worsen autointoxication. This program works best in patients who have been moderately to mildly ill for less than 3 years. This does not preclude other patients from trying it. Success rates may be diminished among those who have been ill for longer than 3 years, but some benefits may be seen and, in those with chronic digestive problems, may well be worthwhile. However, supervision by a physician or nutritionist and prior testing for glutathione levels are a must in these cases.

AVAILABILITY AND COST. UltraClear products are available through nutritionists, physicians, and other health care providers. They are rarely distributed through health food stores. UltraClear and UltraClear Sustain can be directly purchased at a discount from L&H Vitamins (800-221-1132). One 29.4 oz jar of UltraClear Sustain costs $42. Seven jars are needed to complete the 3-month program. One 32.6 oz jar of UltraClear powder costs $50.20. Additional information is available through Health Comm, Inc. (206-851-3943).

Caution: Because of the possibility of severe side effects, the program must be supervised by a physician.

MORE INFORMATION

The *CFIDS Chronicle*, Spring 1995 issue contains an article describing Dr. Rigden's Entero-Hepatic Resuscitation Program. The *CFIDS Chronicle*, Fall 1993 issue includes Dr. Cheney's report on the general suitability of entero-hepatic programs for patients with CFIDS.

ESSENTIAL FATTY ACIDS

DEFINITION. Essential fatty acids are fats (lipids) that are important in a number of physiologic processes. They cannot be produced by the body and therefore must be obtained through dietary sources.

BACKGROUND. The two most important types of essential fatty acids are omega-3 and omega-6. Omega-3 fatty acids are found in fish oil (especially cold water fish) and flaxseed oil (linseed oil). Omega-6 fatty acids are found in many plant oils, including evening primrose oil, borage oil, and black currant oil.

Essential fatty acids are vital to a number of physiologic processes, such as regulating cholesterol levels, keeping the skin moist and supple, and producing prostaglandins (hormone-like substances that affect a variety of body functions). Essential fatty acids are also indispensable in maintaining the structure and function of cell membranes.

Several factors can affect fatty acid metabolism. Poor diet, stress, diabetes, excessive alcohol intake, radiation, and viral infections can disrupt the metabolism of essential fatty acids, making it difficult for the body to produce fatty acid metabolites in sufficient quantities. In such cases, supplementation may be necessary to prevent deficiency states. Supplementation with essential fatty acids has improved such diverse conditions as premenstrual syndrome (PMS), heart disease, rheumatoid arthritis, multiple sclerosis, hyperactivity in children, and mononucleosis.

USES IN CFIDS. In 1987, Dr. Peter Behan, a professor of Clinical Neurology in Glasgow, Scotland, found that patients with CFIDS had a disorder in fatty acid metabolism. Dr. Behan surmised that the disorder was the result of chronic viral infection, much like mononucleosis, a prolonged illness that also produces abnormal serum fatty acid concentration. He conducted a double-blind trial using a fatty acid supplement (Efamol) that contains both omega-3 and omega-6 fatty acids (*Acta Neurologica Scandinavica,* 1990). After 16 weeks of treatment, an astounding 85% of patients showed marked improvement, primarily in the areas of fatigue, dizziness, headaches, depression, and muscle pain. Since then, a number of other researchers have confirmed Dr. Behan's findings, making essential fatty acids one of the most highly recommended supplements for treating CFIDS.

PROS AND CONS. Essential fatty acids are an effective, readily available, and relatively inexpensive supplement. Of the many supplements currently marketed, essential fatty acids are among the most widely used in CFIDS. They produce relatively few side effects. People with schizophrenia, however, should not take evening primrose oil because it may interact with phenothiazine drugs (antipsychotics) and precipitate temporal lobe epilepsy.

Evening Primrose Oil

Evening primrose oil is the most popular and perhaps most effective of the omega-6 essential fatty acids. It comes from the evening primrose (*Oenothera*), a lovely yellow flower that grows wild along roadsides. The seeds contain large amounts of GLA (gamma-linoleic acid), a linoleic acid metabolite. Evening primrose oil has been used to help alleviate the symptoms of premenstrual syndrome (PMS), menstrual cramps, and arthritis, often with dramatic results. It may even lessen the symptoms of endometriosis.

Patients with CFIDS have reported increased energy, improvements in skin disorders (eczema, acne, dry skin), and decreased mood swings. Side effects, although uncommon, include headache, nausea, mild intestinal discomfort, and, rarely, weight gain.

The brand recommended by most patients and clinicians, Efamol, is produced in Great Britain and marketed in the United States by Murdock Pharmaceuticals. A bottle of 90 capsules (500 mg) costs $20.95. Other brands available in the United States can also be purchased through health food stores or the CFIDS and Fibromyalgia Health Resource (800-366-6056), which markets its own brand for the reasonable price of $18 per bottle (100 softgel capsules). The dosage is two to six capsules a day. Efamol Marine, a blend of 80% evening primrose oil and 20% fish oil, was used by Dr. Behan in his study. The dosage for Efamol Marine is eight capsules a day for up to 12 weeks, after which the dose can be reduced. Efamol Marine costs $15 to $30 a month, depending on the dosage.

Borage Seed Oil

Borage seed oil, made from the borage plant, contains the highest GLA content of any currently available seed oil, up to four times more than the GLA content of evening primrose oil. Patients who have gained little benefit from or cannot tolerate evening primrose oil because of food sensitivities often take borage oil with good results. The recommended dose is lower than for evening primrose oil, only one to three capsules a day. GLA-240 (Metabolic Maintenance) costs $17.50 per bottle (60 softgel capsules) and is available in health food stores. Another brand, Max GLA, is available from the CFIDS and Fibromyalgia Health Resource (800-366-6056) and costs about $20 for a bottle of 60 softgel capsules.

Fish Oils

The oil derived from deep-sea fish (sardines, mackerel, salmon, and herring) is the richest source of omega-3 fatty acids. Four ounces of salmon can contain as much as 3600 mg of omega-3 fatty acids (compared with 300 mg in the same amount of cod). Fish oil capsules have been particularly helpful in treating fibromyalgia, often providing immediate relief from pain. Fish oil is so effective that some physicians suggest it in place of Advil (ibuprofen) for pain from inflammation. Because of its anti-inflammatory properties, fish oil can also be used to treat arthritis and colitis. The only side effect reported is indigestion.

High-quality brands of fish oils are available from Kyolic and Cardiovascular Research Ltd. Plain cod liver oil is not recommended because the amount needed to provide sufficient fatty acids might lead to an overdose of vitamin A. Fish oils can range in price from $5 to $15 for a month's supply, depending on the brand, and can be purchased in health food stores or through vitamin catalogs. The usual dose is one to four capsules a day.

Flaxseed Oil

Flaxseed (linseed) is a good plant source of omega-3 fatty acids. It is also high in magnesium and zinc, two important factors in fatty acid metabolism, as well as B complex vitamins, protein, and potassium. Flaxseed oil is low in saturated fat and calories and contains no cholesterol. It has a delicious nutty flavor and can be added to salad dressings or sprinkled over vegetables.

Flaxseed is high in alpha-linoleic acid (ALA), which the body converts to eicosapentaenoic acid (EPA) and docosahexaenoic acid (DHA), the two fatty acids found in fish oils. Some clinicians prefer flaxseed oil to fish oil because it is lower on the food chain and thus contains fewer fat-soluble contaminants. Fish oils, as opposed to vegetable oils, also contain large amounts of vitamin A, which can be toxic in excessive amounts.

Flaxseed oil can be purchased in health food stores and is inexpensive. At 1 to 3 tablespoons a day, a month's supply costs $5 to $10. Flaxseed oil must be stored in the refrigerator to avoid rancidity. It should not be used for cooking.

FURTHER READING

Graham, Judy. Evening Primrose Oil. Rochester, Vt.: Healing Arts Press, 1987.

Rudin, Donald O, and Felix, Clara, with Schrader, Constance. The Omega-3 Phenomenon. New York: Avon Books, 1987.

GLUCOSAMINE SULFATE

DEFINITION. Glucosamine sulfate is a mucopolysaccharide made up of the sugar glucose and the amino acid glutamine. Glucosamine sulfate is the synthetic form of glucosamine, a naturally occurring amino acid compound found in the joints.

BACKGROUND. Glucosamine sulfate has been used for many years in Europe, Asia, and the Philippines to treat osteoarthritis. It appears to stimulate the synthesis of connective tissue and cartilage by aiding in the production of glucosaminoglycans and proteoglycans, the key building blocks of cartilage. Because glucosamine is also one of the main components of the synovial fluids that cushion joints and surrounding tissues, it has been used to treat degenerative joint diseases. It also may have anti-inflammatory properties, thereby lessening the need for anti-inflammatory pain medications.

USES IN CFIDS. Because glucosamine sulfate has only recently gained public attention, it is difficult to determine how useful it may be for people with CFIDS. Its mode of action indicates that, in theory, it may be of benefit to patients with joint pain, fibromyalgia, or interstitial cystitis.

PROTOCOL. Dr. Jason Theodasakis, author of *The Arthritis Cure*, suggests taking glucosamine sulfate with chondroitin, another mucopolysaccharide, for maximum benefits. His daily dosage recommendations are based on patient weight:

- *Less than 120 pounds:* 1000 mg glucosamine sulfate plus 800 mg chondroitin
- *120 to 200 pounds:* 1500 mg glucosamine sulfate plus 1200 mg chondroitin
- *200 pounds or more:* 2000 mg glucosamine sulfate plus 1600 mg chondroitin

Other health care providers believe glucosamine sulfate is effective alone, although some recommend the addition of bromelain, an enzyme derived from pineapple, to help maximize its effects. Standard adult dosage as indicated by the manufacturer is one or two tablets three times a day. Health effects should be noticed within 6 to 8 weeks. If no benefits are apparent by then, glucosamine sulfate should be discontinued.

PROS AND CONS. Glucosamine sulfate is generally considered safe and is well tolerated by most patients. However, some may be allergic to its source (usually crustacean shells). Patients taking blood thinners should consult with their physician before taking glucosamine sulfate because many of the mucopolysaccharides inhibit platelet formation.

AVAILABILITY AND COST. Glucosamine sulfate is available from health food stores and mail-order distributors. The Bronson mail-order brand (800-235-3200) retails for $14.99 (60 600 mg tablets). The CFIDS and Fibromyalgia Health Resource brand (800-366-6056) retails for $22.95 (90 tablets). Health food stores also market glucosamine sulfate.

HERBS

DEFINITION. Medicinal herbs are plants taken orally as teas or tinctures or applied topically as poultices.

BACKGROUND. Plants have always been used as remedies, which makes herbal treatment the earliest form of medicine. (The earliest human graves contain remnants of medicinal flowers.) Even animals eat certain plants when they become ill. Throughout the ages, people have used herbal remedies for an assortment of problems and, until the nineteenth century, herbs were the treatment of choice for most common ailments. Herbs are so ubiquitous that they are regarded as folk remedies. The contemporary medical world, as a consequence, has largely excluded them from scientific investigations, with the exception of the Chinese, who take herbs quite seriously. The government of China has funded research to study the chemical components, action, and efficacy of a number of herbs.

USES IN CFIDS. A large number of patients with CFIDS symptoms use herbs regularly, as herbal substitutes for caffeine-laden coffee and teas or as adjuncts to other therapies. Although many find that a particular herb is helpful for a specific symptom, most report that herbs have limited value in treating CFIDS over the long term. It should be noted, however, that patients who have tried Chinese herbs (usually on the recommendation of an acupuncturist) generally report a higher rate of success.

PROTOCOL. Although herbalists recommend blending herbs for maximum effect, patients with CFIDS frequently have had poor responses to multiple-herb blends. For CFIDS symptoms, herbs are best taken singly in teas or tinctures. Teas are prepared according to the part of the plant used. One teaspoon of herb leaves is steeped in 2 cups of boiling water for 15 or 20 minutes or 1/2 teaspoon of herb root or bark is boiled in 2 cups of water. One to 2 cups of tea per day can be taken for up to 2 weeks. After that, the herb loses its potency. Tinctures are usually purchased from health food stores. Because they are quite strong, tinctures are usually taken a few drops at a time in water. For chronic symptoms, teas are advised. Short-term problems (flu, toothache, etc.) are best treated with tinctures. *Note:* Most tinctures are prepared in an alcohol medium. People with CFIDS are advised to "flash off" the alcohol by adding the tincture to *hot* water.

PROS AND CONS. Herbs are inexpensive, safe, and readily available. However, it is always best to purchase them from a health food store. Culinary herbs from the grocery store are usually treated, seldom organic, and have little medicinal worth. The advantage of herbs for many people with drug and chemical sensitivities is that they can produce the desired therapeutic effects without damage. This is not to say that negative reactions are not possible. People with bladder problems (interstitial cystitis), gastrointestinal symptoms, or migraine headaches may find that all herbs produce adverse side effects.

In general, patients with CFIDS should avoid herbs classified as stimulants (ephedra, lomatium, and ginseng) because these can overtax the adrenal glands. Ephedra (ma huang), used to treat bronchial infections, is a powerful stimulant and can cause high blood pressure, palpitations, and even stroke. Ginseng and lomatium, although not as strong as ephedra, can produce similar reactions in the very ill. Echinacea, because it is an immune system stimulant, might best be avoided by those who are severely ill. Some herbs such as goldenseal and St. John's wort must be used with caution. The antiviral herb, St. John's wort, acts like a monoamine oxidase inhibitor (MAOI) and must be treated with the same care as the drug. (The newsletter of the Center for Specialized Immunology reported a serious reaction in a patient who took St. John's wort concomitantly with an antidepressant.) Chapparal and comfrey have caused liver problems in some people who took too high a dose. In addition to the herbs mentioned, there are many others that can provide temporary, safe relief from numerous CFIDS symptoms. Those interested in persuing herbal remedies should read about herbs before embarking on an herbal therapy program or should consult with an herbalist.

Astragalus

Astragalus *(Astragalus membranaceous)* root has been popularized as an immune system modulator. It reputedly enhances immune system function when it is deficient and downregulates it when overactive. It is also thought to increase energy, stamina, and well-being and supports adrenal gland function. Some use it as a digestive aid. The effects of astragalus are not dramatic in most people, but some CFIDS patients have noted increased energy after taking tincture of astragalus.

Chamomile

Chamomile *(Matricaria chamomila* [German]; *Anthemis nobilis* [Roman]) is a member of the daisy family. It is currently one of the most popular herbs in the United States and is widely used as an herb tea, in shampoos and soaps, and in skin-care products. Chamomile has been known as a sedative and antifever medicine since ancient times and was used by Greek and Roman physicians to treat a variety of ailments. Contemporary herbalists recommend chamomile to treat digestive problems and ulcers, to prevent the spread of infections, and to reduce inflammation. Because chamomile is an antispasmodic, it has also been used to lessen the severity of menstrual cramps. Perhaps the most interesting effect of this herb is its ability to stimulate the immune system. British researchers discovered that chamomile increases the number of macrophages and B lymphocytes. Some patients with CFIDS have chamomile tea before bedtime to help with insomnia and to alleviate gastrointestinal symptoms. In general, the herb is well tolerated. Chamomile tea should not be boiled because boiling makes the tea bitter. Those allergic to ragweed should avoid this herb.

Echinacea

The roots of the purple coneflower *(Echinacea angustifolia, E. purpura)* were used by Plains Indians as a cure for all manner of infections. Although it has been relied on as a topical wound healer since Colonial times, echinacea's antibiotic properties have largely been unexplored until recently. Research conducted in Germany in the 1950s through the 1980s revealed that echinacea has broad antibiotic properties, much like penicillin, due to a substance (echinacein) that counteracts cell-penetrating enzymes. In this manner, echinacea works to strengthen individual cell defenses. Echinacea also acts as an immune system stimulant. Echinacea boosts the macrophage's ability to destroy germs. It possesses antifungal as well as antibacterial properties. As an antiviral agent, echinacea has been used effectively to treat influenza and the common cold and to check herpesvirus infections. People with CFIDS often use echinacea at the first sign of a cold or flu to help lessen the severity of the illness and some even report lessening of all symptoms after using this herb. Because of its immune stimulating properties, however, echinacea may pose some problems for CFIDS patients with upregulated immune systems. Echinacea tinctures are more effective than pills or capsules. An alcohol-free tincture should be used, however, because alcohol dramatically lessens the potency of this herb. Dry echinacea root can be purchased in health food stores and boiled to make tea.

Garlic

The earliest medicinal description of garlic *(Allium sativum)* dates from 3000 BC. Garlic was even found in the tomb of King Tut. It has been used to treat headache, insect bites, menstrual disorders, intestinal worms, tumors, and heart disease. Garlic is a powerful antibiotic and antiprotozoan agent. It kills intestinal parasites, destroys the bacterium that causes tuberculosis, and can be used against various funguses, including *Candida albicans*. Daily ingestion of as little as half a clove of garlic can lower cholesterol. Some people with CFIDS tend to be sensitive to garlic in both its raw and cooked forms. Enteric, deodorized garlic pills can reduce intestinal upset. A commonly recommended brand of deodorized garlic in capsules, Kyolic, is widely available from health food stores.

Ginger

Ginger *(Zingiber officinale)* was used by the ancient Greeks as a digestive aid. It is still used as an antidote for motion sickness, nausea, and numerous digestive disturbances. It soothes smooth muscles, making it useful for alleviating menstrual cramps as well. Ginger can be taken in capsule form or boiled to make tea. Ginger root is available from grocery or health food stores. Ginger powder, however, as found in the spice section of a grocery store, should not be used as a medication because it is usually irradiated. Excessive amounts may cause mild headache. Some people with CFIDS find ginger difficult to tolerate.

Gingko

Gingko *(Gingko biloba)* is a Chinese herb that has been used traditionally as an elixir to promote longevity. Studies have shown that gingko, by increasing blood flow to the brain, helps reduce the risk of stroke. It also can dramatically improve memory and reaction time. In Europe, gingko is used as a conventional drug for treating short-term memory loss, headache, tinnitus, vertigo, and depression. Patients with CFIDS generally use gingko to improve cognitive function. It is taken either in capsule or tincture form. Although gingko is usually well tolerated, some patients with CFIDS have reported increased fatigue. Excessive doses can cause irritability, restlessness, nausea, and diarrhea.

Ginseng

Ginseng *(Panax schinseng* [Chinese ginseng]; *Eleutherococcus senticoccus* [Siberian ginseng]) is an ancient tonic and stimulant. Although it possesses enormous therapeutic potential for common ailments, it is usually not recommended to patients with severe CFIDS. Ginseng stimulates the adrenal glands and can increase production of interferon. Because most patients with CFIDS have excessive interferon production and endocrine abnormalities, ginseng may increase symptoms.

Goldenseal

Goldenseal *(Hydrastis canadensis)* is a North American herb known best for its antibiotic properties. Berberine, a substance found in goldenseal, kills many of the bacteria that cause diarrhea, as well as the protozoa that cause amoebic dysentery and giardiasis. It has been used against cholera bacteria and as a treatment for throat, sinus, and topical bacterial infections. People with CFIDS generally use goldenseal to treat sinusitis and canker sores. It should be used with caution, however. Excessive or lengthy (more than 10 days) treatment can lead to neurologic disturbances and gastrointestinal upset. The safest way to take goldenseal is externally as a paste spread directly over the sinuses or other affected area. Goldenseal should not be used during pregnancy because it stimulates uterine contractions.

Gotu Kola

Gotu kola *(Centella asiatica; Hydrocotyle asiatica)* (also known as sheep rot, Indian pennywort, marsh penny, and water pennywort) was originally used in Sri Lanka as a promoter of longevity. It is a member of the Umbelliferae family, which also includes carrots, parsley, dill, and fennel. Despite the similarity in name, gotu kola is not related to the stimulant kola. In small amounts, gotu kola is taken as a tonic and in larger amounts as a sedative. Gotu kola traditionally has been used in the treatment of leprosy, but it is also noted for its ability to promote blood circulation. Gotu kola has been used to increase memory and mental function by increasing circulation to the brain.

Licorice

Licorice *(Glycyrrhiza glabra)* has long been known as one of nature's most potent healing herbs. It is a popular ingredient in many Chinese herbal remedies and has been used to treat cough, sore throat, ulcers, arthritis, herpes infections, and hepatitis. When combined with other herbs, licorice can increase their effectiveness. In CFIDS, licorice is reputed to alleviate symptoms associated with adrenal insufficiency (intolerance to heat, cold, noise, and other stimuli, low blood pressure, faintness) because the action of licorice's main active chemical, glycyrretinic acid (GA), resembles that of the adrenal hormone aldosterone. The glycyrretinic acid in licorice helps the body retain salt (and water) and ultimately may help raise blood volume and pressure. Because low blood pressure is a problem for many patients with CFIDS, licorice could prove beneficial, especially for those who are sensitive to the drugs normally recommended to correct low blood pressure. In addition, licorice raises serum cortisol levels (commonly low in CFIDS) and stimulates natural killer cell activity.

Dr. Riccardo Baschetti claims that dramatic improvement in CFIDS symptoms can be seen after taking licorice for just 3 days (*New Zealand Medical Journal,* 1995). He recommends 2.5 gm of licorice root a day, in extract or capsules dissolved in milk. The milk enhances the aldosterone-like effects of the licorice. Dr. Peter D'Adamo, a naturopath who also uses licorice to treat symptoms of CFIDS, suggests 1/4 teaspoon (2 gm) of solid licorice extract one to three times a day. He recommends his patients take 500 mg of the amino acid methionine and 99 mg of potassium supplement three times a day along with the licorice to counteract any potassium and sodium imbalances. Patients who have taken licorice report increased energy levels and improvement in symptoms of hypoglycemia; some have noticed that its effectiveness wanes after a few months.

Naturopaths warn that, because of its steroid-like qualities, it is important to monitor licorice intake. Too much licorice, especially without potassium supplementation, can cause serious side effects. If high blood pressure, headaches, lethargy, and water retention develop, the dosage should be decreased immediately. Patients taking drugs that could interact with licorice, such as heart medications, MAOIs, or diuretics, should consult with their physician before embarking on a licorice protocol.

The solid licorice root extract used by Dr. D'Adamo is manufactured by Scientific Botanicals in Seattle (206-527-5521). It is also available from Willner Chemists in New York (800-633-1106) for $14 for a 4 oz bottle. Because of its steroidal effects, licorice supplementation should be supervised by a physician.

Lomatium

Lomatium is a North American herb reputed to have antiviral properties. It has been used to treat influenza, colds, and diseases such as measles. A number of patients who have tried lomatia extract have felt overstimulated. Some have experienced malaise, insomnia, and jitteriness after as little as one drop. Reports from the late 1980s stated that some CFIDS patients have developed severe allergic reactions while taking this herb.

Milk Thistle

The active ingredient in milk thistle *(Silybum marianum)*, silymarin, appears to have a remarkable effect on the liver. It stimulates liver cells to regenerate and is effective in treating jaundice and cirrhosis. Silymarin increases the content of liver glutathione, a tripeptide that activates liver enzymes. As a consequence, milk thistle also helps protect the liver from toxins, including poisonous mushrooms, and various petrochemicals. For CFIDS patients with mild liver dysfunction, milk thistle may provide some relief. It should be used with caution, however, because some patients have reported a worsening of symptoms.

Uva Ursi

A member of the Ericaceae family, uva ursi *(Arctostaphylos uva-ursi)* has been used for more than 100 years as a urinary tract antiseptic. Once in the urinary tract, the arbutin in uva ursi is transformed into an antiseptic agent, hydroquinone. This herb also contains diuretic chemicals (ursolic acid) and astringents. However, uva ursi is effective against urinary tract infections only if the urine is alkaline; therefore, citrus fruits (including tomatoes), vitamin C, and acidic foods should be avoided immediately before and after taking it.

Valerian

Valerian *(Valeriana officinalis)* has long been used as a tranquilizer and to treat epilepsy, nervousness, anxiety, insomnia, headache, and intestinal cramps. During World War I, it was routinely taken to relieve the "overwrought nerves" brought on by artillery bombardment. Valerian is used extensively in Germany, where it is the active ingredient in more than 100 over-the-counter sleep aids. The active ingredients in valerian are chemicals known as valepotriates, which are found in highest concentrations in the roots of the plant. Patients with CFIDS take valerian primarily as a sleep aid. It can be taken as a tea or in capsule form, but because of its odor, capsules are usually preferred. Valerian should be taken with a little milk or food to prevent stomach upset.

FURTHER READING

Castleman, Michael. The Healing Herbs. Emmaus, Pa.: Rodale Press, 1991 (a well-organized introduction to herbs and their uses).

LEM

DEFINITION. LEM *(Lentinus edodes mycelium)* is an extract made from the immature shiitake mushroom.

BACKGROUND. Although shiitake mushrooms have long been appreciated in the East for culinary purposes, they have recently gained attention for their medicinal value. Numerous studies, mostly conducted in Japan, have demonstrated that LEM increases immune system function by stimulating production of lymphocytes and macrophages, the immune system's defense against bacteria, viruses, and tumor cells. LEM may also interfere with the action of reverse transcriptase (an enzyme that aids in viral replication) and block cell receptor sites of viruses. Owing to these properties alone, LEM shows promise in treating cancer, diseases related to immune system dysfunction, and viral infections.

USES IN CFIDS. Most patients with CFIDS use LEM as a general treatment for lethargy, weakness, and exhaustion, the hallmark symptoms of

CFIDS. A number have reported improvement in stamina, energy, and strength, decreased diarrhea, and increased white blood cell count after taking LEM.

PROTOCOL. LEM is taken in tablet form, at a suggested dose of nine tablets a day. As with other medications, patients with CFIDS should start with smaller doses and gradually increase to the full dose.

PROS AND CONS. LEM is one of the few botanical products that affects CFIDS as a whole. A number of patients report general improvement and lessening of some of their worst symptoms.

LEM may provoke a severe allergic reaction in patients with allergies to mushrooms, molds, and other funguses (common in systemic Candida infection). Those with recurring yeast infections, athlete's foot, or thrush should probably delay trying LEM until these problems are resolved.

AVAILABILITY AND COST. LEM is imported from Japan, where the extraction process has been patented, and is not widely available in the United States. LEM is expensive enough to rule it out for many people. The CFIDS and Fibromyalgia Health Resource (800-366-6056) markets a quality brand at a cost of $65 for a bottle of 180 tablets. At the maximum dose, this lasts 3 weeks.

MALIC ACID

DEFINITION. Malic acid, an intermediate of the Krebs cycle, aids in the production of adenosine triphosphate (ATP).

BACKGROUND. Malic acid is found primarily in apples and pears, as well as other fruits. It helps in the breakdown and utilization of fats and glucose in muscle tissue, even in low oxygen conditions.

USES IN CFIDS. Because of the prominent role malic acid plays in the energy-producing Krebs cycle, a deficiency can lead to inadequate breakdown of glucose in muscle tissue, with resulting buildup of lactic acid and other toxins. Increased amounts of malic acid should relieve many of the symptoms associated with tissue acidosis (spasms, cramps, and burning pain). A number of CFIDS physicians recommend malic acid combined with magnesium to treat fibromyalgia-like symptoms. Dr. Guy Abraham, Dr. Jorge Flechas, and Dr. I. Jon Russell have found improvement in pain with supermalic, a combination of malic acid and magnesium (*Journal of Rheumatology,* 1995).

PROTOCOL. As with other supplements, physicians recommend starting with the lowest dose, one tablet daily taken with food and water, to check for possible sensitivities. The dosage can be increased gradually to between 6 and 12 tablets daily, depending on tolerance. If gastrointestinal problems develop, the dosage should be decreased. Although results may be experienced within a few days, most physicians recommend a trial of at least 2 months.

PROS AND CONS. Malic acid as a dietary supplement is relatively risk free. The only reported side effect seems to be diarrhea, most likely due to the added magnesium. Several survey respondents reported almost immediate positive results from malic acid. One patient reported complete cessation of leg spasms, allowing her to rest better. Others have reported less muscle pain and more stamina.

AVAILABILITY AND COST. Malic acid is available without prescription from most health food and vitamin stores. It can also be purchased through the CFIDS and Fibromyalgia Health Resource (800-366-6056) (Ultra ATP+, 1500 mg of malic acid plus magnesium hydroxide) for $16.95 for a bottle of 180 tablets.

MELATONIN

DEFINITION. Melatonin is a hormone produced by the pineal gland.

BACKGROUND. In the past few years, melatonin has been touted as the new wonder aid for chronic insomnia, which affects as many as one third of all people in the United States. Recent studies released by the Massachusetts Institute of Technology showed that it took less than half the time for volunteers given melatonin to fall asleep than those given a placebo. Subjects given melatonin also tended to sleep about twice as long as those given placebo and woke without the hangover normally associated with sleeping pills.

Melatonin is a naturally occurring hormone produced in the pineal gland, the brain's "master gland." It is derived from serotonin, one of the brain's most important neurotransmitters. Serotonin, a neurochemical derived from the amino acid tryptophan, is converted by enzymes sensitive to the diurnal cycle of darkness and light into melatonin. Melatonin, because it is produced in the part of the brain that regulates diurnal rhythms, is essential for maintaining normal sleep patterns. Large amounts of melatonin are produced in children, which is one reason why they sleep so much. As we age, melatonin levels decrease, making it more difficult for the elderly to sleep through the night. Disruption of both melatonin and serotonin production has been implicated in seasonal affective disorder, the treatment of which involves increasing melatonin levels through exposure to full-spectrum light. Low melatonin and serotonin levels have also been implicated as contributing factors to depression. Currently, physicians are exploring the use of melatonin as an antiaging factor. It is possible that supplementation with melatonin in the elderly will help correct the disturbed sleep, poor immune response, and diminished capacity for tissue repair typical of the aging process.

USES IN CFIDS. Sleep disturbance is one of the primary symptoms of CFIDS. Many patients experience persistent insomnia throughout the illness. Even after a full night's rest, patients with CFIDS awaken tired. Many clinicians believe that treating the CFIDS sleep disorder is of primary importance because it also results in lessening of many other symptoms. However, owing to the prevalence of drug and chemical sensitivities in the CFIDS population, it is not always easy to find a safe, effective means of obtaining a good night's rest. Melatonin may offer an alternative.

PROTOCOL. While product labels usually recommend one to two tablets (3 to 6 mg) taken before bedtime, studies at the Massachusetts Institute of Technology indicate 0.3 mg daily is sufficient to raise blood levels to normal. MIT researcher, Dr. Richard Wurtman, claims that serious side effects can be produced by taking standard doses, which can raise blood levels to more than 10 times the norm. Dr. Charles Lapp finds that dosage is highly individualized. He recommends starting with as little as 0.1 mg taken a half-hour before bedtime and increasing the dose until the desired effect is achieved. He also has observed that synthetic (not from animal sources) and sublingual forms of melatonin are safest and most effective (*MEssenger,* 1997).

PROS AND CONS. A number of CFIDS patients have reported that melatonin has given them their best night's sleep in years. Melatonin works quickly (generally within an hour). However, it can lose its effectiveness over time. After working beautifully for a few weeks or months, it can suddenly stop providing the desired results. Some people report paradoxical reactions, such as feeling more awake or experiencing partial or light sleep states. The reason melatonin works for some but not for others may have to do with individual biorhythms. Chronobiologist Benita Middleton and her colleagues at the University of Surrey, England, have discovered that the effectiveness of melatonin varies according to daily temperature fluctuations (*Discover,* 1997). Those whose temperatures rose later in the day experienced extremely fragmented sleep. It is possible that patients with CFIDS whose temperatures rise in the evening may not respond well to melatonin.

Excessive doses of melatonin can cause jitteriness and headaches. A few female patients may experience hormonal disturbances (early onset of periods). Interactions with antidepressant drugs such as Prozac, Elavil, or Zoloft and the pain medication Ultram have been reported. People taking antidepressants should discuss the risks and benefits of melatonin with their physicians because it may be contraindicated. Preexisting depression may be worsened by melatonin.

AVAILABILITY AND COST. Although it is a hormone, melatonin is currently considered a nutritional supplement. Consequently, it can be purchased over the counter from most health food stores and vitamin catalogs. The CFIDS and Fibromyalgia Health Resource (800-366-6056) markets a bottle of 120 2.5 mg sublingual tablets for $16. Allergy Research Group (800-782-4274) and KAL (available through vitamin catalogs and health food stores) also sell melatonin.

FURTHER READING

Bock, Steven, and Boyette, Michael. *Stay Young the Melatonin Way.* New York: Dutton Press, 1995.

MINERALS

Calcium

Calcium is the most abundant mineral in the human body. A 150-pound adult's body contains about 3 pounds of calcium, 99% of which is found in the skeletal bones. The small portion of calcium found in soft tissues and body fluids is essential for maintaining a number of important biochemical functions, including regular heart beat and transmission of nerve impulses. Calcium also prevents muscle cramps and is vital for the formation of healthy teeth and strong bones.

CFIDS patients may take calcium at night to alleviate insomnia. It is also useful for treating muscle spasms. Calcium supplements can be purchased from health food stores, through vitamin catalogs, and at some drugstores. The recommended daily allowance for calcium is 800 mg/day. People ingesting high amounts of protein or phosphorus may want to supplement their intake of dietary calcium because both protein and phosphorus increase calcium excretion from the body. Good natural sources of calcium are milk and other dairy products and green leafy vegetables.

CFIDS patients taking verapamil (a calcium channel blocker) to treat cognitive dysfunction need to be aware that calcium supplements may interfere with the effects of this medication. People with a history of kidney disease or kidney stones should not take calcium supplements because the additional calcium may exacerbate the condition.

Chromium

Chromium is a trace mineral vital for maintaining blood sugar and for metabolizing glucose, which makes this mineral particularly valuable in treating both diabetes and hypoglycemia. CFIDS patients who have taken chromium supplements have noted decreased sugar craving and lessening of appetite surges. Some have even felt mildly increased energy levels. Chromium can be purchased from health food stores, through vitamin catalogs, and most drugstores. It is inexpensive. A bottle of 100 200 µg tablets (standard dosage) costs less than $10. Chromium is naturally present in corn, meat, and whole grains. Brewer's yeast is a rich source of chromium.

Magnesium

BACKGROUND. Magnesium is one of the six major minerals classified as essential for human body functioning. The average human body contains about 25 gm of magnesium salts, about half of which is stored in the bones and one fourth in muscle. Only about 2% circulates freely in the blood. The rest is located within the cells. Blood levels of magnesium are controlled by the kidneys.

Magnesium is necessary for relaying nervous system impulses and for normal metabolism of calcium and potassium. Much like a vitamin, magnesium functions as a coenzyme, aiding in enzyme systems, storage and release of energy generated from carbohydrates, and synthesis of proteins and DNA. Magnesium deficiency can result in anorexia, nausea, learning disabilities, personality changes, weakness, exhaustion, and muscle pain.

USES IN CFIDS. In early 1991, a team of researchers (I.M. Cox, M.J. Campbell, and D. Dowson) published a preliminary study on magnesium levels in CFIDS patients (*Lancet*, 1991). All 22 patients studied had reduced levels of serum magnesium. They followed up their findings with a randomized clinical study in which 15 of the patients received intramuscular injections of magnesium sulfate every week for 6 weeks and 17 received a placebo. Of the 15 patients receiving magnesium, 12 reported improvement in symptoms. Although this study has received subsequent criticism (mostly because of study design flaws), magnesium is still the most frequently recommended mineral supplement for patients with CFIDS. It is chiefly used to relieve pain and muscle weakness and to improve stamina.

PROTOCOL. Magnesium can be administered orally or by injection. Because oral magnesium is difficult to absorb, the forms most frequently recommended are magnesium citrate, magnesium oxide, and magnesium glycinate. Magnesium glycinate causes the least intestinal upset. The usual recommended dosage is 200 to 400 mg/day taken with food, although CFIDS patients are cautioned to start with a smaller dose and increase it gradually. A calcium supplement should be taken along with magnesium to avoid creating a mineral imbalance. Intramuscular injections of 1 gm of magnesium sulfate (50%) can be administered once or twice a week. Because of magnesium's effect on heart function, the first injection should be performed in a physician's office.

PROS AND CONS. Most people who take magnesium, whether oral or injected, report increased stamina and energy. Many include better sleep as an additional benefit (most likely due to magnesium's muscle-relaxing effects). The main drawback of injected magnesium is that the injections are painful. The simultaneous administration of vitamin B_{12} or lidocaine helps relieve the pain of the injection. Because magnesium is a cathartic, high doses can cause diarrhea. In patients prone to gastrointestinal upset, a low dose is normally recommended.

AVAILABILITY AND COST. Oral magnesium is readily available from health food stores, vitamin catalogs, and many drugstores. It is inexpensive. A bottle of 250 tablets costs less than $10. Magnesium sulfate injections cost $10 to $12 for a 6-week course.

Colloidal Silver

DEFINITION. Colloidal silver solution is composed of ultrafine, nonsoluble particles of silver suspended in a liquid medium such as water.

BACKGROUND. Colloidal silver has long been used as a germicide. In the early twentieth century, colloidal silver was used in place of antibiotics. Silver was used orally, intravenously, and intramuscularly (as an injection), as a throat gargle, and in eyedrops. Colloidal silver has been used to treat such varied maladies as tonsillitis, cystitis, ringworm, and dysentery. Over the course of this century, antibiotics have replaced silver as drugs of choice, although silver nitrate is still used to prevent eye infections in newborn infants.

USES IN CFIDS. Some patients with CFIDS report that colloidal silver helps control recurring infections, particularly in the mouth. Silver may be of benefit in treating Candida infection, sinusitis, sore throat, and canker sores.

PROTOCOL. Dosage varies, depending on the concentration of the product used.

PROS AND CONS. It appears that low doses of silver are fairly safe. However, argyria (grayish skin discoloration) may develop when excessive doses of silver are ingested. Because most reports concerning the benefits of silver are anecdotal, patients are cautioned to exercise judgment before choosing silver over a medication whose mode of action and recommended dosage are better known.

AVAILABILITY AND COST. Colloidal silver may be purchased from most health food stores and mail-order distributors. It costs $12 to $45 for a 2 to 4 oz bottle, depending on the brand. Several multilevel or network marketing companies also sell colloidal silver, but discretion is advised when purchasing from unknown companies. Reputable brands such as Source Naturals (800-815-2333) and Futurebiotics (available through health food stores and vitamin catalogs) are preferred.

NOTE: Some of the colloidal minerals distributed by multilevel marketers contain arsenic and lead, which are toxic even in small doses. While many people with CFIDS have reported improvement in energy and stamina after taking colloidal minerals, caution should be exercised. Read labels carefully!

FURTHER READING

Farber, Paul. The Silver Micro Bullet. Houston, Tex.: Professional Physicians Publishing and Health Services, 1977.

Zinc

Zinc is a remarkably versatile mineral. It plays an important role in the more than 70 enzyme systems that regulate most metabolic processes. It stimulates digestion, aids in extracting stores of vitamin A from the liver, helps maintain the mucous lining of the mouth, throat, stomach, and intestines, is vital for the normal growth of hair, skin, and nails, controls sexual maturation and fertility (zinc deficiency in men can lead to infertility), and aids in the healing of wounds. It also helps improve immune responses, although excessive intake of zinc (more than 50 mg) can suppress immune function. Many CFIDS patients take zinc lozenges to help relieve sore throat and other viral symptoms. Zinc is available from health food stores, vitamin catalogs, and some drugstores. As with other mineral supplements, it is not expensive. One hundred 30 mg capsules can cost less than $5 and a bottle of 75 zinc lozenges costs about $8. The recommended daily allowance for zinc is 15 mg. As excessive amounts of zinc can cause severe gastrointestinal problems, zinc should be taken with food to avoid stomach upset. Zinc is found naturally in pumpkin seeds, liver, egg yolks, and seafood (especially oysters).

NADH

DEFINITION. NADH, the reduced form of nicotinamide adenine dinucleotide (NAD), is a coenzyme found in all living cells. It is also called coenzyme 1.

BACKGROUND. NADH was first discovered in the 1930s by an American scientist who observed that NADH played an essential role in the energy production of cells. Not until more than 60 years had passed, however, did Dr. Georg Birkmayer, a biomedical researcher from Vienna, Austria, develop a stable oral form of NADH. Since then, a growing body of research documents that NADH not only acts as a driving force in the production of cellular energy but also acts as a potent antioxidant, is a key component of DNA repair and cellular regeneration, and stimulates the production of the neurotransmitters dopamine, noradrenaline, and serotonin. Ongoing research in the United States and abroad may help define the role of NADH in treating such degenerative neurologic conditions as Alzheimer's disease and Parkinson's disease.

USES IN CFIDS. NADH may be of great benefit in treating CFIDS. When NAD is oxidized (NAD^+) in the cell's mitochondria, energy is released. This energy is preserved in the form of adenosine triphosphate (ATP), a substance required by all energy-absorbing processes in the body.

Researchers have proposed that NADH may help correct the metabolic defect in CFIDS that inhibits the production of ATP. Because low ATP production means less energy, clinicians believe NADH may alleviate CFIDS-related exhaustion and may also improve cognitive function. The three neurotransmitters stimulated by NADH serve critical functions in the central nervous system: dopamine is important for short-term memory; noradrenaline contributes to alertness; and serotonin has a pronounced effect on mood and regulates sleep.

In March 1996, the Food and Drug Administration (FDA) approved clinical trials of NADH in CFIDS patients at the Georgetown Medical Center. Studies began in mid-1996 under the direction of Dr. Harry Preuss, Department of Nephrology, and Dr. Joseph Bellanti, Director of Georgetown's International Immunology Center. The studies are now closed and the CFIDS community awaits word of the results.

PROTOCOL. The suggested dosage of NADH is 2.5 to 10 mg/day, although some people report taking as much as 15 mg. It should be taken first thing in the morning on an empty stomach (about 20 minutes before your first meal).

PROS AND CONS. NADH works rapidly. Benefits may be noticed within days to weeks. One patient reported that it was moderately to mildly helpful, "making bad days somewhat less bad and good days somewhat better" (*CFIDS Chronicle,* Summer 1996). Another CFIDS patient who has had an excellent response to NADH reported increased energy, stamina, concentration, and overall improvement in symptoms.

AVAILABILITY AND COST. NADH is classified as a supplement and therefore does not require a prescription. However, it is not yet widely available in health food stores. There are only a handful of manufacturers. The brand most widely recommended is Enada (Menuco Corp.; 800-636-8261), which costs $50 to $120 a month, depending on the dosage. The CFIDS and Fibromyalgia Health Resource (800-366-6056) also markets NADH for $23.

PROBIOPLEX

DEFINITION. Probioplex is a whey-derived product that concentrates the active globulin (immune) proteins in cow milk.

BACKGROUND. Probioplex is a source of secretory IgA, the immunoglobulin found in external secretions. Secretory IgA is produced in the mucous lining of the intestines and is essential both for maintaining the gut barrier and for "tagging" unfriendly organisms in the gastrointestinal tract. It is used in the treatment of leaky gut, ulcers, and damage to gut mucosa. Secondary benefits include increased immune system efficiency, reduction of yeast overgrowth, and control of enteric viral and bacterial infections.

USES IN CFIDS. Probioplex is recommended for treating digestive tract problems, particularly leaky gut, irritable bowel syndrome, gas, and food sensitivities. It may serve as a substitute for L-glutamine for those who cannot tolerate amino acids as it performs a similar function. Probioplex also stimulates the growth of helpful bacteria in the intestines, making it a useful corollary treatment for Candida overgrowth (systemic yeast infection), common in CFIDS. The secondary benefits of improving immune system function are also highly relevant for patients with CFIDS.

PROTOCOL. Probioplex is a powder that can be mixed with water or juice. Nutritionists recommend 1/2 teaspoon two to three times a day for 3 to 4 weeks. After that, the dosage should be reduced to 1/4 teaspoon once or twice a day and discontinued when benefits are no longer noticeable. Reported benefits include reduced abdominal pain due to gas, reduced bloating, relief of constipation, reduced food reactivity, and improved sleep.

PROS AND CONS. Probioplex is safe, easy to use, relatively inexpensive, and is available without prescription. It resists digestion in the stomach and small intestine and so may be taken with meals. However, because it is a whey product, persons with milk allergies or sensitivities may not be able to tolerate it. Probioplex also contains rice maltodextrin, which may limit its value for those with rice allergies as well.

AVAILABILITY AND COST. Probioplex is available from nutritionists and specialized vitamin stores. A 75 gm bottle (a 2-month supply) costs about $20.

PROBIOTICS

DEFINITION. Probiotic bacteria, primarily *Lactobacillus acidophilus* and *Bifidobacterium bifidus,* aid in many digestive processes and help maintain balance in the intestines.

BACKGROUND. Digestive tract bacteria (intestinal flora) have evolved within humans to aid in completing the breakdown and absorption of many foods. Without the thousands of "friendly" bacteria that inhabit the intestines, malnutrition would develop no matter how much food was eaten. These bacteria not only help in digestion, they are responsible for manufacturing many nutrients that are essential to survival, such as the B vitamin complex. Some bacteria, such as bifidus, live in the small intestine; others, such as acidophilus, live in the large intestine. As long as the intestinal flora are working well, a minimum of digestive problems can be expected. However, once the function of friendly flora is upset, harmful bacteria can move in and cause bloating, stomach upset, poor digestion, constipation, gas, and malabsorption problems. The most common sources of flora upset are recurrent use of antibiotics, oral contraceptives, aspirin, corticosteroids, poor diet, stress, and Candida infections. In these cases, it may be necessary to use a probiotic supplement to reestablish a healthy balance of intestinal flora.

USES IN CFIDS. Patients with gastrointestinal symptoms or recurring yeast infections, or who regularly take antibiotics, nonsteroidal anti-inflammatory drugs (NSAIDs), oral contraceptives, or cortisone are advised to use a probiotic supplement. Products that contain bifidus seem to help with leaky gut. Most patients with CFIDS who regularly take probiotics report easing of gastrointestinal symptoms (especially gas and bloating) and overall improvement in digestion.

PROTOCOL. Probiotics are sold in different forms. Each should be taken according to directions. Enteric-coated tablets, for example, need to be taken only once a day and can be taken with food because the enteric coating protects the bacteria from being destroyed by stomach acids. Powdered forms and capsules generally need to be taken an hour before meals or on an empty stomach. Patients with altered intestinal flora as a result of taking antibiotics need to take a probiotic supplement for a least 2 weeks after finishing the treatment to repopulate the intestines. Single-strain varieties are reported to be more effective than multiple strains.

PROS AND CONS. One of the main advantages of probiotics is that they can be taken daily for months, or even years, without causing any adverse effects or loss of benefits. They rarely cause side effects.

AVAILABILITY AND COST. Many good brands of probiotic supplements can be purchased from health food stores and vitamin catalogs. Probiotics should be kept in a refrigerator because the bacteria may be denatured by heat. Acidophilus can also be found in foods such as yogurt and kefir, although these are used more effectively to maintain intestinal balance once it has been established. Foods such as miso and tofu can enhance bifidus growth, as can a number of supplements that provide intestinal substrate in which the bacteria can flourish, such as Probioplex, fructo-oligosaccharides (FOS), biotin, and lipoic acid. Probiotic supplements are not expensive. A month's supply costs about $14.

PYCNOGENOL

DEFINITION. Pycnogenol (proanthocyanadin) is an antioxidant derived from pine tree bark or grape seed.

BACKGROUND. Pycnogenol is a potent free radical scavenger derived from botanical sources. Studies have shown that, as an antioxidant, pycnogenol is up to 50 times more effective than other antioxidants to clear free radicals created from chemical sources (air pollution and food additives). It is 20 times more effective than vitamin C to scavenge superoxide, hydroxyl, and peroxide radicals. Pycnogenol is reported to enhance immune system function, increase energy, promote healing, and reduce allergic reactions. It is particularly effective in the brain.

USES IN CFIDS. Pycnogenol is frequently recommended by CFIDS clinicians because it is generally better tolerated than other commonly used antioxidants, such as vitamin C, and may be more effective. Patients who have used pycnogenol report small increases in mental and physical energy and better resistance to bacterial and viral infections and stress.

PROTOCOL. The recommended dosage is one to two tablets a day (25 mg), taken with meals with a glass of water.

AVAILABILITY AND COST. A bottle of 60 tablets costs $17 to $20 and can be purchased from health food stores and vitamin catalogs. Bronson (800-235-3200) markets both pine and grape extract pycnogenol for under $20.

ROYAL JELLY

DEFINITION. Royal jelly is a thick, milky substance secreted by young nurse honeybees to nourish the young larvae in a colony, especially the queen larvae.

BACKGROUND. Royal jelly is one of nature's most potent foods. It is rich in B vitamins (especially pantothenic acid), biotin, folic acid, and inositol. It also contains vitamins A, C, D, and E, seven minerals, 18 amino acids, fatty acids, enzymes, and hormones and is the only natural source of acetylcholine, the neurotransmitter that aids in memory. Health-enhancing properties attributed to royal jelly range from reducing cholesterol levels to healing skin disorders.

USES IN CFIDS. Royal jelly has been highly touted for use in CFIDS despite the fact that its mode of action is not well understood. Royal jelly is a natural source of acetylcholine, the neurotransmitter some researchers believe is deficient in CFIDS, which may be why it is effective in some patients with CFIDS. It also provides an easily tolerated form of B vitamins. Many patients with CFIDS who need B vitamins cannot tolerate yeast-based vitamin B products.

Steve Wilkinson, author of *Chronic Fatigue Syndrome: A Natural Healing Guide,* claims that royal jelly can help provide increased stamina and energy, greater mental alertness, and relief from muscle problems. He states that in his case the improvement in muscle pain was "dramatic" after just a few weeks of taking royal jelly. A number of patients with CFIDS have reported that royal jelly seems to increase their energy and stamina. Some women have even reported normalizing of menstrual cycles.

PROTOCOL. One manufacturer (Y & S Royal Jelly Farm; 800-654-4593) recommends taking 1/4 teaspoon of royal jelly daily on an empty stomach. When combined with honey (for preservation), up to 2 teaspoons a day can be eaten. Royal jelly can be taken for months. Some patients need 2 to 3 months before its benefits can be felt. Pure royal jelly (not mixed with honey) requires refrigeration because it spoils easily.

PROS AND CONS. Royal jelly is a safe, inexpensive supplement that may provide some necessary nutrients. Side effects from pure royal jelly have not been reported. However, patients with CFIDS should be sure the royal jelly they use has not been mixed with other products (ginseng, bee pollen) to avoid possible allergic reactions to these additives.

AVAILABILITY AND COST. Royal jelly is available in pure form as a thick liquid, in capsules, or mixed with honey. A 4 oz jar of pure royal jelly costs about $75 and lasts 6 months at the recommended dosage (or about $12 a month). Less expensive royal jelly capsules are available from most health food stores. Montana Big Sky capsules retail at $10 a bottle. Because royal jelly loses its potency when improperly handled or processed, it may be worthwhile to buy the purest form available. The refrigerated section of health food stores usually contains the most potent royal jelly products.

SAMBUCOL

DEFINITION. Sambucol is an extract made from the fruit of the European black elder tree *(Sambucus nigra L.)*, a member of the Caprifoliaceae family.

BACKGROUND. Black elderberry has long been used in Europe to make jams, jellies, soft drinks, and aromatic wines. In addition to its pleasant taste, elderberry is valued as a rich source of B vitamins, bioflavonoids, and minerals such as calcium and phosphorus. Medicinal use of black elderberry has been documented as early as the fifth century BC, when the ancient Greeks described it as a remedy for colds, flu, and upper respiratory tract infections. In the mid-1980s, researchers found that two of the active ingredients in elderberry inhibited the replication of the influenza virus by preventing the virus from entering cells.

In a continuation of this research, in 1992 a group of Israeli scientists and physicians formulated a black elderberry syrup that acted successfully against the influenza virus in a laboratory setting. Soon afterward, a double-blind, placebo-controlled study was conducted in patients with influenza in southern Israel. The results of that study indicated that black elderberry effectively reduced the duration and severity of influenza infections. Flu symptoms (fever, cough, and muscle pain) significantly improved in 20% of the patients within 24 hours, compared with 8% of the control group. Within 3 days, more than 90% of the patients were symptom free, compared with 6 or more days for the control group. Preliminary results of further studies have also shown that elderberry extract can act against herpesvirus and Epstein-Barr virus.

USES IN CFIDS. The fact that Sambucol has such a wide range of antiviral effects may make it particularly useful for the many patients with CFIDS who have frequent colds and flu. It may also be valuable for those who demonstrate reactivation of Epstein-Barr virus and other latent viruses, the effects of which can lead to many of the symptoms typical of CFIDS. CFIDS patients taking Sambucol noted overall improvement (*Mass CFIDS Update*, Fall 1995).

PROTOCOL. The recommended dosage of Sambucol syrup is 4 tablespoons daily in adults and 1 tablespoon daily in children younger than 12 years. Patients with CFIDS should probably start with a smaller dose to check for tolerance. Sambucol should be taken on a full stomach. Dairy products should be avoided for 30 minutes before and after to avoid stomach upset. The manufacturers recommend refrigeration after opening.

PROS AND CONS. Sambucol is an all-natural product, which is an advantage for patients with chemical and drug sensitivities. There are no reported side effects or contraindications associated with its use. Although reports from CFIDS patients have been scant, those who have tried it claim that it hastens recovery from flu and colds. Sambucol is also safe in children, which is good news for parents of children with CFIDS because so few effective pediatric medications are currently available. One reported that Sambucol helped alleviate sore throat in her child with CFIDS, usually within a day, with no side effects.

AVAILABILITY AND COST. Sambucol is currently marketed in the United States, France, Israel, and South Africa through health food stores and drugstores. The liquid extract contains glucose and honey for sweetening and raspberry extract to enhance flavor. If a glucose-free product is desired, Sambucol is available in lozenge form and as a liquid sweetened with sorbitol. A 4 oz bottle of liquid Sambucol or a bottle of 16 lozenges costs about $13.

VITAMINS

DEFINITION. Vitamins are organic (carbon-containing) substances needed in tiny amounts to promote biochemical reactions within living cells.

BACKGROUND. Vitamins, as independent biochemical agents, were discovered around the turn of the century when an English biochemist proposed that diseases such as rickets and scurvy were most likely caused by a lack of "accessory food factors" in the diet. After observing that these diseases could be corrected by adding certain foods (whole rice, which is high in vitamin B, to cure rickets; and oranges, an easy source of vitamin C, to cure scurvy), scientists began to search for chemical compounds in these foods that could produce such extensive changes in the body. When these accessory food factors were finally isolated in food, the name "vitamine" was proposed (from the Latin *vita*, necessary for life, and *amine*, a chemical substance containing nitrogen). Later, when it was discovered that not all vitamins were amines, the final "e" was dropped.

There are 13 known vitamins, all of which act as catalysts, or more specifically, coenzymes; that is, they initiate or speed chemical reactions in cells while remaining unchanged. They accomplish their task mainly by combining with a protein-containing apoenzyme (vitamins contain no protein) to form a complete enzyme. The completed enzyme performs the role of biochemical catalyst, enabling most of the body's vital cell functions to occur in an orderly and efficient manner. Without vitamins, many essential cell functions would cease, resulting in any number of vitamin deficiency–related diseases and problems. Most vitamins must be obtained from food because the body rarely manufactures them in adequate amounts (vitamin K is the exception).

USES IN CFIDS. Most CFIDS physicians and clinicians include vitamin supplementation as a part of a general treatment protocol. The reasons vitamin supplementation is considered such a central part of CFIDS treatment are threefold. First, the ill body consumes vitamins much faster than the healthy body. Patients, particularly those with long-term illnesses, need vitamins in amounts that exceed those which can be derived from food, especially when (as in CFIDS) the illness causes certain metabolic defects. Second, at least 50% of patients with CFIDS have absorption problems (leaky gut, low stomach acid production, or other gastrointestinal difficulties). When food is improperly digested, vitamins are not extracted efficiently, sometimes not at all, necessitating some kind of supplementation. Third, as has been pointed out by a number of researchers, the particular nature of CFIDS immune system activation prevents some vitamins from working properly. The excess cytokine production that blocks vitamin C function, for example, is justification enough for supplementation. The most frequently recommended supplements, however, are not specific vitamins (except, perhaps, vitamin C) but general wide-spectrum supplements. CFIDS clinicians usually recommend a quality, well-tolerated supplement such as Optivite, All 1, Solgar, Schiff, or Reliv, which can be easily obtained from health food stores and vitamin catalogs (Reliv is available through local distributors only; call 800-358-9283). Benefits of vitamin supplementation generally are not apparent for several weeks, but some seriously malnourished patients notice significant effects within a few hours. Many CFIDS patients report overall improvement in vitality, energy level, and stamina with vitamin supplementation. Few report any adverse effects (and these are usually remedied by switching brands).

In addition to a wide-spectrum vitamin supplement, many CFIDS physicians and clinicians recommend taking extra amounts of specific vitamins for the purposes of providing added antioxidant protection, for immune system enhancement, or to compensate for the functional deficits common to the illness. Vitamins are easily obtained from supermarkets, health food stores, pharmacies, or mail-order catalogs. They are inexpensive, ranging from $3 to $15 per bottle. Care should be taken to purchase high-grade vitamins because the excessive heat and poor handling to which low-grade vitamin products are exposed often cause fat-soluble vitamins to become rancid and considerably reduce the efficacy of water-soluble vitamins. With the exception of vitamin E, synthetic vitamin preparations are as effective as natural vitamins.

Vitamin A

Vitamin A (retinol) plays a variety of roles in human metabolism. It helps maintain the health of the skin and all mucous linings of the body (stomach, intestines, bladder, mouth, nose, throat, windpipe, and other air passages). It is essential for vision. Vitamin A also increases resistance to infections and is involved in the maintenance of the adrenal cortex, where cortisol is formed.

USES IN CFIDS. Vitamin A is primarily used to help maintain mucous membranes, which are often compromised in CFIDS. Patients prone to intestinal, respiratory, or ear infections also take vitamin A to maintain resistence. There have been attempts in the past to redefine vitamin A as an "anti-infective agent." However, because its protective capacity is limited to bacterial infections of the mucous membranes, these have been abandoned. The recommended daily allowance for vitamin A is 5000 IU a day. Because vitamin A is fat soluble, it can be stored in the liver, which means it can be taken less frequently in larger doses. A physician or nutritionist should be consulted before taking larger doses, however, to prevent possible negative reactions.

Vitamin A is available from health food stores, many pharmacies, and some supermarkets. The form of vitamin A most easily absorbed is micellized A, a liquid suspension sold in health food stores. Vitamin A intake (unlike water-soluble vitamins) must be monitored to prevent overdose. Loss of appetite, irritability, widespread itching, headaches, and mouth ulcers are all signs of vitamin A toxicity. The best natural sources of vitamin A are animal products (liver, whole milk, butter, and cheese). Fish liver contains huge amounts of vitamin A (200,000 to 1 million IU, depending on the type). Pregnant women should not take more than 5000 IU of vitamin A because higher doses have been associated with birth defects.

Beta Carotene

Beta carotene is the precurser to vitamin A. When foods containing beta carotene (yellow or orange vegetables) are ingested, the liver converts the beta carotene to vitamin A. Unlike vitamin A, however, it cannot be stored in the body and therefore entails far fewer risks of toxicity, although its function remains largely the same. Like vitamin A, beta carotene strengthens mucous membranes. It also helps protect against skin and lung cancer and improves the functioning of the thymus gland (where T cells are produced). There is no recommended daily allowance for beta carotene, but people who take large amounts often notice that certain areas of their skin, particularly the palms and around the fingernails, turn yellowish orange. This condition is called carotenemia and, while benign, is a sign that too much beta carotene is being consumed. Patients with diabetes or hypothyroid conditions should avoid taking beta carotene because they cannot convert it to vitamin A.

USES IN CFIDS. Beta carotene is one of the vitamins mentioned by clinicians as having particular value in CFIDS. Dr. Burke Cunha proposes that one of the chief benefits of beta carotene for CFIDS patients lies in its ability to stimulate the production of natural killer cells (*CFIDS Chronicle,* Fall 1993). He found that among the majority of his patients who tested low in natural killer cells (below 6%; the normal range is 6% to 22%), high doses of beta carotene resulted in an increase in the number of these cells. He also found less fatigue in these patients. (Patients with normal numbers of natural killer cells before therapy showed less improvement, however.) Dr. Cunha postulates that by increasing natural killer cell production, beta carotene may serve as an effective antiviral agent. He recommends a high dose (25,000 to 50,000 IU/day, depending on the patient's needs), but cautions that high doses of beta carotene should not be taken for more than 3 weeks to prevent carotenemia and vitamin A toxicity. Most clinicians recommend a daily dose of 5000 to 10,000 IU in combination with other antioxidants to prevent carotenemia.

Vitamin B$_{12}$

Vitamin B$_{12}$ (cobalamin) is a member of the B vitamin complex. It is naturally found in animal products and is required for proper digestion, food absorption, protein synthesis, metabolism of carbohydrates and fats, myelin synthesis, nerve function, and activation of folic acid (used in the formation of red blood cells). Its name is derived from cobalt, the mineral to which this vitamin is bound. When cobalamin is ingested, contact with stomach enzymes splits it apart, freeing it to join with a special protein called "intrinsic factor," which is secreted by the stomach lining. Only when vitamin B$_{12}$ combines with intrinsic factor can it be absorbed by the body. Because vitamin B$_{12}$ is highly unstable outside the body, two stable forms have been developed—hydroxycobalamin and cyanocobalamin. Oral vitamin B$_{12}$ cannot be absorbed in malabsorptive states such as pernicious anemia.

USES IN CFIDS. Although the traditional use for vitamin B$_{12}$ injections has been limited to the treatment of anemia, Dr. Charles Lapp and Dr. Paul Cheney have observed that such injections are highly beneficial to their CFIDS patients, even in the absence of vitamin B$_{12}$ deficiency or any sign of anemia. They report that some 50% to 80% of their patients demonstrate improved stamina and energy with vitamin B$_{12}$ therapy (*CFIDS Chronicle,* Fall 1993). Dr. Cheney was first motivated to include vitamin B$_{12}$ in his general treatment plan after seeing evidence that vitamin B$_{12}$ injections had been helpful in a number of nonanemic neuropsychiatric patients. These patients had demonstrated some of the symptoms common to CFIDS (paresthesia, sensory loss, loss of coordination, and mood swings), all of which improved with vitamin B$_{12}$ injections. Dr. Cheney theorized that vitamin B$_{12}$ injections work so well among CFIDS patients because the elevated rate of cytokine production in CFIDS may be effectively blocking vitamin B$_{12}$ function in the body. In this case, massive amounts of vitamin B$_{12}$ would be needed to overcome the functional deficiency brought about by excess cytokine production. Vitamin B$_{12}$ may also help correct the red blood cell membrane defects common in CFIDS, as observed by New Zealand researcher Dr. L.O. Simpson (*CFIDS Chronicle*, Fall 1995).

Most patients who try vitamin B_{12} injections report favorable results. Common benefits are increased energy, mental clarity, and stamina, usually lasting for several days after a single administration. Because benefits may not be felt for the first 3 weeks, a month's trial is generally recommended. Although vitamin B_{12} is fairly innocuous, some patients report side effects. One noted a feeling of extreme lassitude followed by a period of hyperactivity (resulting in sleeplessness). Some also report local rashes, which diminish when dosage is reduced, and various allergic reactions (including diarrhea) to the preservatives used in the solution. To avoid potential allergic reactions, a patch test should be performed first. Administration of the first injection in a physician's office is also recommended in highly allergic persons.

The dosage Dr. Cheney recommends is 2000 to 5000 µg/ml (in a 0.5 to 1.0 cc syringe) administered subcutaneously or intramuscularly every 2 or 3 days. Other physicians generally recommend 1000 to 2000 µg (1 to 2 cc syringe) one to three times a week. High doses of vitamin B_{12} must be accompanied by a multivitamin that includes the entire vitamin B complex to avoid B vitamin imbalances. This dosage can be tolerated over long periods, although benefits can wane. In that case, a short period (1 to 2 weeks) without vitamin B_{12} injections is usually enough to reestablish its efficacy. Most physicians prefer cyanocobalamin to hydroxycobalamin (vitamin B_{12a}) because it is the most stable form of vitamin B_{12}. However, some patients who cannot tolerate cyanocobalamin prefer the more expensive, and longer acting, hydroxycobalamin.

Some advantages of vitamin B_{12} are that it is relatively inexpensive (about $6 a vial), safe, and can be self-administered, and the effects are generally felt quickly (within 12 hours). Injectable vitamin B_{12} is available by prescription. If local pharmacies do not compound high-dose vitamin B_{12}, it can be ordered from Giant Genie Pharmacy (704-525-3956) or Pharmacy on the Park (800-654-3115). Vitamin B_{12} injections are often covered by insurance.

Vitamin B Complex

Many patients with CFIDS benefit from taking a vitamin B complex formulation, either in accompaniment with single B vitamins (to prevent imbalances) or alone. CFIDS patients have reported improvement in energy levels, symptoms of premenstrual syndrome (PMS), mood, and sleep disorders after taking vitamin B complex. Most vitamin B complex formulations include vitamins B_1 (thiamine), B_2 (riboflavin), B_6 (pyridoxine, pyridoxal, and pyridoxamine), B_{12} (cobalamin), niacinamide, pantothenic acid, choline, inositol, vitamin C, and folic acid. People with allergies, systemic Candida infection, or digestive symptoms should avoid yeast-based formulations, which may be poorly tolerated. Nature's Life brand (available in health food stores) seems to be fairly well tolerated by people with CFIDS and the CFIDS and Fibromyalgia Health Resource (800-366-6056) also markets a non-yeast–based vitamin B complex.

Vitamin C

Vitamin C (ascorbic acid) is a water-soluble antioxidant found in most raw fruits and vegetables. It serves a number of vital functions in the body, including connective tissue repair (especially collagen), maintaining healthy teeth and bones, promoting the synthesis of anti-inflammatory hormones in the adrenal glands, helping to produce the neurotransmitters serotonin and norepinephrine, healing wounds, maintaining capillaries, healthy adrenal glands, and ovaries, absorbing iron into the blood stream, promoting efficient white blood cells, and maintaining cholesterol balance. It is widely touted as a preventive for the common cold, perhaps because vitamin C increases the production of interferon, an antiviral cytokine. Animal experiments have shown that vitamin C has other immune system–enhancing effects as well, increasing the body's ability to fight off bacterial infections and promoting general immunity. Patients with allergies may want to take special note of vitamin C's function as a natural antihistamine. A research team led by the co-discoverer of vitamin C, Professor Charles Glen King of Columbia University, demonstrated as early as 1940 that it can both prevent and moderate allergy symptoms. In addition to its other wonderful properties, vitamin C is also a natural chelator, helping to remove heavy metals and toxins from the body.

Vitamin C is not stored in the body, as are fat-soluble vitamins, and thus must be constantly replenished. Smoking, drinking (alcohol), illness, and physical or emotional stress all cause rapid depletion of vitamin C.

USES IN CFIDS. Vitamin C is the most widely used of all vitamins, not just because of its role as an antioxidant and free radical scavenger but also because of the numerous other vital functions it performs. Of particular relevance to patients with CFIDS is the role of vitamin C in maintaining healthy capillaries. A number of researchers have remarked on the poor circulation in patients with CFIDS, resulting in corollary illness such as

Reynaud's phenomenon. Even more critical is the reduced blood flow to the brain, which is especially dependent on capillary action for its blood supply. This function alone helps to place vitamin C at the forefront of any vitamin therapy. However, its role in collagen formation and tissue repair, its importance in immune system function, and its place as an adrenal gland support do much to explain why it is one of the most frequently recommended CFIDS nutritional treatments.

Most nutritionists recommend taking vitamin C to tolerance; that is, until the patient begins experiencing diarrhea or burning urine. Considering the broad spectrum of sensitivities among CFIDS patients, tolerance can vary considerably. CFIDS clinicians generally recommend up to 2000 mg/day, taken in divided doses initially. Because vitamin C is rapidly excreted in urine, this dosage may be broken up into smaller, more frequent doses without any loss of efficacy. The most frequently recommended form of vitamin C is ester C, which enters the blood stream four times faster than regular forms of the vitamin and is retained longer in tissues. It is buffered to prevent irritation to the stomach and bladder. Nonetheless, some people with sensitive stomachs have reported problems with ester C. For those with many gastrointestinal symptoms, acid-free C powder may be more tolerable (Allergy Research Group, 800-782-4274; and Bronson, 800-235-3200). Nonacidic C powder has the advantage of being gentle on the stomach and can be measured out in minute doses. Oral nonacid vitamin C in small doses is extremely safe, with virtually no side effects. Nevertheless, it should be noted that some patients do not tolerate vitamin C in any form or quantity. Vitamin C is one of the least expensive vitamins and is widely available at most pharmacies, health food stores, and many supermarkets.

Intravenous drip is another form of vitamin C therapy used in CFIDS. Administering vitamin C directly into the blood stream not only increases the rate at which it is absorbed but enhances its role as a chelating agent. A number of alternative health care practitioners in the United States and Mexico use vitamin C drip to the exclusion of most other forms of CFIDS therapy, claiming it can cause complete remission. Many patients have believed that they made temporary, although much appreciated, improvement with vitamin C therapy, but rarely has anyone claimed long-lasting effects. A few patients have reported worsening of some symptoms, primarily gastrointestinal and bladder problems, as a result of vitamin drip therapy. Intravenous drip therapy should not be administered daily and requires monitoring by a physician. The charge for an intravenous drip is $70 to $125, depending on locale. Insurance usually does not cover the cost.

Vitamin E

Vitamin E (tocopherol) is an antioxidant, fat-soluble vitamin found in butterfat, meats, vegetable oils, and particularly wheat germ oil, from which this vitamin was first isolated in 1936. Like other antioxidants, vitamin E serves to protect cell linings from damage caused by oxidation. It helps to maintain red blood cell membranes and other cell tissues (even the walls of the tiny structures within cells), ensures normal muscle metabolism, and protects essential unsaturated fatty acids and vitamin A from destruction from oxidation. Vitamin E has protective activity against methyl mercury toxicity and increases the activity of glutathione. Zinc is needed to maintain proper levels of vitamin E in the blood; thus, zinc deficiency can lead to low vitamin E levels.

USES IN CFIDS. Vitamin E is recommended chiefly for its properties as an antioxidant. It does not appear to have any specific immune-modulating or antiviral capacity. However, its ability to strengthen cell walls and protect other vitamins from destruction makes it desirable as an adjunct to other vitamin therapies. Because it is fat-soluble, only minimal amounts are needed to produce antioxidant benefits. The standard dosage, 400 IU of natural vitamin E, taken daily with the largest meal is usually recommended for patients with CFIDS. If nausea, diarrhea, or worsening of fatigue or weakness ensue, the dosage should be reduced.

6

Alternative and Complementary Medical and Supportive Therapies

Acupressure	Homeopathy
Acupuncture	Hydrotherapy
Aroma Therapy	Hypnosis
Bach Remedies	Live Cell Therapy
Bed Rest	Massage
Biofeedback	Meditation
Chelation Therapy	TENS
Chiropractic	Visualization and Imagery
Exercise	

ACUPRESSURE

DEFINITION. Acupressure (or G-Jo), a Chinese technique for the immediate treatment of minor ailments, is based on the same principles as acupuncture (see Acupuncture).

BACKGROUND. Acupressure was developed to provide a fast remedy for various symptoms and ailments. Much like acupuncture, it relies on stimulation of certain points on the surface of the body to release *chi,* or life energy. The fingertips are used to apply acupressure. Usually, light pressure for only a few seconds is exerted with the tip of the thumb. Most points are located by placing the fingers along easily identifiable body landmarks. Distance between points is measured in fingerwidths. The technique is easy to learn and requires relatively little exertion.

USES IN CFIDS. Acupressure can be used for short-term relief of mild to moderate CFIDS symptoms, such as minor aches and pains, insomnia, anxiety, shortness of breath, nausea, headache, eyestrain, and tension.

Inner Wrist Point

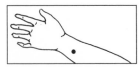

For nausea, insomnia, indigestion, and nervousness

Place your three middle fingers crosswise along the inside of your wrist. The third finger should align with the first crease that separates your hand from your wrist. The inner wrist point is located directly under the index finger, in the middle of your arm.

Inner Shoulder Point

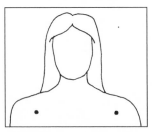

For shortness of breath, chest tension, coughing, and congestion

This point is located on the outer part of the chest near the shoulder, four fingerwidths above the armpit and one fingerwidth toward the chest.

Lower Back Point

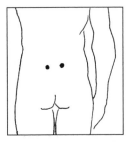

For general muscle tension, anxiety, leg spasms, and insomnia

This point is located at the base of the spine, approximately at the top of the hip bone, four fingerwidths from the spine.

Feet Points
For fatigue, weakness, and pain
The Chinese believe that the lines of *chi,* which run throughout the body, end in the feet. For this reason, the feet are a rich source of acupressure points for all kinds of problems. Many people with CFIDS find that exerting pressure with the tip of the thumb over the entire bottom of the foot provides relief from generalized achiness.

FURTHER READING

Blate, Michael. The Natural Healer's Acupressure Handbook. Falkynor Books, 1983.

ACUPUNCTURE

DEFINITION. Acupuncture is a therapeutic technique in which small needles are inserted under the skin at *chi* points to promote the repair and healing of major organs, regulate body metabolism, and correct physical ailments that result from imbalances in the flow of *chi.*

BACKGROUND. The Chinese invented acupuncture sometime in the third millennium BC, but it was not systematized until 200 BC, when the *Hungdi Neiging Suwen* (The Yellow Emperor's Classic of Internal Disease) was written. Acupuncture is based on the concept of *chi,* or vital or life energy. In the Chinese conceptual system, *chi* flows along channels throughout the body, which can be felt at specific points. When a person is ill, these points become tender. The acupuncturist can discern the nature of the illness and treat it by finding the tender points and stimulating them with small needles inserted just under the surface of the skin. Many years of rig-

orous training, as well as considerable talent, are required to be able to locate these acupuncture points. Since the concept of vital energy, or "life
force," is entirely absent in European conceptions of illness, it is difficult to
say how acupuncture works. The system of meridians does not correspond
to the central nervous system (CNS) or any other physiologic system, inso-
far as anatomists can determine. There has been speculation that some of
the effects produced by acupuncture may result from localized stimulation
of cortisol or perhaps a kind of "distraction" of the CNS utilizing electrical
fields or endorphins; the mechanism, however, is still not readily explained
using the European model of the body. Acupuncture produces distinct effects in about 80% of patients, whereas 20% note no effect. The Chinese
use acupuncture to treat any condition that is reversible. They also use it to
block pain. Since the late 1950s, more than 600,000 operations have been
performed in China using acupuncture analgesia.

USES IN CFIDS. About half of the patients with CFIDS we surveyed
had tried acupuncture, half of whom reported positive results. Improvements were noted in generalized pain, eye pain, overall well-being, mental
clarity, and energy. About a third reported negative results, including overstimulated immune system, severe relapse, and intolerance. A smaller percentage reported no results from acupuncture. Positive results are most often obtained when the treatment focuses on specific problems such as
pain, insomnia, loss of appetite, or nausea. Negative results in many cases
are due to the acupuncturist's mistaken idea that patients with CFIDS have
depressed immune systems and, as a consequence, require immune system
stimulation. In CFIDS, the excess stimulation may cause a profound exacerbation of symptoms.

PROTOCOL. During acupuncture, the patient lies on a table while the
acupuncturist places small sterile needles under the skin. (Needle inser-
tion is painless.) Usually the acupuncturist will first "pulse" you, that is,
measure the flow of *chi*. The effectiveness of the treatment is determined
by the size of the bore of the needle, how long it is left in place, the depth
of penetration, how much it is moved, and how often the treatment is repeated. Sometimes one treatment is all that is needed to achieve the desired effect. For complicated or severe problems, therapy may be needed
two or three times a week. Often acupuncturists are trained in Chinese
herbal medicine. Certain Chinese herbs may be recommended as part of
the acupuncture therapy. Moxa (herbal incense sticks) is also used to provide localized heat. Many people with CFIDS, particularly those with
chemical sensitivities, cannot tolerate the odor of Moxa. Be sure to discuss
sensitivities with your acupuncturist *before* Moxa treatments.

PROS AND CONS. Acupuncture generally provides an alternative to drug treatment for pain. This may be of particular value to patients with numerous allergies and environmental sensitivities. However, acupuncture is not necessarily innocuous. An inexperienced or misinformed acupuncturist can provoke a relapse. Check the acupuncturist's credentials, how long he or she has been practicing acupuncture, and whether he or she has any experience with CFIDS. If possible, talk to another person with CFIDS who has been a patient.

AVAILABILITY AND COST. Acupuncture is available in most urban centers in the United States and is becoming increasingly more so, owing to the recent attention given alternative healing practices in the media. Fees vary, but most acupuncturists charge $30 to $65 per treatment. Insurance may cover the cost, especially if the acupuncturist is also a physician.

MORE INFORMATION

American Academy of Medical Acupuncture
5820 Wilshire Blvd., Suite 500
Los Angeles, CA 90036
213-937-5514 (telephone)

International Foundation of Oriental Medicine
42-62 Kissena Blvd.
Flushing, NY 11355
718-321-8642 (telephone)

AROMA THERAPY

DEFINITION. Aroma therapy involves use of the distilled essential oils naturally found in plants for healing and cosmetic purposes.

BACKGROUND. For centuries, aromatic oils have been recognized for their medicinal properties. In biblical times, oil of myrrh, which is a powerful antiseptic, was revered for its power to quickly heal surface wounds (hence the significance of the gift of the Magi). When Tutankhamen's tomb was opened in 1922, scent pots of frankincense were found. The range of uses for essential oils appears limitless. Essential oils can be used to induce sleep (jasmine), calm the nerves (valerian, clary sage), clean wounds (lavender), reduce aches and pains (rosemary), relieve gas pains (peppermint), and open respiratory airways (basil). The mode of action of aromatic oils is complex. A single oil can produce a number of different, and even opposing, effects. Lavender, for example, sedates in small quantities but stimulates in larger quantities. It is not known how plant oils produce these effects in people, but it has been theorized that smell, our most primordial sense, stimulates a complex set of central nervous system (CNS) reactions that can culminate in emotional and physiologic changes. It is well-known that the ketones, esters, aldehydes, and alcohols found in plant oils can serve as insect repellents, fungicides, and bactericides. Many oils also have hormone-like properties (for example, hops, fennel, and anise contain estrogens).

Production of essential oils is a long, arduous process involving oil-based extraction and repeated distillation (alcohol is never used). It takes many pounds of flowers, leaves, or bark to produce 1/3 oz of concentrated essential oil, which is why only a drop or two produces the desired effect (and also accounts for the expense).

USES IN CFIDS. Aroma therapy may hold promise for the alleviation of some CFIDS symptoms because odors readily cross the blood-brain barrier. Because the olfactory bulbs tie in directly to the limbic system (that part of the brain that processes emotion), essential oils may be useful in alleviating emotional symptoms such as anxiety, anger, and fear. Essential oils can also be effectively used to relieve insomnia and muscle aches. A number of patients who have tried aroma therapy have reported good results in treating anxiety, "jitters," and insomnia, with no negative side effects. To relieve chronic, severe stress, Valerie Worwood, author of *The Complete Book of Essential Oils and Aromatherapy,* recommends use of hypnotics such as narcissus (hyperactivity), jonquil (anxiety), jasmine (depression), carnation or valerian (insomnia), and vanilla. Oils that can help relieve muscle fatigue include rosemary, thyme, and marjoram. To treat insomnia, a blend of sandlewood, clary sage, lemon, and chamomile may be helpful. In *Chronic Fatigue Syndrome: A Natural Healing Guide,* Steve Wilkinson recommends the following oils to treat symptoms of CFIDS: lavender (tension), lemon (to calm the mind, night sweats), peppermint (fever, night sweats, digestive disorders), basil or orange (to lift the spirit), rosemary (lethargy), clary sage (invigoration), and geranium (sluggishness, emotional upset).

PROTOCOL. Essential oils are used by the drop. (Measurements are precise, so you should have a "recipe." Either consult a book on the topic or see an aroma therapist.) The oils are not meant to be taken internally. They can be rubbed on the skin (after thorough cleansing), inhaled, or floated in a bath. When applied directly to the skin, they must be mixed with vegetable oil. To make a rub for the skin, warm slightly 2 tablespoons of pure vegetable oil (corn, safflower, sunflower, peanut, or soy oils are all readily obtained and make good mediums) and add four or five drops of essential oil (or of each of several oils if you are making a blend). You can also run bath water and simply add the oils to it before getting into the tub and soaking. One or two drops of lavender is all that is needed for a relaxing bath. To treat insomnia, try placing one or two drops of clary sage, jasmine, or any of the hypnotics on a handkerchief and place it near your pillow. The oils are strong, so not much is needed. Breathing the vapor from a single drop of peppermint floated in a glass of hot water can relieve gas pain instantly, and help clear the sinuses, too!

PROS AND CONS. Essential oils are usually benign when used externally and in small amounts. Aroma therapy can prove particularly useful for treating gastrointestinal problems because the oils are not processed through the digestive tract. Oils also may be a good therapy option for those who are sensitive to chemicals because they generally do not provoke reactions. Because the oils act synergistically, you may want to purchase a book on aroma therapy for the most effective blends.

AVAILABILITY AND COST. Essential oils can be purchased at health food stores. They are sold in 1/3 oz quantities and range in price. One of the least costly (about $5 per bottle), and perhaps most useful, is lavender. One bottle can last for years. The more exotic and rare oils can cost $15 or more per bottle.

MORE INFORMATION

For a list of registered aroma therapists in the United States, write:
    American Aromatherapy Association
    PO Box 1222
    Fair Oaks, CA 95628

In Europe, write:
    International Federation of Aroma Therapists
    Department of Continuing Education, Room 8
    Royal Masonic Hospital
    Ravens Court Park
    London W6 0TN, England
    081-864-8066 (telephone)

BACH REMEDIES

DEFINITION. Bach remedies involve use of herbal essences (principally from flowers) to remedy specific physical or psychological complaints.

BACKGROUND. Bach remedies were devised by Dr. Edward Bach, a British bacteriologist, in the 1930s. In the 1920s, he proposed the theory that altered mental and emotional states were brought about by disharmonies that could be corrected with the use of plant essences. Dr. Bach collected these essences, at first, by gathering the dew that had collected on the underside of leaves and flower petals. Because this method proved arduous, he later tried putting plant parts in a bowl of pure spring water, which he left in the sun for a few hours. He then preserved the water in alcohol. To make his remedy, he took a few drops from the bottled essence and added them to an ounce of pure water. He administered four drops in a little water four times a day. By the time of Dr. Bach's death in 1936, he had discovered 38 such herbal remedies. Dr. Bach claimed that his flower remedies cured various common physical ailments, but primarily the remedies were used to treat emotional problems. For example, he treated fearfulness with mimulus, obsessional thoughts with white chestnut, lack of faith with gentian, and general ailments with a blend of five of the essences, which he called "Rescue Remedy."

USES IN CFIDS. Some patients report success using scleranthus to control night sweats. Given the low risk associated with Bach remedies, scleranthus might be worth trying if night sweats are severe or resistant to other treatment. Rescue Remedy, a blend of several essences that alleviates many symptoms simultaneously, is popular among those who use Bach remedies to relieve stress and improve sleep.

PROTOCOL. Standard dosage is three to seven drops placed under the tongue, or in a small glass of water, taken four times a day.

PROS AND CONS. Bach remedies are generally well tolerated. Patients who are highly reactive, severely ill, or have multiple allergies may want to start with one drop. Keep in mind that the more essences you use the less effective the mixture will be. Try to focus on one or two problems rather than several.

AVAILABILITY AND COST. Bach remedies can be purchased at most health food stores for less than $10 a bottle or can be ordered through Ellon Bach.

MORE INFORMATION

Ellon Bach USA, Inc.
644 Merrick Road
Lynbrook, NY 11563
516-593-2206 (telephone)

BED REST

DEFINITION. Bed rest means lying down and *resting*.

BACKGROUND. Resting was an integral part of daily life until the last generation. The Spanish siesta, the dinner hour, teatime, the evening cigar, and afternoon snooze all acknowledged the need to take a break from long periods of activity. Rest charges our batteries, so to speak. Bed rest was an essential part of every therapy until the middle part of the twentieth century. Conscientious physicans (and mothers) have recognized throughout the ages that the body needs adequate rest to recover from daily wear and the insults of infectious disease. Given the frequent occurrence of serious infectious diseases that characterized life in the earlier part of this century, the sickbed was a place where everyone would no doubt spend time at some point in a lifetime. Since the discovery of antibiotics, however, we have become rather overconfident. We get sick, take a pill, and keep going. In contemporary society, resting is regarded as a luxury rather than a necessity, much to the detriment of our health. We seem to have forgotten that the human body is material and, like any material object, it wears down with continual use.

USES IN CFIDS. Virtually every CFIDS patient recommends bed rest as an essential part of coping with the illness. As one patient points out, "Nothing cures better than rest." Resting seems obvious when you are tired, but all too many times we "push on." Patients with CFIDS learn quickly that pushing past their limit exacerbates symptoms. Both those who are well into recovery and those who are recently ill learn this lesson over and over again. *Rest is essential.*

PROTOCOL. There is a method to resting. Simply lying down is not enough. In order for your body to rest, your mind must rest, too. If you use rest time to study, or do taxes, or some other task, you will not reap the benefits of rest. When you rest, lie as comfortably as you can. Listen to relaxing music or do relaxation exercises. Do nothing else. The important thing is to allow your body some time for self-repair. Resting may be considered "doing nothing" in our achievement-oriented world, but as far as your body is concerned it is "work." Your body needs rest to reestablish a normally functioning metabolism and immune system. If you are severely ill or relapsed, you will need to rest all the time. Even if you are nearly fully recovered, include rest time during the day. Remember, rest time is not wasted time; it is healing time.

BIOFEEDBACK

DEFINITION. Biofeedback is a technique in which physiologic processes are monitored by computer to enable a person to exercise control over previously unconscious body functions.

BACKGROUND. Biofeedback is a relatively new technique, although the concept of using the mind to control the body is an ancient one. Tibetan lamas and Indian yogis achieve tremendous control over unconscious functions through the practice of simple meditation techniques. In biofeedback, the patient actually sees or hears a representation of brain waves. Different brain wave patterns can be represented by fish swimming, abstract designs, or music. The object is to change the pattern—make it grow or shrink, make the fish swim faster, make the music play louder—through the power of concentration.

Biofeedback has been a topic of great interest in the medical community since the 1950s. Biofeedback devices have been used to help patients regulate heart beat, eliminate migraine headaches, and control elevated blood pressure. Ultimately, any medical problem that is affected by stress hormones can be influenced by biofeedback techniques. In CFIDS, biofeedback may be useful in reducing symptoms exacerbated by disregulation of the hypothalamus-pituitary-adrenal axis because adrenal hormones are sensitive to brain wave output.

USES IN CFIDS. Myra Preston, Ph.D., a biofeedback therapist practicing in Charlotte, North Carolina, has patented a neurofeedback technique that in some patients has resulted in a significant decrease in cognitive problems (*CFIDS Chronicle,* Winter 1996). She uses the basic biofeedback apparatus together with an EEG to correct the excess delta wave (slow wave) anomaly found in people with cognitive difficulties. Dr. Preston argues that when the brain wave pattern reverts to normal, many central nervous system (CNS) symptoms will recede, including difficulty in concentrating, headaches, and insomnia. Michael Tansey, a researcher in Somerville, New Jersey, successfully used neurofeedback techniques to reduce cognitive confusion, pain, headaches, and cold extremities in a CFIDS patient who had had severe symptoms for 2 1/2 years (*CFIDS Chronicle,* Fall 1993). He placed sensors along the top of the skull, just above the supplemental motor area (SMA) of the brain, with the idea that because that area controls limbic outflow and the flow of sensory information, resolution of abnormal brain waves in the SMA would result in cessation of cognitive, verbal, and motor control problems.

PROS AND CONS. Biofeedback is safe and effective for most people.

Patients with CFIDS have successfully used it to treat cognitive problems, headache, cold hands, and for relaxation. Because the technique is noninvasive and seems to address one of the core CFIDS problems, it may hold great promise for those with severe CNS and cognitive problems.

AVAILABILITY AND COST. Myra Preston charges $1100 for diagnostic tests, and $90 per session for 20 weeks of twice-weekly sessions. Insurance often covers the cost.

MORE INFORMATION

American Association of Biofeedback Clinicians
2424 Dempster Street
Des Plaines, IL 60016
847-827-0440 (telephone)

Myra Preston, Ph.D.
10620 Park Road, Suite 230
Charlotte, NC 28210
704-543-0427 (telephone)

CHELATION THERAPY

DEFINITION. Chelation therapy involves use of intravenous EDTA (ethylenediaminetetraacetic acid) to bind and remove metal molecules from the body.

BACKGROUND. Chelation was developed in the late 1940s to treat lead poisoning. It had been discovered about a decade earlier that EDTA, a synthetic amino acid compound, had the ability to bind with calcium. (EDTA is, as a consequence, classified as a calcium channel blocker.) The resulting calcium combinations then bind with heavy metals in the blood stream and remove them by way of the kidneys and bladder. Although the only approved use of chelation in the United States is to treat lead poisoning, chelation therapy has also been used to treat chronic degenerative diseases such as hardening of the arteries, diabetes, stroke, cataracts, senility, Parkinson's disease, and osteoporosis.

USES IN CFIDS. Because of the American Medical Association's reluctance to accept chelation as a valid form of treatment for conditions other than lead poisoning, no studies from the United States support its use in CFIDS. However, Dr. E.C. Boergman of South Africa reported a 100% improvement rate in 16 CFIDS patients using EDTA chelation (*CFIDS Chronicle,* Summer 1994). One of Dr. Boergman's patients recovered totally after 10 infusions. The others reported 60% to 90% recovery from physical and mental symptoms. (However, it is important to note that Dr.

Boergman's study was quite small and has not been replicated. Other patients have not substantiated his claims.) In theory, chelation could offer considerable benefit to patients in whom CFIDS was triggered by exposure to pesticides or other toxic chemicals. In these cases, chelation could remove heavy metals, which continue to cause symptoms and exacerbate immune system irregularities.

PROTOCOL. To be effective, EDTA chelation must be administered by intravenous drips. Each treatment takes approximately 4 hours. The recommended frequency of treatment is once a week. The main chelating ingredient used in this therapy is EDTA, but other chelators such as vitamin C, vitamin A, and selenium may be added to the infusion to boost the chelating power of the mixture. Chelation can also be accomplished orally with natural chelating agents such as vitamin C (4000 mg/day). Oral chelation usually is not as effective as intravenous chelation.

PROS AND CONS. Side effects of chelation include decreased blood pressure, hypoglycemia, joint pain, fatigue, weakness (due to potassium depletion), and peeling of the skin (due to decreased zinc and vitamin B_6 levels). Because the chelated compounds are excreted through the kidneys, chelation can damage those organs. Chelation is contraindicated in patients with a history of kidney, liver, or bladder disease (such as interstitial cystitis). Chelation also depletes the body of vitamin B_6 and minerals such as potassium, zinc, magnesium, and chromium. In patients with low concentrations of these vitamins and minerals, a long course of chelation therapy can cause considerable damage. Before starting chelation therapy, nutritional status should be checked and corrected if necessary. In any case, nutritional supplementation is necessary during chelation therapy. Be sure your physician is familiar with the American College of Advancement in Medicine protocol before chelation therapy is started.

AVAILABILITY AND COST. Each chelation treatment costs $50 to $100, depending on where it is performed (costs are higher on the east and west coasts) and whether other supporting therapies are included. With additional tests and supporting treatments, an entire course of treatment may cost more than $1000. Insurance companies usually require a predetermination for this treatment to establish "medical necessity," so check with them first.

MORE INFORMATION

American Board of Chelation
70 W. Huron
Chicago, IL 60610
312-787-2228 (telephone)

American College of Advancement in Medicine
23121 Verdugo Drive, Suite 204
Laguna Hills, CA 92653
800-532-3688 (toll-free telephone)
714-583-7666 (local telephone)

CHIROPRACTIC

DEFINITION. Chiropractic is the technique of manipulating the spinal column and body joints to alleviate back or joint pain.

BACKGROUND. Although hands-on manipulation of the joints and spine was practiced in ancient Egypt and Assyria, the technique was not popularized in the United States until the late 1800s. The central premise of traditional chiropractic is that subtle deviations of the spinal column, called subluxations, can interfere with nerve transmissions causing various health problems. The chiropractor, by manipulating the vertebrae back into their normal position and giving recommendations about exercise and posture improvement, can remove irritation to the nerves that may be causing pain.

USES IN CFIDS. Chiropractic is normally used to treat back and neck pain, although it also helps alleviate a broad range of related symptoms such as insomnia, headaches, and sciatica.

PROTOCOL. Most chiropractors like to see their patients two or three times a week. In the majority of patients, improvement is noted in 9 to 12 sessions.

PROS AND CONS. Results in CFIDS are mixed. Some patients claim relief from headaches and muscle pain, which, in turn, has helped them sleep. An equal number say chiropractic worsened their pain. The muscles and other tissues surrounding the spine are exquisitely sensitive. The traditional form of chiropractic, in which the spine is abruptly "popped" with a sharp hand movement, may place too much strain on these tissues, causing injury. The pain generated by such treatment lasts for days, sometimes weeks. Patients interested in trying chiropractic for the first time might want to locate a more gentle form of chiropractic (such as "network").

AVAILABILITY AND COST. Chiropractic adjustments usually range between $25 and $45 per visit. Initial visits, which may include taking a history and x-ray examination, cost more, depending on the amount of time the chiropractor spends. Many insurance companies cover the cost of chiropractic treatment.

MORE INFORMATION

American Chiropractic Association
1701 Clarendon Blvd.
Arlington, VA 22209
703-276-8800 (telephone)

Association for Network Chiropractic
PO Box 147
Yonkers, NY 10710
718-891-4077 (telephone)

EXERCISE

DEFINITION. Exercise includes any systematic program of body movement that is designed to strengthen, tone, or stretch muscles.

BACKGROUND. Exercise has been an important component of school health programs since the early 1960s when President Kennedy called for a new era of "vigor." Since then, exercise has become a perpetual preoccupation for health-conscious Americans, many of whom incorporate jogging, running, swimming, and regular visits to a health club into busy work schedules. Moderate exercise produces many health benefits, such as increased strength and sense of well-being, lowered risk for heart disease, reduced arthritic pain, increased mental alertness, and improvements in digestion and metabolism. For most people, exercise is "good for what ails you."

The three basic types of exercise are aerobic, subaerobic, and anaerobic. Aerobic exercise induces systemic changes. In practical terms, aerobic exercise is any exercise that lasts at least 12 minutes, involves deep breathing, and uses major muscle groups (thighs and buttocks). Jogging and biking are good examples of aerobic exercise because they affect heart rate and breathing and utilize major muscle groups. Some metabolic changes that occur as a direct result of aerobic exercise are increased utilization of oxygen, increased production of ATP (adenosine triphosphate), and increased utilization of the Krebs cycle (tricarboxylic cycle).

Subaerobic exercise is what most clinicians mean by "gentle" exercise, such as walking, golfing, nonstrenuous hiking, light weight lifting, and swimming. All of these can be done without pushing the heart rate past 50% of its maximum capacity. None of these forms of exercise will produce metabolic changes unless the person is out of shape or is ill. However, they help build muscle strength and endurance. Subaerobic exercise also elevates mood, improves cognition, enhances immune system function, and improves circulation.

Anaerobic exercise is any form of aerobic exercise that pushes heart rate to its limit. A runner who reaches a point of breathlessness is running anaerobically. Metabolic changes induced by anaerobic exercise are increased production of lactic acid (causing burning pain in muscles), lowered ATP production, and decreased dependence on the Krebs cycle.

USES IN CFIDS. One of the ongoing debates among CFIDS clinicians, as well as their patients, is whether exercise is good or bad for patients with CFIDS. The Centers for Disease Control and Prevention (CDC) maintains that patients with CFIDS need to maintain a steady, low-impact exercise regimen to avoid becoming deconditioned. Indeed, some physicians recommend exercise as one of their chief CFIDS therapies. Other clinicians disagree, noting that exercise is contraindicated in viral illnesses (witness poliomyelitis). They point out that exercise intolerance is a hallmark symptom of the illness and that symptoms invariably worsen after any form of exercise.

Which position is correct? Both. According to Dr. Charles Lapp, exercise is the proverbial "double-edged sword." On the positive side, people mention that exercise increases their strength and helps keep them mentally alert. It also seems to have beneficial effects on the immune system. Some physicians believe gentle exercise can help reverse some of the immune system malfunction of chronic CFIDS. Dr. Benjamin Natelson, of the New Jersey CFS Center, points out that natural killer cells decline with inactivity (*CFIDS Chronicle,* Winter 1996). He contends that with a "very, very gentle training program," immune markers may improve. On the negative side, single-photon emission computed tomographic (SPECT) scans have shown that in patients with CFIDS who exercise, brain blood volume is reduced 1 to 3 days after exercising. In patients who are acutely or seriously ill, this could have profoundly negative effects on immune and endocrine system regulation. In patients with CFIDS, exercise also lowers cortisol levels, which makes it more difficult for the body to control inflammation. In addition, it increases erratic breathing and leads to a rapid progression to anaerobic metabolism, which produces ammonia and lactic acid. These negative results are the opposite of what would normally be expected.

In short, a simple answer to the exercise question is, if you are severely or acutely ill, exercise can make matters worse—in some cases, much worse. The time to discuss an exercise program with your physician is when the illness is stabilized and clear signs of recovery are noted.

PROTOCOL. Most CFIDS clinicians advise a *gradual* reintroduction of exercise. Subaerobic exercise, that is, exercise that does not cause the body to heat up or increase heart rate, is often recommended. This form of exercise helps keep muscles conditioned, increases stamina, and helps with blood circulation. It also puts little strain on ATP production, making it appropriate for people with CFIDS-induced metabolic disturbances. Walking and swimming are probably the best forms of exercise for this purpose. Patients who have been severely ill or have had relapses should begin exercising at extremely low levels, walking slowly for 2 or 3 minutes at most. The amount of time spent walking can be increased in gradual increments over weeks or months (not days). It is good to begin exercising only twice a week to make note of any negative effects over the following 3 days (keep a diary).

Once you are able to walk for 6 or 7 minutes without feeling short of breath, you can consider "weightless" weight training to strengthen specific sets of muscles. CFIDS patients have had some success using weight-lifting equipment set at zero to help improve and tone muscles that have been inactive for months or years.

Once you begin to exercise, it is important to remember that you are not in a contest. How fast you go, how many laps you swim, how many blocks you walk, or how many weights you lift is not only irrelevant, but can be counterproductive. As Dean Anderson, a former ski racer put it, "Most important was learning to enjoy exercise without succumbing to the urge to 'train,' which meant I had to give up on any idea of progressing—of doing more push-ups or of jogging farther or faster. . . . Had I set training goals, as healthy people do, I would have invited not only a succession of relapses, but also discouragement and perhaps demoralization" (*CFIDS Chronicle,* Winter 1996). In other words, learn your limits, which may very well fluctuate from day to day, and stick to them.

FURTHER READING

Bailey, Covert. Smart Exercise. New York: Houghton Mifflin Co., 1994.

RESOURCE

A videotape designed to provide gentle conditioning and stretching for fibromyalgia patients has been prepared by Dr. Robert Bennett and Dr. Sharon Clark. The cost is $19.95 and can be purchased from:

    The Oregon Fibromyalgia Foundation
    1220 SW Yamhill, Suite 303
    Portland, OR 97205
    503-228-3217 (telephone)

HOMEOPATHY

DEFINITION. Homeopathy (from the Greek *homeos,* similar, and *pathos,* suffering) is a system of medicine based on the principal that "like cures like"; that is, substances that produce symptoms similar to those manifested by the illness will act as remedies for that illness.

BACKGROUND. The basic principles of homeopathic medicine date from the fourth century BC, when Hippocrates first articulated the idea that a remedy which produces specific symptoms in a healthy person will cure the same symptoms in a sick person. It was not until 1810, however, that homeopathic remedies achieved wide popularity in Europe and America. In the early part of the nineteenth century a young German physician, Dr. Samuel Hahnemann, discovered that chinchona bark gave him malaria-like symptoms. What surprised him was that chinchona bark was used to *treat* malaria. Over the years, Dr. Hahnemann experimented with a number of other plant extracts, drugs, and chemicals that produced symptoms of various illnesses. He discovered that minute quantities of these substances served to cure the illnesses whose symptoms they mimicked. Larger quantities of these plants were poisonous so Hahnemann devised a system of repeated dilutions, or titrations, to preserve effectiveness without injury to the patient. Homeopathic remedies are so diluted as to leave no perceivable trace of the original plants from which they are derived. The effectiveness of the substance, even in molecular traces, is due to its ability to stimulate the body's natural healing mechanisms along certain specific lines, the symptoms produced by the remedy acting as a set of instructions to the immune system.

USES IN CFIDS. Homeopathic remedies have been used successfully in CFIDS, although they may be better used for treating specific or acute problems such as headache, sinusitis, or insomnia than as a primary treatment for CFIDS.

PROTOCOL. Classic homeopathic remedies are usually taken either all at once or over a short time. Because they are incompatible with allopathic, or pharmaceutical, remedies, you must make a choice as to which approach you think will work best for you. You cannot take homeopathic remedies and drugs at the same time, although you can try taking them serially. The decision as to which remedy is best is based on careful, lengthy evaluation of symptoms by a homeopath, who must choose wisely because only a single remedy is prescribed. Often the remedy will provoke a "healing crisis" or worsening of symptoms, after which the homeopath will re-assess the situation and recommend a different remedy (or none, if the problem is resolved).

Although classic homeopathy includes a limited number of remedies (about 20), modern, "eclectic" homeopathy can make use of hundreds of solutions. Homeopathic blends and remedies for specific problems can also be purchased in health food stores, although these tend to be less reliable. The dosage is usually "as needed" or as indicated on the package. This type of homeopathic remedy may be taken in conjunction with pharmaceutical agents, which is an advantage for patients who must take certain medications on a regular basis. Homeopathic remedies are taken on an empty stomach in pill, liquid, or sublingual form.

PROS AND CONS. Homeopathic remedies are generally less expensive (especially single-dose remedies) than drugs and are usually regarded as having fewer side effects. Homeopaths refer to these remedies as "suggestions" that the body may take or ignore. This may be true for the most part, but does not always seem to be the case in CFIDS. The reason may simply be that because homeopathic remedies stimulate the body to self-repair, they can also stimulate the immune system. Because many CFIDS symptoms seem to arise precisely because of an overactive immune system, it is possible that homeopathic remedies can exacerbate the problem. Consult with a trained homeopath before embarking on this type of therapy.

AVAILABILITY AND COST. Homeopathic remedies range from $10 to $25, although imported remedies (usually German) can cost more. Office visits are comparable to those to a physician and sometimes include the cost of the remedy. As some homeopaths are also physicians, insurance may cover the cost of a consultation.

MORE INFORMATION

International Foundation for Homeopathy
2366 East Lake Avenue E, Suite 301
Seattle, WA 98102
206-324-8230 (telephone)

National Center for Homeopathy
801 N. Fairfax Street, Suite 306
Alexandria, VA 22314
703-548-7790 (telephone)

HYDROTHERAPY

DEFINITION. Hydrotherapy is the use of water for healing.

BACKGROUND. The idea of using water to heal is not new. For centuries, people have immersed themselves in therapeutic baths as a means to prevent and cure illness. The ancient Romans and the Incas built sumptuous tiled baths to acknowledge the importance placed on the restorative powers of water. Healing waters can be found all over the world, from Lourdes in France to the Ganges River in India. Spas and hot springs have long been popular in the United States as well. Saratoga Springs, New York, and Hot Springs, Arkansas, still enjoy a reputation for restoring health and vigor. Although spas are no longer as popular as they were a century ago, the effects of water on the body should not be underestimated. The body is, after all, 70% water. Water, in one form or another, supplies most of the nutrients our bodies need to maintain life. Our permeable skin allows substances in mineral-rich water to pass into our bodies. And various water temperatures and pressures can have a profound effect on the way our metabolism and immune system function.

USES IN CFIDS. Warm-water baths can help reduce pain associated with lactic acid buildup in muscle tissues. This is the pain so often experienced by patients with fibromyalgia-like symptoms. The water temperature should be at about body temperature. Many people have reported that warm-water baths help loosen tight muscles, reduce leg pains, and in general create a feeling of relaxation.

Cool-water baths can also be beneficial. One woman reported that a daily 20-minute bath at a very cool 61° F (16° C) helped her feel better overall. The effectiveness of this strategy is most likely due to the fact that the body, when immersed in cold water, automatically shuts down the blood supply to the skin, shunting it instead to vital organs. The additional blood supply to the brain, liver, and other organs affected by CFIDS could theoretically have a profound impact on reducing symptoms.

Dr. Paul Cheney has also used cool-water hydrotherapy with good results. Vertical immersion up to the neck in water at about the temperature of a heated swimming pool has reduced symptoms in a number of his patients. The rationale behind this novel form of hydrotherapy is that the increased pressure at the feet forces lymphatic flow to reverse itself, up the body to the thoracic duct (just below the left clavicle), where it is infused into the blood stream. The presence of the extra lymph tissue signals the immune system that cytokines are already circulating and the immune system automatically downregulates. In patients experiencing the effects of excess cytokine production, downregulation of immune system chemicals can provide tremendous relief. Whether due to the additional blood supply provided to vital organs or to downregulation of the immune system, cool-water hydrotherapy may offer considerable benefits to a number of people with CFIDS.

PROTOCOL. Dr. Cheney's hydrotherapy protocol requires almost complete immersion in water at 80° to 86° F (swimming pool temperature). For the process to work, it is important that the patient remain vertical and immersed up to the neck, which means a flotation device is necessary. Initially, immersion time is 15 minutes and is increased by 5 minutes per session to 1 hour (at about 3 weeks). The entire treatment plan calls for 16 weeks of hydrotherapy, with three sessions per week.

PROS AND CONS. Dr. Cheney's hydrotherapy program may be a particularly good treatment option for people with pain because it appears to have a positive effect in relieving fibromyalgia-type symptoms. It seems to have minimal side effects, although some severely ill patients have experienced temporary worsening or relapse of symptoms, no doubt due to the increased concentration of cytokines in the blood stream. These symptoms decrease over time. Patients who stopped treatment before the 16-week period have had relapses. Once you embark on this treatment, you are committed to finish it. Another problem that could occur is chilling. Dr. Cheney recommends that if you start to shiver, get out of the pool, but do not take a hot shower. If necessary, purchase a wet suit to help maintain body heat.

AVAILABILITY AND COST. Most forms of hydrotherapy are not expensive. Warm or cool baths, for example, can be taken at home. A membership to a facility with a pool (such as a club or a community center) may be necessary to follow Dr. Cheney's hydrotherapy program, however. For his program, you will also need to purchase a flotation device to rest on while you are in the water.

MORE INFORMATION

The Cheney Clinic
10620 Park Road, Suite 234
Charlotte, NC 28210
704-542-7444 (telephone)
> The clinic provides a detailed description as well as adjunct recommendations for Dr. Cheney's hydrotherapy protocol.

HYPNOSIS

DEFINITION. Hypnosis involves inducing a trance-like state, somewhere between sleep and wakefulness, to produce greater suggestibility in a patient.

BACKGROUND. Although the technique of producing physiologic and psychological effects by means of deep trances has been used by yogis, mystics, and oracles since earliest times, it was not until the eighteenth century that Europeans regarded the hypnotic trance as useful for medical purposes. In the 1760s, Franz Anton Mesmer popularized hypnosis in Europe via a series of theatrical demonstrations of what he called "animal magnetism." Mesmer believed that illness was the direct result of an imbalance in animal magnetism and that hypnosis could correct these imbalances. Because Mesmer's subjects did rather silly things while "mesmerized," hypnosis initially acquired the reputation as a form of entertainment rather than a therapy. The current practice of hypnosis has discounted Mesmer's theory of animal magnetism and eliminated the theatrical aspects of hypnosis to provide a unique means of influencing normally inaccessible physiologic functions, namely, those controlled by the autonomic nervous system. By accessing the body's ability to produce heat, dilate or constrict blood vessels, speed or slow metabolism, and so forth, the hypnotist can utilize the body's own mechanisms to control pain, reduce anxiety, relieve phobias, and cure addictions.

USES IN CFIDS. Hypnosis can be beneficial in reducing the effects of anxiety and stress brought on by illness. It can also help increase blood flow to the brain, thereby alleviating headaches, insomnia, and some cognitive problems. One person reported successfully breaking the smoking habit through the use of hypnosis. Most describe hypnosis as "very relaxing."

PROTOCOL. A standard visit to a hypnotist involves evaluation of a particular problem (insomnia, smoking, anxiety). After assessing the problem, the hypnotist will ask you to sit back in a reclining chair and focus your eyes on a point on the ceiling or a light while he or she speaks to you in a low, monotonous voice. After a short time, your body will relax, and the hypnotist will suggest that you close your eyes. While your eyes are closed, the hypnotist will read from a script specifically designed for your particular problem. After listening, you will be asked to open your eyes on the count of 10 and come back to the office setting. The hypnotist may ask you what you felt or "saw." The visit usually takes 1 hour.

AVAILABILITY AND COST. Licensed hypnotists generally charge $50 to $90 per hour session, depending on their degree of training. Hypnotherapists, who usually hold an advanced degree in psychology, may charge more.

MORE INFORMATION

International Medical and Dental Hypnotherapy Association
4110 Edgeland, Suite 800
Royal Oak, MI 48073
313-549-5594 (telephone)
or
11824 Lyon Rd.
Delta Vancouver, BC V4E 2S9 Canada
604-597-4264 (telephone)

LIVE CELL THERAPY

DEFINITION. Live cell therapy involves implantation of healthy cells, usually derived from calf fetuses, into humans to revitalize vital organs and reverse the course of degenerative diseases.

BACKGROUND. Live cell therapy, or cellular therapy, was devised in the 1930s by a Swiss surgeon, who discovered that he could help regenerate organs that had been damaged by disease and the aging process by injecting cells obtained from healthy unborn animals. (He used unborn animals to minimize the effects of immune system rejection of foreign material.) The theory behind the therapy is that cells from healthy organ tissues injected into the body will migrate to the same organ in the patient, replacing or rejuvenating damaged cells. Consequently, live cell therapy is appropriate for treatment of diseases that affect specific organs. Live cell therapy also enjoyed considerable popularity among men who hoped to prolong sexual vitality and youthful vigor. Notable among these were Winston Churchill, Dwight Eisenhower, Charles DeGaulle, Charlie Chaplin, and Bob Hope. Live cell therapy is currently unlicensed in the United States, but can be obtained in clinics in Switzerland and Mexico.

USES IN CFIDS. Live cell therapy is one of the CFIDS treatments offered by the American Biologics Clinic in Tijuana, Mexico, as well as other alternative health care clinics abroad. In general, live cell therapy provides short-term relief of some CFIDS symptoms, particularly exhaustion. Given the nature of the therapy, however, it does not hold much promise for affecting the general course of the illness.

PROTOCOL. Live cells are administered by injection, usually once every few months. The cells to be injected can come from any part of the endocrine or exocrine system of the calf, but for CFIDS the recommended organs are the hypothalamus, thymus, adrenal glands, brain, pituitary gland, intestines, and umbilical cord.

PROS AND CONS. Some patients report that live cell therapy helps provide an energy boost and improves overall immune function. Patients who tend to be reactive, however, have reported side effects such as sweating and heart palpitations. Because live cell therapy is not available in the United States, it can be expensive. Live cell therapy is short-lived, which means the injections must be repeated to be effective. Injections are painful, although not unbearable. Due to the unpredictability of its effect on the immune system, some clinicians regard live cell therapy as extremely risky in patients with CFIDS.

AVAILABILITY AND COST. Depending on duration of treatment, live cell therapy can cost $500 to $2000. Although it is not available in the United States, some extracts (such as thymus) can be ordered from Canada and Germany.

MASSAGE

DEFINITION. Massage therapy involves manipulation of soft tissue by rubbing, stroking, kneading, compressing, or vibration.

BACKGROUND. Massage techniques are as old and as varied as the cultures that originally devised them. As a consequence, it is almost impossible to make a general description of massage therapy. Some techniques such as Swedish massage are vigorous and cover the entire body. Others such as shiatsu apply pressure to specific areas. All massage techniques share the principle that the body can be healed through mechanical means. Massaging the body can produce profound metabolic changes. A vigorous massage stimulates the sympathetic nervous system, which speeds up the metabolism, increasing blood circulation, heart rate, respiration, and surface temperature. A light massage, especially over the lower back, stimulates the parasympathetic nervous system, decreasing heart rate and blood pressure and increasing digestive action. Any relaxation of muscle knots and spasms enhances the ability of the vascular system to cleanse the lymphatic system and to clear stagnant tissue fluid, toxins, and the excess lactic acid buildup that causes acidosis and muscle pain.

USES IN CFIDS. Most CFIDS patients use massage to relieve the pain associated with fibromyalgia, headaches, and muscle spasms. A number of patients have reported that firm massage of the soles of the feet has a profound beneficial effect throughout the body.

PROS AND CONS. While it may seem like the logical therapy for pain, a vigorous massage can paradoxically make pain worse. A number of people have reported worsened pain after general massage. The reason for the aggravation of pain is probably due to the practice of placing excessive pressure on nerve endings to relieve knotty muscles. Nerve compression only exacerbates the pain created by an already irritated nervous system. Vigorous massage can also release accumulated toxins into the system. Patients with CFIDS may feel general malaise after massage because of the sluggish elimination of these toxins. On the other hand, gentle massage is often beneficial. Those who want to try massage to treat chronic or severe pain may want to consider starting with some of the less vigorous techniques. Vigorous massage is contraindicated in patients with osteoporosis, hypertension, inflammation, arthritis, varicose veins, thrombosis, aneurysm, skin, muscle, or bone disease, unhealed bone fracture, torn ligaments, tendons, or muscles, diabetes, tumors, and frostbite, and in pregnant women.

AVAILABILITY AND COST. Massages cost $40 to $60 per hour. Sometimes massage schools offer less expensive, apprentice rates. If performed by a licensed physical therapist, the cost of massage may be covered by insurance (usually a physician referral is required).

Craniosacral Massage

Craniosacral massage is a gentle form of massage focusing on the spinal cord and skull. It was developed in the 1970s by an American osteopath, John Upledger, who noticed that spinal fluid made rhythmic pulsations as it traveled up the spinal column. He speculated that alterations in the pulses could be used for diagnosis and devised a system by which illnesses could be treated by subtle readjustments. Craniosacral massage is used to treat head injuries, learning difficulties, balance disorders, dyslexia, hyperactivity, whiplash, ear and eye problems, and temporomandibular joint (TMJ) syndrome.

Lymphatic Drainage

The Vodder method of manual lymphatic drainage is a gentle, rhythmic European massage technique designed to increase and accelerate the movement of lymphatic fluid through the body. It was developed in France in the 1930s to treat a variety of conditions that might be caused or aggravated by congested lymph tissue, including sinusitis, acne, edema, inflammation, and arthritis.

Reflexology

Reflexology is based on the idea that reflex points (or zones) located on the hands and feet correspond to every organ in the body. Steady, even pressure applied by the fingers to these zones is said to remedy any imbalances in the corresponding organs. Reflexology promotes improved circulation and contributes to a sense of relaxation and well-being. Because reflexology may be practiced easily on one's own feet and hands, it is an ideal form of self-massage. In contrast, zone therapy, a more complex form of reflexology, can be performed only by a practitioner. Unlike self-administered reflexology, zone therapy is quite painful.

Shiatsu

Related to acupuncture, shiatsu is an ancient form of massage that dates to the third millennium BC. The basic technique consists of the application of pressure by the fingers over some 600 neural trigger points located on lines (meridians) throughout the body. The points are said to be places where lymph vessels tend to congregate. By releasing the point with gentle sustained pressure, energy blocks are removed and the body can better eliminate waste products such as lactic acid and carbon monoxide that have accumulated in body tissues.

Therapeutic Touch

The gentlest of all massages, therapeutic touch, is derived from the ancient practice of laying on of hands. It was devised in the 1960s by Dolores Krieger, a nurse, and Dora Kuntz, a clairvoyant. Technically, therapeutic touch is not massage but "energy work" because it does not involve direct contact with the body. Instead, the body's "energy fields" are manipulated to promote healing. Therapeutic touch is reported to be very relaxing and can help relieve pain.

MORE INFORMATION

American Massage Therapy Association
National Information Office
1130 W. North Shore Avenue
Chicago, IL 60626
773-761-2682 (telephone)

MEDITATION

DEFINITION. In meditation, a particular state of consciousness is achieved by means of concentration, contemplation, or visualization techniques.

BACKGROUND. Meditation is an ancient practice that has been used throughout the ages to reach an inner state of quiet. Meditation techniques form the backbone of Buddhism, one of the world's major religions. Because meditation was, and still is, practiced to achieve an altered or "higher" state of consciousness (a drawing closer to a divine state of being), the practice of meditating is less a therapy than a way of being. Meditation is as much a way of looking at the world as it is a technique, as much a philosophy as a practice. In meditation, the means and the ends are as one. One meditates for its own sake, not to achieve a specific goal but to let go of all goals. In the process of letting go, a different person emerges. A different body may emerge, as well. Meditators have been known to achieve lowered blood pressure, relief from pain and migraine headaches, and greater mental clarity and alertness through the simple act of gazing within.

USES IN CFIDS. A significant number of patients with CFIDS meditate. All report an increased feeling of calm and improved outlook on life. Meditation is also effective in controlling the pain generated by an overreactive nervous system. Like rest, meditation seems to cause no damage and results only in a general sense of improvement. Patients with CFIDS, especially those who find themselves plagued by depression, anxiety, fear, and anger, can benefit greatly by the practice and philosophy of "letting go."

PROS AND CONS. There is no "right" way to meditate, but some practitioners may try to convince you there is. Of the many meditative traditions, not all are conducive to healing long-term illnesses. Zen, for example, was developed for healthy, young, Japanese monks. Sitting for several hours staring at a blank wall (and getting roused when you drift off to sleep) is perhaps not the best meditation technique for ill people. When you begin to meditate, especially if you are quite ill, do it your own way. Lie down, in the comfort of your bed, and listen to your favorite relaxing music. Remember, meditation is a state of mind. How you get there is up to you.

AVAILABILITY AND COST. You can meditate at home for free or you can join a meditation group. Classes in meditation and yoga centers are not usually expensive ($5 to $8 per class). Meditation retreats are more expensive. You can teach yourself to meditate easily and painlessly by listening to tape series made for that purpose or by reading a book on meditation techniques.

RESOURCES

Borysenko, Joan. Minding the Body, Mending the Mind. New York: Addison-Wesley Publishing Co., 1987.

Sounds True audiotape catalog (800-333-9185). Included in this catalog are several excellent tape series on meditation by authors who have written books on the topics of meditation and healing. These can serve as useful introductions to Eastern meditation and the philosophy that inspired it. Examples include the following:
- "The Inner Art of Meditation" (insight meditation as taught by clinical psychologist Jack Kornfield is a meditation course complete with practice periods and question-and-answer sessions).
- "The Higher Self" (control of body and mind through Ayurveda and Indian meditation as taught by endocrinologist Deepak Chopra).
- "The Art of Mindful Living" (the art of bringing mindful awareness into daily life, as taught by meditation master and Nobel Peace Prize Nominee Thich Nhat Hanh, a Vietnamese Buddhist, Zen master, and practitioner of the Art of Peace).

TENS

DEFINITION. TENS (transcutaneous electrical nerve stimulation) is the topical application of an electrical stimulus to a peripheral nerve in order to control pain.

BACKGROUND. The TENS machine was developed after the "gate" model of pain became popular. Pain researchers believed that when nerves are overstimulated the pain message stops (the assumption being that the brain cannot process sensory input from so many "gates"). The stimulation from TENS is supposed to "drown out" the pain felt in a nerve. Some have also proposed that the reason TENS works is not because the nerve is overstimulated but because the electrical stimulation prompts the release of pain-killing endorphins. Whether the relief is through nerve overstimulation or chemistry, the result is the same—pain is relieved.

USES IN CFIDS. TENS has been recommended for patients with fibromyalgia-type pain, that is, pain generated by trigger points and nerve irritation.

PROTOCOL. The TENS unit is a small machine that generates electrical current, which is conveyed along wires to small rubber-tipped electrodes. The unit can be worn on a belt. The electrodes are placed on specific sites on the skin by a physician or physical therapist and are held in place with adhesive tape. The amount of stimulation is regulated by the physician.

PROS AND CONS. TENS is nonaddictive, has no damaging side effects, and, in many cases, is an effective form of pain control. However, it does require a visit to the physician's office and can be expensive if many treatments are required.

AVAILABILITY AND COST. The TENS unit is expensive ($300 to $500) and must be ordered by a physician; therefore, they usually are used in the context of an office visit. The cost of the application varies, depending on the supervising clinician. In some cases, insurance covers the cost.

VISUALIZATION AND IMAGERY

DEFINITION. Visualization (or guided imagery, creative visualization, creative imagery, or mental imagery) is the use of mental images to produce changes in the body.

BACKGROUND. The use of imagery for healing first drew attention in the 1950s when a cancer patient went into remission after visualizing the disappearance of a tumor. This case fueled great interest in the medical community and eventually led to the development of visualization techniques geared specifically to certain diseases. While visualization has enjoyed a reputation as a "miracle cure," it should be remembered that spontaneous remissions are possible with any illness. Those who question the curative powers of visualization point out that its "healing powers" are coincidental at best. Despite its limitations, visualization can serve as a useful coping technique.

Visualization works by mobilizing the immune system, which is not normally under conscious control, through the efforts of higher brain functions. The act of voluntarily creating images (as opposed to hallucinations or dreams) is controlled by the cortex, whereas the immune system is regulated, at least in part, by structures in and around the limbic system, notably the hypothalamus. Since the nerve fibers that connect the limbic system to the cortex flow through the hypothalamus, allowing for a two-way interchange between thought and autonomic nervous system and, hypothetically, immune system function, it is argued that thought can also direct the outcome of illness.

USES IN CFIDS. Visualization techniques can be helpful in maintaining a sense of calm. This can be useful for patients who are severely ill or are experiencing a relapse. Some have reported that, much like hypnosis and meditation, visualization helps them control pain and anxiety.

PROTOCOL. To visualize, you must begin by relaxing. Get comfortable, take three or four deep breaths (if you practice meditation or self-

hypnosis, you can use any of those techniques), and concentrate on the desired images. For CFIDS, images that have been suggested include the following:
- Imagine you are surrounded by a bubble of pink light through which nothing can pass. You are completely protected.
- Breathe in light through the crown of the head. Feel that the light's energy is going through every cell and every tissue, bringing feelings of love and well-being to every part of your body.
- See the light perfectly balancing your immune system and restoring it to the way nature intended.

If "seeing" does not work for you, try kinetic imagery. Kinetic, or motion, imagery techniques are more primal than techniques that rely on vision alone. As a consequence, they may be more useful to patients who are acutely ill or cannot make a visual image. Some patients have imagined they are gently rocking in a boat, floating down a stream, or traveling around a sideways figure of eight. These movement-oriented images are useful to alleviate headaches, panic, vertigo, and episodes of nonlocalized pain.

PROS AND CONS. Visualization is inexpensive (all you need is a book to explain the theory and you can invent your own images) and it might help you feel more in control. Visualization, however, does not seem to work against the disease process itself. Patients who are led to believe that skillful use of imagery will rid them of all their ills invariably are disappointed. However, if your goal is short-term alleviation of pain, anxiety, or stress-related symptoms, guided imagery, like hypnosis or meditation, can serve a purpose.

MORE INFORMATION

International Imagery Association
PO Box 1046
Bronx, NY 10471
914-423-9200 (telephone)

The National Institute for the Clinical Application of Behavioral Medicine
Box 577
46 King Hill Road
Storrs, CT 08268
203-429-2238 (telephone)

FURTHER READING

Collinge, William. Recovering From Chronic Fatigue Syndrome. New York: The Body Press/Perigee Books, 1993 (includes many guided imagery techniques).

IV

COPING
AND MANAGEMENT
STRATEGIES

C oping with chronic illness presents quite a challenge. A patient with diabetes, cancer, multiple sclerosis, allergies, high blood pressure, or any other condition that does not resolve itself has to make lifestyle adjustments. Some illnesses require constant accommodation, while others may require fewer changes in thinking and behavior. For example, for those with high blood pressure, changes in medication and diet may be the only adjustments the patient has to make. CFIDS, unfortunately, does not fall into this category. Patients with CFIDS must make profound adjustments in the way they see themselves in the world and modify the way they live accordingly.

The keys to coping with CFIDS consist of first acknowledging the illness, and then adjusting to its limitations. Acknowledging the illness must be the first step. If you cannot accept that you have an illness, making the necessary practical adjustments will be difficult indeed.

Acknowledgement and acceptance of CFIDS are formidable tasks for most patients. The majority of people diagnosed with CFIDS had been healthy until they contracted the illness. According to statistics, most CFIDS patients are individuals who had led normally productive lives prior to becoming ill. As a consequence, a diagnosis of CFIDS may be received with as much shock as relief. The physician who makes the diagnosis may be as likely to hear, "This can't be happening to me!," as "Thank you for clearing up the mystery." Even after the diagnosis is made, the process of accepting it may take years.

Dean Anderson, a former skier and manager of renewable energy projects in the United States, conveys the process of acceptance eloquently:

> In America we are taught from early childhood that succeeding in life is important and that striving is the key to achievement. I initially viewed the healing process as one in which I would succeed through determination and hard work. . . . I believe today that a certain kind of acceptance may be important to recovery. It is not a resignation to one's fate as a sick person. Rather, it is an acceptance of the reality of illness and of the need to live a different kind of life (*CFIDS Chronicle*, Winter 1996).

Acceptance of the reality of one's illness implies that this new life is going to be quite different from one's former life—a scary thought for most individuals. In this new reality all the rules are different. They are also unknown. CFIDS, unlike better researched ailments, is new territory for clinicians as well as patients, making expert advice difficult to obtain. The rule book for living with CFIDS is yet to be written, for even after the illness has been diagnosed and acknowledged, there still remains the task of figuring out how to live with it.

Dr. Paul Cheney remarks that "patients with this disease must, for many of them for the first time, place limits on their workstyles and lifestyles. Proper limit-setting, which is *always* individualized, is the key to improvement in this syndrome" (*CFIDS Chronicle*, March 1991). This comment comes after observation of thousands of patients, many of whom denied their illness for extended periods before adjusting to its limitations. Dr. Cheney has seen not only the successes inherent in making these adjustments, but the failures that resulted from attempting to ignore them. But first, we must address the question of what is meant by "proper limit-setting."

To set proper limits, we must start with a basic awareness of how CFIDS affects the body and the mind. CFIDS affects the ability to maintain homeostasis; that is, once the illness is established, it alters the body's ability to adjust to changes in the environment. For example, a person with CFIDS climbs a set of stairs and feels like he or she has just climbed Mount Everest. The out-of-breath, depleted feeling is the result of sluggish heart rate, which, in CFIDS, does not respond in time to the greater demands for oxygen required by exertion. As a result, not enough oxygen is available, and a person with CFIDS feels winded after even minimal strain. This type of delayed reaction also results from temperature changes. People with CFIDS often remark that when they become cold, "it takes forever to warm up." The same is true for heat. Both temperature extremes produce symptoms as the body attempts to adjust.

People with CFIDS often comment that they are either "on" or "off." Once they stop, they can't get going again; and once they start, they can't stop. In *The Clinical and Scientific Basis of ME/CFS*, Dr. Byron Hyde, a well-known clinician and researcher of myalgic encephalomyelitis (ME) describes taking a walk with one of his patients. Dr. Hyde noticed that when he stopped to look in a store window, his companion kept going. When asked why, Dr. Hyde's companion replied that if he stopped, he would never get going again! Once embarking on a project, a task, or a plan, it is difficult to stop. Even when performing formerly easy activities such as taking a walk or balancing a checkbook, patients with CFIDS often pass the point of endurance, and symptoms rapidly develop as a result.

Learning when we are "overdoing" it is how we define our own particular limits. This takes awareness, skill, and practice. Each person has limits that are defined by the severity of the illness. For a person who is bedbound, limits will be very different from those of someone who is able to work. Patients who are bedbound may find that extended telephone conversations, standing in the shower, or tackling stressful tasks such as filling out disability application forms produce exhaustion and a general exacerbation of symptoms. These patients may find that sitting in a plastic chair while showering, limiting conversations to 10 minutes, and resting before and after doing necessary paperwork are ways to conserve energy. A patient who is mildly ill and able to work may wish to cut back on work hours, take naps, and forego activities that place excessive or inflexible demands on the body (such as team sports or other activities that do not allow the participant to "listen" to the body).

A former airline pilot refers to limit setting as living in a box. "As long as I'm in the box, I do alright. If I cross the margins of this box, I don't do very well" (*CFIDS Chronicle,* March 1991). Defining the limits of your own particular box is the key to developing good coping strategies. Whatever produces symptoms on any particular day or at any particular hour is where you should define your limits, not by an abstract assessment of what you think you should be doing or a comparison with former capacities. Dean Anderson sees this process as a form of discipline:

> It is the discipline to recognize and adhere to one's known limitations and to follow a strict regimen without lapsing. It is the discipline not to succumb to family or societal pressures to get back into the rat-race. It is the will to protect oneself, to not over-do and to find ways to be productive and find fulfillment under unfamiliar and difficult circumstances.

By setting limits and staying within them, a person can learn to live with, and in spite of, CFIDS.

Chapters 7 through 9 discuss some of the main pitfalls of CFIDS in three of the areas that require considerable adjustment: coping with stress, the home environment, and dietary limitations. Each offers a series of useful coping suggestions based on the experiences of patients with CFIDS and related conditions, as well as those of the clinicians who specialize in these areas.

Children with CFIDS present a special challenge. Chapter 10 offers some suggestions for helping children and their parents cope with the unique problems CFIDS creates for children and their families.

7

Stress Reduction and Elimination

One of the most common observations made by CFIDS patients is that stressful situations become harder to handle after becoming ill. Difficulty coping with stressful situations may arise as one of the earliest symptoms of CFIDS and, depending on the circumstances, can be one of its more problematic aspects. Many people with CFIDS remark that a stressful job or home environment during the early stages of the illness contributed to the severity of the illness at onset; patients in the recovery phase often note that emotional stress can bring on relapse; and those who are severely ill experience profound exacerbation of symptoms when placed in stressful situations or environments.

The relationship between stress and relapse is striking enough to have garnered the attention of psychologists and therapists who specialize in CFIDS. In 1994, Fred Friedberg, a psychologist who has both researched and treated CFIDS for the better part of his professional life, conducted an investigation of relapse triggers in CFIDS. In a study group of 300 CFIDS patients, he found that in the majority, physical or emotional stress was likely to trigger a relapse.

The controversy surrounding the relationship between stress and exacerbation of CFIDS symptoms has generated considerable discussion among researchers. The proposed correlation between prolonged stress states and certain physiologic problems has led a number of health care professionals to conclude that prolonged stress can produce CFIDS. This, in essence, is the origin of the misnomer "yuppie flu," a disease believed (by journalists mostly) to result from the hectic lifestyle and inflated expectations of young, upwardly mobile professionals. The treatment recommendation for "yuppie flu" was to "take it easy," with the assumption that once the stress was removed the body would return to normal.

287

FACTORS THAT TRIGGER CFIDS RELAPSE*

Relapse Trigger	CFIDS Patients (%) (n = 300)
Physical stress (doing too much)	97
Exercise	85
Emotional stress (upset)	80
Other infections	75
Emotional trauma	65
Exposure to chemical or air pollutants	56
Physical trauma	60
Humidity	57
Allergens	56
Hot weather	47
Barometric pressure	45
Certain foods	43
Cold weather	41
Medications	32
Vaccinations or immunizations	25
Pregnancy	13
Birth control pills or estrogen replace- ment therapy	9

*Adapted from Friedberg, Fred. Coping With Chronic Fatigue Syndrome: Nine Things You Can Do. Oakland, Calif.: New Harbinger Publications, 1995.

For patients with CFIDS, taking it easy, while helpful, does not fix the problem. Inexperienced physicians treating this puzzling illness, though quick to recommend "taking a break," have been at a loss to understand why their patients do not bounce back after a week or two of vacation. A little distraction or a vacation does not bring a complete restoration of body and mind because CFIDS is not a stress-*induced* illness. Rather, it is a stress-*sensitive* illness; that is, stress does not cause CFIDS, but it can prolong, or worsen, the disease process (as with most illnesses). This is the real difficulty faced by most patients with CFIDS.

The many negative consequences of stressful situations make managing stress one of the most important of the coping and lifestyle changes that a CFIDS patient can make. Most clinicians recommend reducing or eliminating stress as part of their general CFIDS treatment plan. Stress, however, is an unavoidable fact of life. Whether it's losing a job or a loved one, moving to a new home, being injured, having a baby, or becoming ill, everyone experiences stress during the normal course of a lifetime. It is difficult to plan for such life events, let alone avert them. However, numerous other stressful situations are predictable and can be effectively controlled. This chapter explains how stress control can be accomplished with a minimal amount of effort, through methods that have withstood the test of time.

THE STRESS RESPONSE: A BRIEF OVERVIEW

The study of the physiology of stress did not gain significant attention in the medical world until Hans Selye popularized the term in the 1930s. At that time, Selye, a young endocrinologist studying ovarian hormones, discovered that when rats were subjected to various environmental stresses (prolonged heat or cold, rough handling, forced exercise), they developed peptic ulcers, adrenal enlargement, and atrophy of the immune system. Selye concluded that the physiologic effects of prolonged stress cause damage to the endocrine system and, consequently, the immune and nervous systems. He formalized this concept with the term "general adaptation syndrome." This syndrome is characterized initially by enlargement of the adrenal glands, to compensate for an increased stress response, followed eventually by shrinking of adrenal tissue, leading to an inability to handle stress.

Although Selye's perceptive conclusions have since been modified (most researchers no longer believe that prolonged stress causes adrenal gland atrophy), stress remains an area of medical interest. Physicians are well aware that prolonged stress can increase the risk of heart disease, hypertension, chronic headache, and numerous other conditions. Stress exacerbates the effects of many illnesses. The reason stress has such far-reaching effects is that its mechanisms are complex, diffuse, and involve nearly every system in the body. Stress affects the vascular system, digestive system, endocrine system, central nervous system, and most metabolic processes. It also affects the immune system in ways that are sometimes subtle or contradictory, but which, nevertheless, have profound consequences.

What happens when a person experiences stress such as news of illness in the family or experiences a near accident on the highway? In response to emotional stresses, the cortex (that part of the brain responsible for thinking and reasoning) signals the limbic system (that part of the brain that governs raw emotions) that something is wrong. The limbic system recognizes a threat and produces the appropriate emotions of fear and

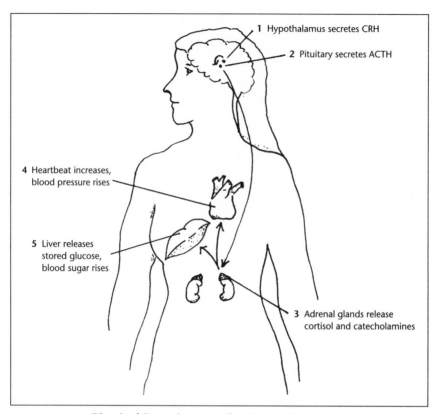

1 Hypothalamus secretes CRH

2 Pituitary secretes ACTH

4 Heartbeat increases, blood pressure rises

5 Liver releases stored glucose, blood sugar rises

3 Adrenal glands release cortisol and catecholamines

Physical Reactions to the Stress Response

anxiety. The hypothalamus, located in the center of the limbic system, sends chemical messages to the pituitary gland to speed metabolism. The pituitary gland signals the adrenal glands to release stress hormones, the catecholamines epinephrine (adrenaline) and norepinephrine (noradrenaline), and the physiologic effects of stress become manifest.

As stress hormones are released throughout the system, certain changes occur that enable a person to respond to a potentially dangerous situation. This is called the "fight-or-flight" response. After the sympathetic nervous system is aroused, the heart rate increases to supply extra blood to major muscle groups. The heart may pound and the chest may feel constricted as breathing control shifts from the diaphragm to the upper chest. Catecholamines as well as glucocorticoids (cortisol) are released from the adrenal glands. These release stored glucose from the liver, raising blood sugar levels and providing extra energy to muscles. The additional norepinephrine in the brain increases alertness and the ability to focus in order to make quick responses.

In addition to speeding up the endocrine system, the stress response slows all competing systems to maximize the amount of energy available for either fighting an enemy or fleeing. Because digestive processes utilize a lot of blood and energy, the appetite is suppressed, and digestion and salivation are slowed. During stressful events, a dry mouth and difficulty swallowing may be experienced, as well as "butterflies" in the stomach. Production of the reproductive hormones, estrogen and testosterone, is inhibited and metabolic processes involving cell repair and growth are halted since these too are expensive in terms of energy requirements. The net result of all these changes is that the body is now at its maximum readiness to face danger.

What happens when the danger does not require the numerous physiologic changes necessary for the fight-or-flight response? Say a person is driving a car during rush hour, or dealing with a grouchy boss every day, or coping with a difficult domestic situation. The final outcome could be a stress response that goes awry, or what Hans Selye termed the "stress syndrome," a set of physiologic responses that, if unchecked over time, create havoc. The prolonged arousal of the sympathetic nervous system can lead to high blood pressure, increased sensitivity to environmental changes, and various gastrointestinal disorders. Worse still, the continued release of stress hormones leads to depression of the immune system, paving the way for opportunistic infections and increasing susceptibility to a host of transmissible diseases. Whereas short bursts of stress hormones can be beneficial and, indeed, may be crucial in circumstances in which running from danger will guarantee survival, the long-term results can be disastrous. This is part of the problem patients with CFIDS encounter when their stress response triggers symptoms.

THE STRESS RESPONSE IN CFIDS

In CFIDS, there is ample demonstration that something is amiss in the processes through which the body normally handles stress. In early 1990, Dr. Peter Behan, a neurologist and professor at the Institute of Neurological Sciences in Glasgow, Scotland, observed that patients with CFIDS seemed to have abnormal endocrine responses. Although he found that many symptoms, and even test results, were similar to those of Addison's disease (a disorder in which low tolerance to heat, cold, and other stressors results from decreased production of adrenal hormones), the symptoms did not resolve with administration of adrenal hormones (steroids), as they do with patients with Addison's disease. Dr. Behan suggested that these abnormal adrenal responses indicate some subtle problem in brain regulation.

The interesting puzzle of adrenal function was considered again 2 years later when a research team headed by Dr. Mark Demitrack published the results of a study concerning the production and response to cortisol, adrenocorticotropic hormone (ACTH), and corticotropin-releasing hormone (CRH) in 30 CFIDS patients and 72 healthy volunteers (*Journal of Clinical Endocrinology and Metabolism,* 1991). It is the orchestrated release of each of these hormones that provides adequate responses to environmental stress.

Cortisol, a glucocorticoid steroid produced in the adrenal cortex, helps reduce inflammation, inhibits immune system activity, and serves a variety of systemic functions, including blood sugar regulation. The adrenal cortex is stimulated by the pituitary gland to release cortisol through pituitary ACTH. The hypothalamus, by releasing CRH, stimulates the pituitary gland to release ACTH. Primary adrenal insufficiency (such as Addison's disease) reflects a defect in the adrenal gland's ability to respond to ACTH, no matter how much ACTH is released. In secondary adrenal insufficiency, the problem lies not with the adrenal glands but with the glands that control it—the pituitary and hypothalamus. Dr. Demitrack and colleagues found that whereas the basal cortisol level was lower in CFIDS patients than in healthy controls, responses to low levels of ACTH were exaggerated. When higher levels of ACTH were administered, the adrenal glands *slowed* production rather than responding with a greater output of cortisol. In other words, the adrenal glands overreacted to a mild stimulus and underreacted to a greater stimulus. Because these findings are incompatible with primary adrenal insufficiency, Dr. Demitrack's team concluded that CFIDS patients demonstrate secondary adrenal insufficiency, probably originating in the hypothalamus.

These findings help explain why patients with CFIDS respond poorly to stress. If the adrenal glands overrespond to minor stresses, the cumulative effects of daily stress can be as difficult to endure physiologically as a major stressful event. On the other hand, the blunted responses to ACTH indicate that with major stress, the body is unable to adjust accordingly. Both the constant state of arousal provoked by an oversensitive stress response and the underactive state of adrenal competency produce symptoms. Therefore, the person with CFIDS may feel worse under stress, which makes reduction of stress such an integral part of the healing process.

COPING WITH STRESS

As stress accumulates, so does the damage. A person who must endure the constant stress of a demanding job or social life while ill with CFIDS may find it difficult to recover. This does not prevent people from "carrying on," or at least attempting to, even while quite ill. Letting go of obligations, responsibilities, and activities that have provided the framework for a productive life is a hard task, and one that many CFIDS patients, particularly those with mild cases, would rather not face. Those who are severely ill have no choice. In either case, some adjustments are necessary because CFIDS rarely accommodates the patient's former lifestyle.

Two important stress-reduction strategies involve *avoidance* and *minimization*. Very ill patients probably should concentrate on avoiding as much stress as possible; those who are moderately to mildly ill and who cannot escape stress because of continuing work or family obligations should concentrate on methods to minimize the effects of stress.

Avoidance of Stress

Avoidance strategies are appropriate for stress you can control, such as how much work you do and when. The goal is to avoid putting yourself in stressful situations in order to forestall a stress response. The longer you avoid the cascade of stress hormone effects, the more time your body has to rest and repair itself.

- *Just say no.* You can do it politely if you wish, but when people call you on the telephone to participate in surveys, organize block parties, contribute to clothing drives, donate to worthy causes, subscribe to newspapers, or anything that contributes to your overall stress load, you need to let them know that you are not available. If it is something important, tell them you will do it when you feel better. If it is a stranger calling, insist that your name be removed from the calling list. Although it may be difficult, it might also be wise to ask annoying or demanding acquaintances not to call at all.
- *Set limits.* Make sure close friends and family members know when not to disturb you (nap or rest times). They should also be informed as to what you can and cannot do. Sometimes it is hard for people who used to depend on you to realize that you have limits now. Life will be easier for you, and for them, if you let them know that you cannot lift or carry, go out dancing, or anything else you formerly did

but cannot do now. Be clear; set some rules. You can set these rules without causing too much friction by inviting people to help you with your recovery. For example, by not calling after 8:00 PM, not asking you to do strenuous work, and so on, your friends can help you get necessary rest.

- *You don't have to finish what you start.* This important piece of advice was given to a person with CFIDS by a therapist who worked with cancer patients. No doubt you were involved in a number of projects when you became ill. Let them go. Tell yourself that the world will just have to wait for you (it will, believe it or not). You can decide whether these projects merit finishing when you have recovered. Meanwhile, have somebody pack up your work and store it away.

- *Ask for help.* For self-reliant individuals, asking for help feels like an admission of weakness. However, this is no time for false bravado. Ask your friends and family to help you. Pass on as many chores to them as you can. Friends can make appointments for you and then drive you there, pay your bills (you just need to sign the checks), clean your house, make your bed, take care of your children, cook, fend off salesmen, and perform numerous little daily chores that are a constant source of aggravation to you. If friends are not available, many churches have volunteers whose mission is to help shut-ins.

- *Buy an answering machine.* Answering machines were invented to record messages when you are out. For people with CFIDS, they are most useful for recording messages when you are in. They are a wonderful aid for people who need a break from the demands of conversation during "down time" or who need to go to bed early or sleep late but do not want to miss an important call. To screen calls, investigate the Caller ID option now offered by telephone companies. Caller ID displays the name and number of the person who is calling. The service costs about $6 a month. Many companies offer a free display box; if they do not, the display box costs about $30.

- *Be selective about television programs.* Television can be either a detriment to your health or a lifesaver, depending on how you use it. Sensationalist news programs, specials on serial killers, tense thrillers, frenetic commercials, and the general rapid pace and constant screen changes may produce anxiety and tension in anyone who is ill. In general, it may be of greater benefit to watch light comedies, mysteries, nature programs, old movies, and programs designed to relax or inform rather than arouse.

Minimizing the Effects of Stress

Many stressful situations cannot be avoided, such as the death of a family member, loss of a job or spouse, and accidents. But even comparatively minor stresses such as an unavoidable family visit or a medical appointment are guaranteed to produce symptoms in patients with CFIDS. If avoiding the situation is simply not possible, learn how to deal with the cascade effects that a stress reaction produces, and how to stabilize your system as soon as possible.

- *Practice stress reduction exercises.* Stress reduction exercises are invaluable to reduce the amount of stress you feel, calm adrenal responses, gain perspective, and give yourself a break from pressures and demands. Meditation, hypnosis, biofeedback, deep breathing, relaxation tapes, and yoga are all excellent methods for reducing stress. Remember, the mind-body connection goes two ways. When the body begins to churn out anxiety-producing hormones, the mind can limit the extent of its arousal. Many patients with CFIDS have observed that even during severe illness and relapses, stress reduction techniques are invaluable for maintaining a sense of calm.
- *Take a break.* The first thing to remember when confronting any stressful situation is that the natural tendency is to overdo. Try not to give in entirely to the impulse and plan rest time. Lie down whenever you have a chance, and try to take your mind off situations that can easily become all-encompassing. Reducing stimulation also helps: turn off the television or radio, tell your children to play outside, turn off the lights, and turn on the answering machine.
- *Develop a routine.* CFIDS produces internal chaos; therefore, anything you can do to promote external order will be helpful. Following a routine can provide a sense of security and stability that can make stressful situations easier to handle. The routine can be simple. For people who are quite ill, a daily routine can consist of getting up, getting dressed, washing, eating breakfast, and lying down again. It is not particularly important when or how you perform your routine. The idea is to develop a regular and predictable routine that helps structure your day.
- *Find distractions.* Mental distraction is important and should be pursued when outside demands become overwhelming. Mystery or romance novels, soap operas, knitting, watching fish swim in a tank . . . in short, anything that takes your mind off your problems and

puts the focus on something that requires no effort (and generates no anxiety) helps maintain tranquility.

- *Search for humor.* Norman Cousins, in his best-selling account of his own healing experience, *Anatomy of an Illness,* recommended humor as the best possible distraction. Cousins maintains that watching funny movies (and taking large doses of intravenous vitamin C) turned the course of ankylosing spondylitis (a disease in which the connective tissue of the spine disintegrates). Cousins asked himself, "If negative emotions produce negative chemical changes in the body, wouldn't the positive emotions produce positive chemical changes?" He observed that putting positive emotions to work was not as simple as "turning on a garden hose. But even a reasonable degree of control over [the] emotions might have a salutary physiologic effect."

- *Express yourself.* When humor is not possible or appropriate, another good way to deal with stressful situations is to share your thoughts and feelings with someone who understands. A sympathetic ear can help alleviate many of the helpless, trapped feelings that CFIDS patients have when cornered by a stressful event and can eliminate some of the endless mental rehashing that accompanies decision-making under stress. If another person is not available, writing letters, keeping a journal, and drawing can be good forms of self-expression. Support groups, therapists experienced with CFIDS, and services such as the Center for Attitudinal Healing (check your phone directory for a local chapter) can also provide a healthy outlet for stress-related emotions. The best strategy is to find someone with CFIDS who has shared your experience. If you are housebound and no one is close by, a computer can provide access to the world. Many people find support through the Internet (CFIDS Bulletin Boards can be lifesavers).

- *Herbs and supplements.* A number of herbs can help mitigate the effects of stress hormones. Valerian root, a plant that produces a mild sedative effect, is perhaps the best known. Some people find it produces digestive tract distress, however. Skullcap is also calming and works well for the jitters and anxiety. Chamomile, hops, and passion flower are other calming herbs. Some of the essential oils, especially jasmine, clary sage, and lavender, can ease a stress reaction. Many people also find calcium, magnesium, and B vitamins soothing, but these are not generally useful in emergencies.

- *Pharmaceuticals.* Stress responses so severe that a person is unable to sleep or eat may require pharmaceutical intervention. A small dose of a benzodiazepine (Valium, Xanax) may be helpful to reestablish equilibrium. The excess adrenaline produced by stress is not cleared from the body for about 3 days so small doses over several days may be required.

A FINAL WORD ON COPING WITH STRESS

The most intense source of stress for patients with CFIDS is being ill. Lying in bed for several years, in pain, with little hope for a cure from the medical establishment, while you watch livelihood, friends, family, career, and dreams slipping away is devastating. There is no "best" way to cope with a long-term illness such as CFIDS. If the above suggestions make life easier for you, this chapter will have accomplished its purpose. However, whether they accomplish their purpose or not, perhaps the most effective stress remedy, designed just for people with CFIDS, is to seek support from others with CFIDS.

There is simply no substitute for the experience of others. For people newly ill, advice from others is essential, not just in terms of which medications to try, who to see, and what tests to undergo, but how to cope. Knowing that other people have had your symptoms and have survived them, and discussing how they have learned to live with them (if not recover from them) is a source of immeasurable comfort to people with CFIDS. Even if you are so ill that you cannot get out of bed, seek out others. Jeanette, a severely ill 65-year old woman (see Chapter 1), expressed how valuable this type of support can be when she described her friend:

> She has been such a help to me. I cannot tell you how wonderful she's been. She is very encouraging. I try to be upbeat. But once in a while I have just had it. I call her up on the phone and I scream, "No more! I will not be sick anymore! I can't take it!" She brings me out of it; she understands. She says she used to be that way also, and reassures me that I will feel better . . . maybe next year. I always come out of our phone conversations feeling much, much better.

If you have not written to the national CFIDS Association for a list of support groups in your area, do so. Someone out there in the CFIDS community will be willing to hold your hand through the worst and encourage you to "hang in there," as she or he already has.

FURTHER READING

Chrousos, George P, and Gold, Philip W. The Concepts of Stress and Stress System Disorders. Journal of the American Medical Association 267:1244-1252, 1992 (somewhat technical but thorough review of the physiologic and behavioral responses to stress).

Cousins, Norman. Anatomy of an Illness. New York: Bantam Books, 1981.

Friedberg, Fred. Coping With Chronic Fatigue Syndrome: Nine Things You Can Do. Oakland, Calif.: New Harbinger Publications, 1995 (discusses the effects of stress and offers relaxation exercises tailored to CFIDS).

Sapolsky, Robert. Why Zebras Don't Get Ulcers: A Guide to Stress, Stress-Related Diseases, and Coping. New York: W.H. Freeman and Co., 1994 (provides a good overview of how stress works).

SEE

- Chapter 4: Benzodiazepines.
- Chapter 5: Herbs, Minerals, Vitamins.
- Chapter 6: Acupuncture, Aroma Therapy, Biofeedback, Hypnosis, Meditation.

8

Cleaning Up: Eliminating Toxins in the Home

Sensitivity to chemicals is common in patients with CFIDS. In a 5-year study of 690 patients conducted by Dr. Dedra Buchwald, more than 50% of those with CFIDS reported having chemical sensitivities. Some clinicians claim that a majority of CFIDS patients develop sensitivities to the chemicals encountered in daily life, petrochemicals in particular. Car exhaust, diesel fumes, glues, dyes, inks, and perfumes are among those most commonly mentioned as producing headaches, dizziness, faintness, nausea, and malaise. Detergents, solvents, aerosol propellents, wood preservatives, and paints all contain petroleum derivatives, which, while generally regarded as safe unless used in large amounts, can provoke severe reactions in those with multiple chemical sensitivities, even in minute quantities.

Even those who do not experience the severe reactions typical of multiple chemical sensitivity should be careful to avoid exposure to synthetic chemicals. The metabolic disturbances that have been described by CFIDS researchers not only produce cellular fatigue but also affect the body's ability to remove toxins. Alpha ketoglutarate and glutathione, two of the most powerful components of the body's detoxification system (see Chapter 5), are frequently found to be deficient in CFIDS. To complicate the picture, many patients with CFIDS have suboptimal liver function (the liver is the body's main detoxification organ). Through these reductions in the effectiveness in the body's detoxification system, CFIDS can compromise the body's natural capacity to break down and eliminate toxins.

By far, the most important coping strategy for chemical sensitivities is avoidance. In a survey of multiple chemical sensitivity (MCS) treatments conducted by a DePaul University research team, all but one of the 304 respondents reported that "adopting a practice of avoiding exposures to chemicals which could cause MCS reactions" was helpful. The majority of the respondents reported that avoidance was of "enormous help" (*CFIDS Chronicle*, Winter 1996). Direct exposure to toxins can be significantly reduced by eliminating chemical offenders in the home, the environment that poses the most risk to individuals who are partially or completely housebound.

The following discussions on cleaners, pesticides, and personal care products provide safe alternatives to the numerous harmful ingredients found in many commercial products.

CLEANERS

Some of the most toxic chemicals we are routinely exposed to are found in the kitchen and bathroom. Many of us are unaware that household cleaners may contain substances that are carcinogenic (cause cancer), mutagenic (cause gene mutations), or teratogenic (cause birth defects). In addition, a number of the chemicals added to general cleaners, spot removers, metal polishes, and other such products are listed by the Environmental Protection Agency (EPA) as "Priority" toxics. In other words, they are powerful poisons. You may be unaware of the hazards associated with these products because manufacturers are not legally required to state their ingredients.

Fortunately, most cleaners commonly found in American homes have safe, easy-to-use substitutes.

CHEMICALS COMMONLY FOUND IN HOUSEHOLD CLEANING PRODUCTS

The following chemicals commonly found in household cleaning products should be rigorously avoided:

- *Ammonia.* Ammonia is an eye and respiratory tract irritant that can cause conjunctivitis, laryngitis, and burns. Because ammonia is toxic to the brain, breathing ammonia fumes is dangerous. The combination of ammonia with chlorine produces a deadly gas. CFIDS patients need to be particularly careful to avoid ammonia because the anaerobic cell metabolism characteristic of CFIDS produces ammonia as a by-product. Products that contain ammonia include window cleaners, all-purpose cleaners, tub and tile cleaners, furniture and floor polish, and laundry detergents.

CHEMICALS COMMONLY FOUND IN HOUSEHOLD
CLEANING PRODUCTS—cont'd

- *Benzene.* Benzene (carcinogen) attacks the central nervous system (CNS), blood, bone marrow, eyes, and respiratory tract. Benzene is found in spot removers and dishwashing detergents.
- *Chlorine.* Chlorine (potential carcinogen) causes erosion of mucous membranes, skin eruptions, severe respiratory tract irritation, and vomiting. Those with cystitis should be especially cautious to avoid chlorine because it can irritate the bladder. Chlorine is found in bleach, tub and tile cleaners, and spot removers.
- *Cresol.* Cresol (corrosive) affects the CNS, liver, kidneys, lungs, pancreas, spleen, and can be absorbed through skin and lungs. Disinfectants, air fresheners, and deodorizers can contain cresol.
- *Detergents.* Detergents can cause dermatitis, asthmatic episodes, flu-like symptoms, and severe eye damage. Tub and tile cleaners, bleach, dishwashing detergents, furniture and floor polish, oven cleaners, and rug and carpet cleaners contain detergents.
- *Ethanol.* Ethanol can cause CNS depression, nausea, and vomiting. Air fresheners, tub and tile cleaners, dishwashing detergents, glass and window cleaners, laundry detergents, metal polishers, and rug and carpet cleaners contain ethanol.
- *Formaldehyde.* Formaldehyde (mutagen and likely carcinogen) can cause respiratory problems, headaches, rashes, tiredness, and insomnia. Formaldehyde is found in air fresheners, disinfectants, mold and mildew cleaners, and water-resistant paper (such as paper towels, napkins, and toilet tissue).
- *Methylene chloride.* Methylene chloride (carcinogen) has been known to cause cardiac arrest. Shoe polish and paint strippers contain methylene chloride.
- *Naphthalene.* Naphthalene (carcinogen) can cause skin irritation, headache, and confusion. It attacks the kidneys, liver, red blood cells, and CNS. Air fresheners and deodorizers, glass and window cleaners, laundry detergents, rug and carpet cleaners, and spot removers contain naphthalene.
- *Petroleum distillates.* Petroleum distillates (carcinogens and poisons) can be found in drain cleaners, furniture and floor polish, glass and window cleaners, and metal polishes.
- *Phenols.* Phenols (carcinogens) cause skin eruptions, burning, numbness, gangrene, vomiting, and convulsions. Air fresheners and deodorizers, disinfectants, laundry detergents, and mold and mildew cleaners can contain phenols.
- *Toluene.* Toluene (carcinogen) causes nervous system changes, irritability, depression, and damage to the liver and kidneys. Toluene is found in spot removers.
- *Xylene.* Xylene (hazardous waste) causes nausea, cough, tinnitus, headache, mental confusion, and eye damage. Xylene can be found in air fresheners, spray paint, and shoe polish.

Safe Cleaners for Specific Circumstances

The five nontoxic items needed to keep your home and belongings clean are salt, baking soda, soap, white vinegar, and borax. These can be found in most grocery stores and supermarkets and are surprisingly effective, safe, and easy to use.

AIR FRESHENERS
Note: Commercial air fresheners do not "freshen," but merely mask odors.
- *Carpet odors* — Sprinkle baking soda liberally (several pounds per room), and vacuum.
- *Toilet bowls* — Clean with borax to eliminate odors as well as disinfect.
- *Garbage pails* — Sprinkle the bottom with baking soda. Rinse with borax and water to disinfect.

DISHWASHING SOAP. Use liquid soap to wash, and vinegar to cut grease. For machines, buy biodegradable dishwasher soap.

DISINFECTANTS. Borax in water is a great disinfectant. In fact, hospitals that use it have discovered that borax disinfects as well as any commercial antiseptic product. A machine-washable chemical-free cloth is available that kills bacteria on contact (Real Goods; 800-762-7325).

DRAIN CLEANERS. Pour a mixture of 1/2 cup salt and 1/2 cup baking soda, followed by a quart of boiling water, in blocked drains. If that doesn't work, call a plumber.

LAUNDRY DETERGENTS. Presoak laundry with soap and borax for 1 hour before washing. For the ultrasensitive, Laundry Disks, a Japanese product that eliminates the need for soap or detergents, is available through mail-order catalogs.

METAL POLISHERS
- *Aluminum* — Soak in lemon juice or vinegar and boiling water.
- *Copper and brass* — Rub with a mixture of salt and vinegar (or lemon juice).
- *Chrome* — Rub with lemon peel, rinse, and polish with a soft cloth.
- *Gold* — Wash in warm, soapy water, dry, and polish with a clean cloth.

- *Silver* — Soak in salted water in an aluminum pot (a nonaluminum pot with aluminum foil can be substituted). Or boil for 3 minutes in 1 quart of water with 1 tablespoon each of salt and baking soda.

OVEN CLEANER. Dissolve 2 tablespoons of liquid soap (not detergent) and 2 teaspoons of borax in enough warm water to fill a spray bottle. Spray the sides of the oven and leave for 20 minutes. Scrub with baking soda. Pumice can be used for hard, baked-on spills.

RUG CLEANERS. Mix two parts cornmeal and one part borax. Sprinkle liberally over carpet and let stand for 1 hour. Vacuum.

SCOURING POWDER. Baking soda is a mild abrasive and can be used for any cleaning job that requires scouring.

SHOE POLISH. Clean shoes with a damp cloth. Apply walnut oil and buff with a chamois cloth.

SPOT REMOVER
- *Blood* — Soak cotton items in cold water. Blot spots on wool with hydrogen peroxide.
- *Coffee* — Mix egg yoke with water and rub on stain.
- *Chewing gum* — Rub with ice.
- *Fruit and wine* — Pour salt or hot water on the stain; soak in milk.
- *Grease* — Pour boiling water over stain and sprinkle baking soda on it.
- *Ink* — Soak in milk.
- *Mildew* — Pour soap and salt on spots and place in sunlight. Repeat if necessary.
- *Rust* — Saturate with lemon juice, rub with salt, then place in direct sunlight until dry.

TILE CLEANERS. Use baking soda on a sponge as an abrasive. Use borax and water to disinfect. For mold, sponge on a mixture of vinegar and borax.

WINDOW CLEANER. Make a mixture of vinegar or cornstarch (about 1 tablespoon of either) and 1 quart of water and spray or wipe on windows with a clean sponge. Dry with newspaper or a clean lint-free cloth.

WOOD POLISH. For wood furniture or floors, make a mixture of three parts olive oil and one part lemon juice or vinegar and apply with a soft cloth.

• • •

If you are unable to make your own mixtures, it may be more convenient to purchase nontoxic cleaners. Many brands are available from mail-order suppliers (see Appendix D).

PESTICIDES

Pesticides such as Raid and other vermin destroyers are often found in supermarkets in the same aisles as cleaning supplies. Their proximity to sponges and dishwashing liquid may lead the shopper to think they are no more toxic than soap. Yet household pesticides, because of the frequency with which they are used, combined with the fact that they are used indoors, where their fumes will be inhaled, are more a risk than the 1.67 billion pounds of chemicals U.S. farmers use on crops every year.

Exposure to household pesticides is not only dangerous, it is widespread. According to figures compiled by the Pesticide Action Network, some 69 million American households used pesticides in 1995. That means that nearly every man, woman, and child in this country has been exposed to pesticides in their homes.

What is so dangerous about pesticides? Most pesticides work by directly interfering with the insect nervous system. They either prevent a key neurotransmitter from being broken down, producing a state of terminal excitement in the nervous system synapses, or they prevent the neurotransmitter from operating by binding to its receptor sites so that the nervous system ceases to function. In the first instance, the insect dies of convulsions. In the second, the insect dies of paralysis. In both cases the principal mode of action is the disruption of the neurotransmitter acetylcholine.

Acetylcholine is also one of the most important neurotransmitters found in humans. One of its major functions is to connect muscles to nerves, allowing nervous system control of movement. Acetylcholine also affects memory. (Patients with Alzheimer's disease demonstrate a deficit of this important neurotransmitter.) Human exposure to neurotoxins that disrupt acetylcholine function (such as the nerve gas poisoning in Gulf War veterans) produces myriad harmful effects, including loss of appetite, urinary frequency, sweating, excess salivation, diarrhea, jitteriness, emotional instability, combativeness, headache, and mental confusion.

Patients with CFIDS should make a concerted effort to avoid pesticides. CFIDS produces disruption of normal nervous system activity, which itself can affect the cholinergic (acetylcholine) pathways in the brain. At least one researcher, Dr. E. Snorrason of University Hospital in Reykjavik, Iceland, believes that upsets in the cholinergic system play a primary role in the development of CFIDS symptoms. Further upsets in brain function, through exposure to neurotoxins in pesticides and other chemicals, only worsen the condition.

Safe Pesticides for Specific Insects

ANTS. Pour a thin line of talcum powder at the point of entry. Wipe the surrounding area with a wet sponge to erase the ant trail.

BEETLES. Place a bay leaf in flour containers. Keep food containers tightly closed.

COCKROACHES. Mix sugar and boric acid and sprinkle on a piece of cardboard around garbage cans or wherever roaches gather. Boric acid causes gases to build up in the roaches' bodies so that they explode.

FLIES. Hang sticky paper made with honey on cardboard. Pierce and hang orange peels (flies do not like citric acid).

HEAD LICE. Coconut oil contains dodecyl alcohol, which is lethal to lice. Wash hair with a bar soap or shampoo that contains coconut oil or coconut oil derivatives (cocamide, sodium lauryl sulfate). Leave shampoo in hair for 30 minutes. Rinse with a half-and-half mixture of white vinegar and water to loosen egg cases. Comb hair thoroughly, one section at a time, with a metal lice comb to remove nits (allow 2 hours for this process). Repeat in 10 days.

MOTHS. Hang sachets of rosemary and other strong-smelling herbs in closets or place cedar chips in drawers. The aromatic oils in cedar kill moth larvae. Avoid cedar if you have allergies.

TERMITES. Remove rotting wood from around property. Kill termites with a heat lamp at 140° F.

TICKS AND FLEAS. Wash and dry animal. Spray with rosemary tea to deter insects. Garlic and brewer's yeast added to pet food also help repel fleas.

GENERAL INSECT REPELLENT. Pennyroyal tea sprayed on skin and clothes will deter most biting and stinging insects.

GARDEN AND PLANT PESTS. Numerous techniques can safely eliminate garden pests, including hosing down plants to prevent spider mites, planting chives around plants to discourage aphids, and purchasing beneficial predators such as ladybugs. Hot-pepper or soap spray will discourage most insects. For specific problems, consult an organic gardening manual (available in most libraries).

PERSONAL CARE PRODUCTS

According to the Food and Drug Administration (FDA), a cosmetic includes anything that can be "rubbed, poured, sprinkled or sprayed on . . . the human body . . . for cleansing, beautifying, promoting attractiveness, or altering the body's appearance without affecting the body's structure or functions." Any cosmetic packaged after 1977 must include a list of ingredients on the label. However, there are some exceptions, notably deodorant soaps, hair dyes, fluoridated toothpastes, antiperspirants, sunscreens, and antidandruff shampoos. In addition, a number of products contain ingredients that do not have to be specifically detailed (such as the 4000 ingredients that make up "fragrances"). Anyone with chemical sensitivities should be aware that the petrochemical components of cosmetics and personal health and hygiene products can provoke severe reactions because they are absorbed directly through the skin.

Some of the more noxious ingredients of cosmetic and health products include aerosol propellants (propane, methylene chloride), BHA/BHT (butylated hydroxyanisole/butylated hydroxytoluene), BNPD (reacts with amines on the skin to form carcinogenic nitrosamines), ammonia, coal tar colors, cresol, detergents, ethanol, formaldehyde, hexane, lead, mineral oil (blocks vitamin absorption), paraffin, phenol, plastics, quaternium 15 (releases formaldehyde), toluene, and xylene. Products that contain any of these, are scented, are applied by means of aerosols, or are artificially colored should be avoided by CFIDS patients.

Safe Personal Care Products

Many alternatives to commercial personal care products can be purchased from health food and vitamin stores, specialty shops, mail-order suppliers, and buyers' clubs. Following are suggestions for some commonly used personal care products.

DEODORANTS. Commercial deodorants can contain triclosan, a liver toxin. Numerous nontoxic alternatives (such as crystals and plant-based products such as Weleda and Desert Essence) are available from health food stores. The very sensitive can apply baking soda to absorb odors and moisture after bathing.

HAIR DYES. Commercial hair dyes are completely exempt from regulation and, as a result, contain numerous toxins. If you color your hair, use henna for red or walnut hull infusion for brown (available in health food stores).

LOTIONS AND HAND CREAMS. Commercial lotions may contain ethanol, phenol, and mineral oil (which is more toxic when absorbed through the skin than when inhaled). Pure vegetable oils (olive, sesame, canola) or vegetable oil–based products such as those made by Nature's Gate can be substituted.

MOUTHWASH. After brushing and flossing teeth, rinse mouth with baking soda and water to eliminate odor and reduce plaque. For those with gingivitis, an occasional rinse with hydrogen peroxide solution (10% peroxide, 90% water) will disinfect the mouth. Be careful not to overdo, because peroxide also destroys beneficial mouth flora.

SHAMPOO. Many shampoos are relatively free of unnecessary additives (Dr. Bronner's, Raintree, and Kiss My Face, for example, all make gentle, fragrance-free shampoos). Or, a shampoo can be made by blending one part olive oil with four parts liquid castile soap and then adding two parts distilled water. Use this mixture like concentrated shampoo. To treat dandruff, use pure baking soda. (Dandruff shampoos contain selenium sulfide, a liver toxin.)

SHAVING CREAM. Use petrochemical-free soap or shaving cream such as Tom's or The Body Shop.

SOAP. Numerous soaps are made from vegetable oils, including Kiss My Face, The Body Shop, Conti Castile, Pears Transparent Soap, and The Soap Opera. Use scentless varieties.

TOOTHPASTE. You can make toothpaste with salt, baking soda, and a drop of mint essential oil. Tom's, Desert Essence, or other pure toothpaste brands can also be purchased. Most commercial toothpastes contain saccharin, ethanol, mineral oil, or formaldehyde.

OTHER HOUSEHOLD TOXINS

Air Quality

According to the Environmental Protection Agency (EPA), some 50% of all illnesses can be caused or aggravated by polluted indoor air. Viruses, mold, pollen, bacteria, dust mites, and other contaminants can build up in air conditioning and duct systems, creating health problems in otherwise healthy individuals. For CFIDS patients air quality is of particular concern, especially for those with allergies. Recirculating dust and pollens can exacerbate allergic reactions, which in turn may lead to relapses. Even if you do not have allergies, it is important to make sure that the air you breathe is pure and free from common household contaminants such as carbon monoxide, dust, mold, and other irritants. Following are some steps to take to make sure your indoor air is pure.

- Have gas appliances and gas lines checked for leaks. In most cases your gas company will perform this service free of charge. Make sure gas appliances are properly vented. If you have the choice, opt for electrical appliances. They burn cleaner than gas and leave less residue in the air.
- If you suspect your duct system harbors molds, have it cleaned out. Many heating and air conditioning companies will clean and purify ducts, grills, blowers, and humidifiers for a fee.
- If you have allergies, purchase a high-efficiency particle air (HEPA) filter.
- An ultraviolet light, which kills bacteria and viruses, can be installed in the cold air return. These can be purchased at some health food stores. Be sure to install the light where it cannot be seen because ultraviolet light damages the eyes.

The numerous neurotoxins, fumes, corrosives, carcinogens, and systemic irritants we are constantly exposed to are not good for *anyone*. People with illnesses, and in particular those with chemical sensitivities, should make every effort to avoid these ubiquitous poisons to diminish their harmful effects.

Water Quality

The quality of the water we drink has a profound effect on our well-being because water is needed for every metabolic process in the body. Our drinking water, however, much like the air we breathe, contains numerous contaminants that can have adverse effects on health. The EPA has identified more than 700 pollutants in drinking water, ranging from heavy metals that leech from old plumbing to chemical runoff from industry and agriculture. Many CFIDS patients find that with the advent of the illness they become more sensitive to the pollutants and additives commonly found in drinking water, particularly to chlorine, which is added as a disinfectant to most municipal drinking water supplies. Fortunately, a number of affordable water purification systems are available to help alleviate this problem (see Appendix D).

ACTIVATED-CARBON FILTERS. These filters remove asbestos, bacteria, viruses, chlorine, heavy metals, and most organic compounds. The filter needs to be changed at least every 6 months to be effective. Many countertop and under-the-sink models are available, as well as screw-on filters for shower heads. Manufacturers generally recommend using cold water from municipal sources for drinking water models. Granulated carbon is preferable to powdered carbon.

REVERSE-OSMOSIS FILTERS. Reverse osmosis purifies water by passing it through a fine membrane to remove asbestos, some bacteria and viruses, fluoride, heavy metals, minerals, nitrites, salts, and some organic compounds. Chlorine, however, is not removed. Reverse-osmosis filters are best used in conjunction with carbon filters. Filters should be changed every 2 years or as suggested by the manufacturer.

WATER DISTILLATION. Water is boiled and the steam is condensed to produce water free of most contaminants. Boiling effectively kills bacteria and viruses, and the evaporation process removes heavy metals and trace minerals that are too heavy to rise with the vapor. This method does not remove chlorine.

• • •

The best type of filter to use depends in part on the quality of the water. Before choosing a water purification system, it is wise to obtain a water analysis, which will indicate the hardness of the water, total dissolved solids, and pH level. If you cannot purchase a water filter, you can buy bottled water. The drawback to bottled water is that unless the company will provide a water analysis, you cannot be sure that the water is pure. In addition, a number of people cannot tolerate water bottled in plastic containers. Glass containers, while more difficult to find, do not leech by-products into the water. The following are some home methods to reduce contaminants in tap water.

- Boil water for 10 minutes to kill bacteria and viruses and to remove most chlorine, chlorine by-products, and pesticides.
- Add a little vinegar, lemon juice, or vitamin C. The acid in a small amount of vitamin C or white vinegar neutralizes the effects of chlorine.

ORGANIZATIONS

American Academy of Environmental Medicine
PO Box 16106
Denver, CO
303-622-9755 (telephone)

Chemical Injury Information Network
PO Box 301
White Sulphur Springs, MD 59645-0301
406-547-2255 (telephone)

Environmental Health Association
1800 S. Robertson Blvd.
Suite 380
Los Angeles, CA 90035
301-837-2048 (telephone)

Environmental Health Network
PO Box 1155
Larkspur, CA 94977
415-541-5075 (telephone)

Human Ecology Action League
PO Box 49126
Atlanta, GA 30359
404-248-1898 (telephone)

Multiple Chemical Sensitivities Referral and Resources
2326 Pickwick Road
Baltimore, MD 21207
410-448-3319 (telephone)

National Center for Environmental Health Strategies
1100 Rural Avenue
Voorhees, NJ 08043
609-429-5358 (telephone)

National Foundation of Chemical Hypersensitivities and Allergies
PO Box 222
Ophelia, VA 22530
804-453-7538 (telephone)   *or*   517-697-3989 (telephone)

WEBSITES

Colorado Health Net: Multiple Chemical Sensitivities
http://bcn.boulder.co.us/health/chn/site/idx—mcs.html
http:// rohan.sdsu.edu/staff/hamilto/mcs

FURTHER READING

Dadd, Debra Lynn. Nontoxic and Natural. Los Angeles: Jeremy P. Tarcher, 1984 (an easy-to-use reference and guide to safe alternatives for 1200 of the most commonly used household products; also includes a mail-order source list for nontoxic products).

Dadd, Debra Lynn. The Nontoxic Home. Los Angeles: Jeremy P. Tarcher, 1986 (offers an in-depth look at sources of toxins in the home and offers a broader range of solutions).

Wittenburg, Janice Strubbe. The Rebellious Body: Reclaim Your Life From Environmental Illness or Chronic Fatigue Syndrome. New York: Insight Books, 1997 (a valuable reference guide providing medical explanations, diet recommendations, coping tips, and information on supplements).

SEE

- Chapter 3: Allergies (chemical sensitivities) for further discussion of the role of chemical sensitivities in CFIDS and for treatment suggestions.
- Appendix D for a list of mail-order suppliers of nontoxic products.

9

Food and Diet

Diet is one of the most obvious places to begin making the necessary accommodations to the demands of a chronic illness. However, it is not always the easiest. For many people with CFIDS, choosing a diet poses numerous difficulties. About one third of the CFIDS population have recurring or chronic gastrointestinal symptoms caused by food sensitivities such as heartburn, gas, nausea, diarrhea, constipation, and cramps. Others may have concurrent problems such as interstitial cystitis or migraine headaches that require certain dietary constraints. The remaining group, although perhaps free from gastrointestinal symptoms, food sensitivities, or concurrent conditions, still have the demands of a chronic illness to attend to. Although free from the necessity of maintaining strict dietary restrictions, they need to maintain a diet as wholesome as possible, if only to address the complicated problem of how best to help an ailing body heal.

The disruptions in cell metabolism, immune function, and endocrine system brought on by CFIDS can lead to numerous nutritional deficiencies, including decreased concentrations of zinc, potassium, carnitine, and B and C vitamins. These deficiencies, in and of themselves, can decrease the degree to which the body can absorb and make use of nutrients. Problems caused by disruptions in cell metabolism, malabsorption, and food sensitivities make it all the more important for CFIDS patients to maintain an appropriate diet; that is, following a diet that will maximize the nutrients available to a healing body while minimizing any harmful effects that specific foods or food additives may produce.

DEVISING A CFIDS DIET

"What should I eat?" is a question asked by most CFIDS patients, and, although the question makes a great deal of practical sense, it is not easily answered. Diet is an important consideration for anyone who is ill; in the case of CFIDS, however, what constitutes an appropriate diet? Should we follow a special regimen (macrobiotic, vegetarian, wheat grass, raw, ash-free, fat-free, carbohydrate-free, yeast-free) or can we just throw caution to the wind and eat what we please since we feel so bad anyway?

These questions have no simple answers. CFIDS patients react to foods with the same frustrating inconsistency as they do to medications. Whereas one person can maintain a vegetarian diet, another needs to eat meat at every meal. (Such was the case of one ardent vegetarian who found that after contracting CFIDS she could not get through a day without eating several portions of red meat.) Some feel better after cutting back on carbohydrates and eliminating fruit. Because each person's digestive system reflects one's own unique case of CFIDS (complicated by allergies, food sensitivities, bladder sensitivities, blood sugar problems), there can be no single "best diet."

CFIDS patients need to watch their diet, but not necessarily severely restrict their food choices. Many people with CFIDS have experienced setbacks, including severe weight loss, increased fatigue, and pain, from adopting highly restrictive diets, especially diets that eliminate many of the important food groups.

As not everyone needs the same foods, finding an appropriate diet may at first create some frustration or discouragement. Finding a good diet, however, even in the most difficult circumstances, is not impossible. Most people proceed by trial and error, noting which foods make them feel better or worse. The following are some simple guidelines that may be helpful in devising your particular CFIDS diet.

- *Listen to your body.* This is, perhaps, the most important rule for people with CFIDS. If a particular food item makes you feel worse, don't eat it, even if it is supposed to be "good" for you. Even "good" foods, such as salad, broccoli, nuts, fruit, and spinach can be irritating if you cannot digest them. Your body will, in most cases, give you clear signs when it can't. Nausea, insomnia, headaches, anxiety, gas, diarrhea, and constipation are some of the side effects produced by the digestive system when it manufactures ammonia, indole, and greenhouse gases from food instead of usable vitamins, minerals, and proteins.

- *Eat sensibly.* Patients with CFIDS need to consume a healthy, balanced supply of nutrients to provide the basic raw materials required to make them well. For those whose diet is not already restricted by food sensitivities, maintaining a broad, varied diet will provide the best basis for improvement.
- *Eat simply.* Try not to mix a lot of different ingredients. This will help with digestion and make it easier to identify food reactions. Use plain vegetables, starches, and proteins.
- *Eat wholesome foods.* If possible, eat whole-grain foods for complex carbohydrates, vegetables for vitamins and minerals, and low-fat meat products for proteins. Avoid all processed foods, which contain artificial additives (even when advertised as "natural"). Be sure to check labels. Buy organic foods, whenever possible, to eliminate the extra burden of pesticides, hormones, and antibiotics abundant in most commercial produce and meats.

Foods to Avoid

Some foods should be avoided because in most patients they will exacerbate symptoms. The following are the five foods most commonly implicated by CFIDS clinicians and patients.

1. STIMULANTS (coffee, tea, caffeinated sodas, cola, some herb teas, including ginseng, lomatium, mate, and ma huang). When energy levels are low, it is tempting to resort to "pick-me-ups" such as coffee, cola, or strong tea to boost energy. For most people, stimulants provide a temporary boost, enabling them to get through a hard day or a crisis. However, because stimulants cause the adrenal glands to work harder, taking them will eventually result in a "crash." Often the long-term result of a short-term energy boost is simply not worth it. Caffeine also worsens ongoing insomnia, leading to even greater exhaustion. Some nutritional supplements that provide good substitutes for stimulants are malic acid (with ATP), alpha ketoglutarate, CoQ10, vitamin B_{12}, royal jelly, blue-green algae, DHEA, and NADH (see Chapter 3: Fatigue for further suggestions).

2. ALCOHOL (wine, beer, hard liquor). Alcohol intolerance is one of the most common CFIDS symptoms. Most people with CFIDS find out rather early in the illness that even a small glass of beer or wine makes them quite ill. The reasons for alcohol intolerance are twofold: (1) alcohol acts on the central nervous system, which in CFIDS patients can be hyperreactive; and (2) alcohol is toxic to the liver. Because many CFIDS patients have suboptimal liver function, ingestion of alcohol should be avoided. Those who are especially sensitive should also avoid herbal tinctures and alcohol-based mouthwashes.

3. SWEETENERS (sugar, corn syrup, sucrose, glucose, dextrose, brown sugar, fructose, aspartame, saccharin). Many people with CFIDS crave sweets, especially when blood sugar levels fall in the late afternoon and before the onset of menstruation. Most researchers agree that this is due to faulty carbohydrate metabolism and subsequent low levels of ATP and blood glucose. Eating foods loaded with simple carbohydrates (sugars), however, only exacerbates the problem.

Blood sugar levels rise after the consumption of carbohydrates. This leads to an increased production of serotonin (the neurotransmitter responsible for inducing a state of relaxation and sleep). In CFIDS patients, however, the release of serotonin can create unwanted effects. Serotonin inhibits the release of cortisol, the hormone responsible for reducing inflammation and releasing stored glycogen from the liver. Thus, when cortisol is inhibited, inflammation (a perennial problem in CFIDS) increases. The problem becomes even more complicated when carbohydrate metabolism is disturbed (as is the case in CFIDS) and not enough glucose is formed from carbohydrates to maintain blood sugar levels. In that case, blood sugar levels plummet after the temporary elevation caused by the flood of sugar. The result is physical and mental exhaustion.

A young man with CFIDS from New Jersey describes this problem succinctly: "I feel hung over when I've eaten a lot of sugar. I can't even get up the next day. I've been following a low-carb, no sugar, high-protein diet for a couple of years, and realize I must stay on it. For me, no sugar equals life. I'm much better on this diet."

If you have acute candidiasis or hypoglycemia, dried fruits (dates contain an enormous amount of sucrose) and starchy vegetables should also be avoided, particularly in the evening because they may worsen insomnia. Avoid aspartame (Nutra-Sweet), which breaks down into wood alcohol in the blood stream and can cause serious metabolic problems in people with CFIDS.

4. ANIMAL FATS. Fat is the best source of energy, better than carbohydrates, sugars, or proteins. To serve as an energy source, fat must be metabolized, then transported into cells for use by the mitochondria. Patients with CFIDS commonly have deficits in fat metabolism. Liver and gallbladder function (both organs are vital for breaking down fats) is frequently impaired. Even more significant, CFIDS patients have been shown to have deficiencies in the transport molecule acylcarnitine, which enables the body to use fats at the cellular level. Use fats in moderation. Avoid rich foods and sauces. If you eat meat, use very lean cuts and remove the skin from chicken and other fowl. Of the fats, butter and light, pure vegetable oils such as canola or olive oil seem to be best for CFIDS patients. It is worth the effort to experiment. Buy a high-quality brand; cheap oils become rancid quickly.

5. ADDITIVES (artificial colors, artificial flavors, preservatives, MSG). Sensitivities to petrochemicals and their by-products are common in CFIDS patients. People may not realize that many food additives are derived from petrochemicals. Allergic reactions such as inflammation, itching, pain, insomnia, depression, hyperactivity, and headache caused by common food additives can be severe and can even contribute to CFIDS relapses. Although all synthetic food additives should be avoided, the following are particularly problematic for patients with CFIDS.

- *Artificial colorings (lake colors, tartrazine, AZO dyes, FD&C, or "coal tar colors")* — These are derived from petroleum, and although described as "food" colors, are primarily used to dye cloth. The toxic compounds in FD&C colorings have been linked to cancer, bladder polyps, adrenal damage, impairment of thyroid function, and kidney lesions. Artificial colorings also block the enzyme phenolsulphotransferase-P (PST-P). PST-P deficiency has been noted in hyperactive children and in patients with migraine headaches.
- *MSG and MSG-containing substances (monosodium glutamate, monopotassium glutamate, hydrolized vegetable protein [HVP], hydrolized plant protein, sodium caseinate, calcium caseinate, and Flavorings)* — Glutamic acid, from which MSG is derived, is an amino acid found in most plant and animal proteins. When the glutamic acid is separated from the proteins that would normally inhibit or slow its absorption, the blood stream is flooded. Since glutamic acid acts as an excitatory neurotransmitter, a number of neurologic and allergy-type symptoms can result, including sneezing, itching, hives, rashes, headache, asthma attacks, acid stomach, excessive thirst, bloating, restlessness, balance problems, chest pain, joint pain, and severe depression. CFIDS patients have reported all of these symptoms, and others. Read product labels for MSG before buying. In restaurants, ask the chef to prepare your food without MSG.

It is a good idea, in general, to read labels before you buy. Many foods labeled "natural" contain numerous additives that can cause reactions in people with sensitivities. Prepared foods are notorious in this regard, so try to stick to simple foods with ingredients you can pronounce.

FOOD SENSITIVITIES

Sensitivities and allergies to various foods are common enough in CFIDS to merit special mention. Food sensitivities, while not as dangerous as allergies, can produce such a wide array of symptoms, including restlessness, anxiety, panic attacks, migraine, joint pain, insomnia, nightmares, rashes, and malaise, that they might not be recognized as such in a person with the usual broad spectrum of CFIDS symptoms. To complicate matters, food sensitivities are rarely detected on standard allergy tests. For that reason, many patients may be unaware that some of the worst symptoms they experience may be due to the food they are eating, especially since sensitivities tend to fluctuate over time (true food allergies are lifelong).

Since awareness that diet may be leading to symptoms may come as a surprise to a person who has not had any previous experience with food intolerance or allergies, the initial search to find well-tolerated foods may, at first, seem daunting. For a subset of patients, reactions may be so severe that food intake is drastically restricted. One person described herself as "living on Cheerios" for the first few months of her illness. Another reported that the only food that did *not* create symptoms was celery. People with extreme sensitivities may have to resort to heroic measures such as intravenous feeding to get some nutrition into their bodies. If you are among the very sensitive, food supplementation will be a necessity.

For most CFIDS patients with sensitivities, however, food intake need not be so restricted. A number of CFIDS physicians have noted that eliminating a few offending foods from the diet can improve symptoms dramatically. Dr. Robert H. Loblay and Dr. Anne R. Swain, two clinicians working on CFIDS research in Australia, discovered that about one third of their patients considered themselves "much better" after eliminating offending foods from their diets. These patients reported significant improvement in specific symptoms such as headache, muscle pain, malaise, depression, and irritability after adopting a modified diet. Treatment surveys conducted by a DePaul University research team and by Dr. Fred Friedberg also confirm that about one third of patients who adopt antiallergy diets experience moderate to major improvement in CFIDS symptoms.

The task of identifying offending foods is made easier by the fact that most food sensitivities tend to fall into groups that, among CFIDS patients, can be fairly predictable. The following list, compiled with the help of numerous individuals with CFIDS, may help you to identify the most common symptom-producing foods.

NIGHTSHADE FAMILY (eggplant, pepper, tomato, potato). All members of the nightshade group contain atropine, an alkaloid that is an anticholinergic (inhibits acetylcholine) and produces inflammation. A number of people with CFIDS report alleviation of joint pain after eliminating these foods from their diets. Some patients find they can eat potatoes that have been boiled in water (with the liquid discarded).

MILK PRODUCTS. Dr. David Bell reports that most of his patients have sensitivities to milk products. Many people, even in the general population, develop a deficiency in lactase, the enzyme that breaks down lactose. Lactose intolerance can produce bloating, gas, and discomfort. In addition, milk thickens mucus, which can worsen symptoms for patients with allergies. Some people who cannot consume whole milk (or cheese) find they can drink skim milk. Others find they can substitute nonfat yogurt or cheeses that are not aged (cream cheese, cottage cheese, farmer's cheese) for full-fat or aged dairy products.

FRUITS. Fruits contain large amounts of fructose. People with severe problems from defective carbohydrate metabolism experience less fatigue and general malaise with a fruit-free diet. Those with fewer problems sometimes find they can eat fruit after a meal rather than on an empty stomach. Some people also report that some fruits (citrus, for example) are harder to digest than others.

GAS-PRODUCING FOOD (onions, cabbage, brussels sprouts, broccoli). People with gastrointestinal problems should avoid gas-producing foods. Sometimes negative effects are mitigated by cooking these foods thoroughly.

SPICY FOODS (black pepper, curry, garlic). Many people with food sensitivities seem to do best with a bland diet, especially in the acute phase. Avoid spicy foods if you have gastrointestinal problems.

RAW FOODS. Even though salads provide necessary roughage, many CFIDS patients experience discomfort after eating raw vegetables. Eating well-cooked vegetables and grains usually mitigates digestive disturbances.

YEAST-CONTAINING FOODS (brewer's yeast, fermented products, mushrooms, aged cheese, B vitamins). Patients with systemic yeast infections (Candida) should avoid yeast products, not because yeast products cause Candida to grow, as is commonly believed, but because people with Candida overgrowth tend to become allergic to yeasts and molds.

ACID FOODS (fruits, tomatoes, vinegar). Patients with interstitial cystitis or recurrent gastritis should avoid acidic foods, which usually exacerbate symptoms (see Chapter 3: Urinary Tract Problems).

NUTS. Nuts contain large amounts of arginine, the amino acid needed for herpesviruses to replicate. For this reason, they should be avoided. They also tend to produce allergic reactions in those who are sensitive.

SOY PRODUCTS. Soy products sometimes provoke reactions such as headache or gastrointestinal pain in sensitive individuals.

FOOD ROTATION

People with many food allergies and sensitivities may want to rotate their foods. The rationale behind food rotation is, if your body takes a rest from the chemical components of the food you are eating (which it can do only after constant exposure to those chemicals), it will not mount an immune attack. Supposedly, the body will "forget" its first exposure to a food after 4 days. Thus a rotation diet calls for a 4-day delay betfore eating a suspected food a second time. Some very sensitive people may want to wait a week before repeating foods. Foods that produce strong reactions (diarrhea, acid stomach, nausea, headache, hives, itching, any other allergic response) should be strictly avoided. If your diet is very restricted, a 4-day interval may not be possible. In that case, allow as much time as you can between foods. It is also very helpful if you can address the problems of allergies and leaky gut syndrome directly (see Chapter 3: Allergies, Digestive Disturbances). Supplement your diet, if you can, with an easily absorbed liquid or powdered vitamin compound (see Chapter 5: Vitamins) to avoid nutritional deficiencies.

COOKING TIPS

Anything you can do to lessen work in the kitchen will help you improve your diet because you will have more energy to plan and eat meals. If you are acutely ill or bedbound, make it a priority to get some help in the kitchen. People who feel too tired or sick to cook may not eat, which creates problems above and beyond those caused by CFIDS. If friends offer to help, ask them to prepare meals. If you are alone, try some of the following suggestions to cut down on your work load.

- *Prepare meals in advance.* Cook during periods of higher energy or ask someone to prepare food and freeze it in individual portions.
- *Buy frozen food.* Many organic and natural foods are available from health food stores. Cascadian Farms makes frozen organic corn, potatoes, carrots, and other vegetables. You can also purchase frozen organic meats and main dishes that do not contain artificial additives.
- *Order food by phone.* Many grocery stores will deliver for a small fee. Call to see which will take orders by phone.
- *Contact volunteer services.* Many churches and local organizations have volunteers to help you shop and cook meals.

A FINAL WORD ON FOOD AND DIET

Experiment with your diet to find one that works best for you, but remember to use common sense. Many nutritionists, chiropractors, naturopaths, and countless authors of best-selling diet books have special regimens they claim will produce immediate health gains. Often the pressure to adopt one of these diets can be intense, especially if your friends or acquaintances have heard rumors of cases in which people with cancer, diabetes, heart disease, or other conditions have been cured simply by following a particular diet. Special diets can certainly *help* people with CFIDS, but we have yet to see a case of anyone who has been *cured* by using any of the diets that have been popularized over the past decade. Quite the contrary. A number of CFIDS patients have experienced setbacks as a result of rigorous dieting. Several of those we surveyed reported rapid weight loss with diets that severely restrict carbohydrates. Others have reported exacerbation of weakness from diets that eliminate proteins. Make diet changes slowly, proceed with caution (much as you would with any new treatment), and keep in mind that you are the best judge of what is "good for you."

ORGANIZATION

Food Allergy Network
4747 Holly Avenue
Fairfax, VA 22030-5647
800-929-4040 (telephone)

FURTHER READING

Brostoff, Jonathan, and Gamlin, Linda. The Complete Guide to Food Allergy and Intolerance. New York: Crown Publishers, 1989 (guide to symptoms, causes, and management of food sensitivities).

Dumke, Nicolette M. Allergy Cooking With Ease. Lancaster, Pa.: Starburst Publishers, 1992 (a compilation of recipes accommodating every type of allergy).

SEE

• Chapter 3: Allergies (food), Candida, Digestive Disturbances, Hypoglycemia, Urinary Tract Problems for diet suggestions and treatments pertaining to specific symptoms.

10

Special Needs of Children With CFIDS

Maya . . . At age 7 years Maya was a lively, gregarious child, always ready for an "adventure" and full of laughter. She was bright, did well in school, and had a lively interest in all her subjects, especially math. Her parents thought the world of her. In the spring just before her eighth birthday, Maya began complaining of stomachaches and headaches. Her mother had become ill with CFIDS the previous fall, but because she had been told (erroneously, as it turned out) that children could not contract CFIDS, the family attributed Maya's symptoms to flu, which was going around. Maya's stomachaches and headaches did not go away, however, and friends began suggesting that Maya was imitating her mother to get attention. That summer her symptoms seemed to clear up, and Maya went to spend a month with her grandparents. During this time Maya started sleeping excessively. Her grandmother was accustomed to letting children sleep until they awakened naturally, but when Maya was asleep half the day, she realized something was wrong. When Maya returned home just before school started again, she seemed in good spirits and eager for school to begin.

In the week before the start of the school year, Maya began complaining again of stomachaches and headaches. Now she also had diarrhea. The doctor thought she might have worms and gave her medication, but instead of going away her symptoms worsened. Sore throat and low-grade fever developed. Maya was reexamined by the family physician, who noted that the lymph nodes under her jaw were enlarged and prescribed an antibiotic. Maya's condition did not improve with the medication and soon other problems developed. In contrast to her long hours in bed during the summer, she now had insomnia and often stayed awake the whole night. She said that even when she did sleep it felt as though she hadn't. Sometimes before going to bed she would hold her chest and say she "couldn't breathe." When she did finally sleep, her rest was punctuated by nightmares, and she would awaken terrified and crying. Her ankles hurt her so much in the morning she could barely walk, and she lost interest in school. She said math gave her a headache, and she did not do her assignments. Her teachers became frustrated when she said she could not remember spelling and other material she had previously learned and labeled her a "problem." Her appetite disappeared, and she complained that foods tasted bad. Maya lost several pounds. When her friends came to call, she told them to play without her. Within a season, Maya had been completely transformed from a lively little girl to a thin, pale recluse. Her last words at night before she went to bed were always, "I can't believe how bad I feel."

At that point her mother was almost certain that Maya also had CFIDS. She consulted with a CFIDS expert and the family physician, who was already familiar with her mother's case. Both were of the opinion that Maya indeed had CFIDS. The news was devastating to Maya's parents.

The following day, Maya's mother removed her from school. The family physician consented to recommend her for home tutoring through the public school system. For the next 8 months, Maya rarely left home. She went to bed early in the evening, slept as late as she could in the morning, and took naps or rested during the day. Mornings were always hard for her. The tutor came three times a week to keep Maya current with school work, but after a few weeks began berating her for not concentrating on her tasks. The parents requested another tutor, but the director refused to supply one, citing the tutor's opinion that Maya had "school phobia" and was not really sick. Her mother withdrew Maya from the program and home schooled her.

This period was difficult for both mother and daughter. The mother, also ill, had very little energy to cope with a sick daughter. To confound matters, Maya had become extremely volatile and seemed to be either perpetually angry or weeping. Maya herself was confused by her outbursts and, when asked what was wrong, would cry out, "I don't know!" She had become an intractable little girl, and her mother found herself losing patience with Maya. However, despite all their difficulties, the two grew quite close. Maya's frightening symptoms were understood and explained by her mother. Maya never had to endure the skepticism of doctors, friends, and family because her parents were already familiar with the illness. Perhaps most important, Maya learned how to take care of herself. She learned she could paddle around the pool a little, but not ride her bike. She remembered to take her vitamins daily and voluntarily gave up sweets. She came to recognize her own limits and stop activities before they caused a relapse. She learned to talk about how she was feeling. Best of all, she learned patience.

Fifteen months after Maya left school, she returned. The school day always left her tired, but she was able to keep up with her work and, within 2 months, she made the honor roll, despite severe anxiety about taking tests. Her mother wrote a note to the gym teacher to request that Maya be excused from running and all other aerobic activities. A tutor came once a week to help Maya with spelling, handwriting, and math—three areas that caused her particular problems. After-school activities were still curtailed, but Maya's cheer and zest for life had returned, and she was eager to get on with things. Her mother steered her toward quieter activities, such as crafts, languages, music, and art lessons, that did not tax her strength but helped boost her self-confidence. Although she was clearly less energetic than other children and experienced a flare-up of symptoms when she overexerted herself or caught a cold (a frequent occurrence), she was still able to participate fully in most activities and events.

Maya's story demonstrates that children do indeed get CFIDS. In fact, they do so in significant numbers. In early community-wide outbreaks of CFIDS, children were among the most frequently affected. In the Lyndonville, New York, outbreak, Dr. David Bell noted that children younger than 18 years represented 30% of the total number of individuals affected.

In contrast to the adult population with CFIDS, in which women predominate, the illness seems to affect boys as often as girls. Dr. Bell has reported a nearly equal gender distribution in his practice. He also has reported that 45% of his pediatric patients have a family member ill with CFIDS.

While, in most regards, CFIDS in children is indistinguishable from CFIDS in adults, there are some important differences. According to Dr. Bell, the pattern of onset seems to be more age related in children. In children between the age of 8 years and the onset of puberty, CFIDS usually develops gradually. After puberty, CFIDS generally begins with acute onset of symptoms, usually resembling the flu or mononucleosis. In children younger than 8 years old, CFIDS is nearly impossible to diagnose because of the diffuse, transient nature of the symptoms and the difficulty most young children have in giving a detailed description of symptoms. This is not to say that younger children do not contract CFIDS. Parents of children 4, 5, and 6 years of age have reported CFIDS-like symptoms in their children. However, most clinicians will not venture to make a diagnosis for a very young child.

Symptoms in children closely parallel those in adults, although children tend to experience more gastrointestinal problems (manifested as stomachaches) and flu symptoms (sore throat and swollen glands). Children also tend to experience all symptoms with equal severity. Dr. Bell has noted that, whereas adults generally report certain symptoms as consistently more severe than others, children experience severe headaches and stomachaches one day, severe leg pains and insomnia on another, and severe joint pains on a third. Because gradual onset of the illness in young

---

CRITERIA FOR DIAGNOSING CFIDS IN CHILDREN*

- Activity limitation that causes disruption of normal lifestyle for at least 6 months
- No obvious physical or emotional cause of fatigue
- At least 8 of the following 12 symptom criteria:
    Fatigue
    Headache
    Abdominal pain
    Lymph node pain
    Recurrent sore throat
    Muscle pain
    Joint pain
    Sleep disturbance
    Eye pain, photophobia, or both
    Depression
    Neurologic symptoms (lightheadedness, balance disorder, paresthesia)
    Cognitive difficulties (short-term memory loss, attention deficit disorder)

*From Bell, David. Special Bulletin. *CFIDS Chronicle*, November, 1993.

---

children exempts it from the Centers for Disease Control and Prevention (CDC) definition of CFIDS, and because some symptoms tend to predominate in children, Dr. Bell has proposed an alternate set of criteria for diagnosing CFIDS in children.

Routine test results tend to be normal for most children with CFIDS, although low sedimentation rate, slightly elevated white blood cell count, and low titers of antinuclear antibodies are common. Because most doctors order only routine tests for children who come to their offices with flu-like symptoms, a family physician will rarely make the diagnosis of CFIDS, even if the child is seen in the office every few weeks. More specific immune testing is not usually ordered. As in the case of adults with CFIDS, more complex immune system tests (natural killer cells, T and B cells) may reveal abnormalities. Tests for viral involvement (Epstein-Barr virus or human herpesvirus 6) may be unpredictable.

If symptoms are severe and prolonged, the doctor will probably look for other causes, such as ulcers, Crohn's disease, childhood migraine syndrome, atypical epilepsy, food allergies, rheumatoid arthritis, rheumatic fever, diabetes, or attention deficit disorder. The child may even receive a diagnosis of "school phobia" when results of these tests are negative. In this case, the child needs extra support from family members and most likely needs a new doctor.

The persistent attitude on the part of doctors and teachers that the child is "faking" symptoms for psychological reasons causes profound damage to children with CFIDS. Misdiagnosing CFIDS as school phobia, depression, or separation anxiety or chalking it up to family problems places the blame squarely on the shoulders of the child. When adults experience this kind of skepticism, they usually are able to defend themselves against the mistaken ideas of others. Children are unable to do so; they depend on adults for information, explanations, sympathy, and advice. To throw disbelief in the face of a child who not only has all the physical symptoms of CFIDS but is terribly frightened and in profound need of reassurance is not only cruel, it is detrimental to the child's future emotional growth.

Parents of a child with CFIDS should keep in mind that even though school officials and doctors may attribute their child's complaints to psychological causes, they seldom can back up their opinions. School phobia, for example, is a manifestation of separation anxiety. Children with separation anxiety display symptoms when anticipating separation but which resolve when separation does not occur. In CFIDS, symptoms are present not only during school hours, but after school and on weekends as well. Also, symptoms such as fever, lymph node pain, night sweats, and muscle and joint pain are not features of school phobia. Those who are apt to diagnose depression run into the same inconsistencies: lymph node pain and fever are not typical of primary depression. Children with CFIDS can become depressed, but usually do so because no one believes they are ill. No study to date has revealed primary depression among children with CFIDS.

Another difficulty parents may encounter is that some doctors insist that withholding the diagnosis of CFIDS is better for the child. They argue that making the diagnosis will encourage self-identification as a "sick person." This is a fallacious argument. A sick child certainly is aware of the fact. Denying reality will only produce more psychological stress.

It is important to note that the prognosis for the majority of children with CFIDS is good. Many recover within 3 years. In some children, however, severe cases can last for many years. These are marked by neurologic symptoms such as seizures, myoclonus, and paresthesia. Children with severe or long-term neurologic symptoms most certainly need to be under the continuing care of a CFIDS specialist.

TREATMENT TIPS

Treatments for children with CFIDS are more restricted than for adults and, as a consequence, clinicians tend to be somewhat more cautious in their approach. Dr. Bell, for example, does not recommend giving children many of the drugs commonly prescribed for adults, particularly antidepressants (personal communication, 1993). The justification for a more conservative approach is that the child's normal neurologic growth might be affected. Nor do most doctors recommend experimental CFIDS treatments such as Kutapressin in children who have not finished growing (although adolescents may benefit considerably from this treatment).

Many alternative treatments and supportive therapies, however, can be beneficial for children. In fact, some of these gentler therapies (herbs and vitamins, especially) have been more successful in children than in adults. Dr. Charles Lapp, a well-known pediatric CFIDS specialist, recommends valerian root (500 to 750 mg nightly) to help with insomnia. He also uses a mild antihistamine such as Benadryl (25 to 50 mg; a clear liquid is available for those with sensitivities to dyes), Tylenol PM, or Excedrin PM to help children sleep. Children also respond well to supportive therapies such as hydrotherapy, massage, and acupuncture (for pain).

Cognitive problems in childhood are particularly troubling because these are crucial years for intellectual development. Children with CFIDS often experience particular difficulties in maintaining attention (attention deficit disorder), retaining information (memory formation), and focus (concentration). Often they lose confidence in their ability to learn. Dr. Linda Iger, a psychologist who has worked extensively on neurocognitive aspects of CFIDS, has outlined the following useful strategies to help children with CFIDS cope with school tasks.

- *Limit periods of concentration.* The average adult can concentrate for only 50 minutes at a stretch. Children with CFIDS generally lose their ability to concentrate after about 20 minutes (or less, depending on the severity of the illness). Dr. Iger recommends that children time themselves to discover their concentration "ceiling," or limit of concentration. Whatever that amount of time—15 minutes, half an hour—is as much time as should be devoted to a single topic. When concentration wanes, Dr. Iger recommends taking a break for about 10 minutes. Children should get a glass of water, look out the window, or close their eyes and "kick back." In other words, they need to give the brain a break. This work-rest pattern should be repeated twice, then take a long break.

- *Use passive learning.* Often, focusing on a topic makes it harder to absorb. Children with CFIDS may find the task of learning new information easier if they don't concentrate directly on it. For example, a random list of geographic features may be impossible to memorize if tackled directly. The same information is much easier to process if encountered in the form of a story or video. Your local library may have entertaining materials (PBS video series are particularly helpful) that might help the child absorb information indirectly.
- *Limit information.* It is difficult for most people to remember long strings of facts or numbers. For people with CFIDS the task is nearly impossible, Most children (and adults) with CFIDS simply find themselves "going blank" after too much input. Try to limit information input to small increments. For example, a string of numbers such as 4358962 may be difficult to retain. When this set of numbers is broken up into two sets, for example, 435-8962, it is like a phone number. Sets of three and four numbers are much easier to retain than sets of seven digits. Try to use this strategy when faced with memorizing numbers or facts.
- *Eliminate distractions.* Studying with music or television in the background is not a good idea for children with CFIDS. The additional input of music or talking makes it difficult to concentrate. Find a quiet, nondistracting study place for them.
- *Reduce anxiety.* Anxiety can have disastrous effects on attention span, focus, and retention. For this reason, many children with CFIDS find themselves unable to take tests. Children who feel themselves becoming anxious (for example, during a test) should practice deep-breathing and stress-reduction exercises. Self-hypnosis and meditation techniques can also be quite helpful (see Chapter 6: Hypnosis, Meditation; Chapter 7).

Unfortunately, it is still difficult to find pediatricians knowledgeable about CFIDS. Many doctors are unaware that children can contract CFIDS, even when they know it occurs in adults. If you suspect your child has CFIDS, it might be well worth a trip to consult with a specialist, to both confirm a diagnosis and devise a treatment plan best suited to your child's symptoms and age. A pediatrician who is open-minded will follow the specialist's recommendations. Having a supportive physician can make a world of difference to both the child with CFIDS and his or her parents.

Of equal importance to finding a supportive physician is giving careful attention to managing the illness at home. Children with CFIDS spend the majority of their time at home with their families, which means that proper home management of CFIDS is vital for recovery. The following management tips can help provide a basis for dealing with CFIDS in a child and can help make the experience considerably easier for all involved.

Managing CFIDS at Home

PROVIDE SUPPORT AND UNDERSTANDING. Support and understanding are the most important aspects of helping a child with CFIDS. Suspicions of malingering will invariably cause self-esteem problems in children. It is important to show children that you believe them, that what they are feeling can be explained, and that you will do everything in your power to help them. Make sure your doctor demonstrates the same attitude.

MAINTAIN SOCIAL INVOLVEMENT. It is crucial for children with CFIDS to maintain relationships with friends, even if they are out of school. Brief play times for younger children or visits for older children are essential to keep up flagging spirits. To avert depression, don't let your child become too isolated.

REQUEST FREQUENT DIAGNOSTIC REEVALUATION. Though CFIDS rarely leads to other diseases, some symptoms are similar enough to those of anemia, heart, and lung disease to warrant reappraisal. There is one published case of a child in whom juvenile diabetes developed after the onset of CFIDS. New or worsening symptoms should always be investigated.

INSIST ON ADEQUATE REST. Children are more active than adults, and the amount of activity a child with CFIDS can sustain is normally greater than in an adult. Children should be encouraged to be active, but not beyond their limits. An observant parent can judge a child's limits by early warning signs such as paleness, darkness around the eyes, hyperactivity, talkativeness, restlessness, lethargy, crying and irritability, loss of appetite, and sensitivity to light and noise—all signs that the child must rest immediately.

PROVIDE SCHOLASTIC SUPPORT. Home tutors are useful, whether the child is being taught at home or in school. According to federal law (Public Law 94-142, the Education of All Handicapped Children Act of 1975), all children ill for more than a few weeks are eligible for tutoring by teachers from the public school district. A form must be filled out by your doctor to verify that the child is chronically ill. A teacher is then assigned to come to your house, usually three times a week. If the school district balks at sending a teacher (they often have numerous excuses, none of them legal), cite the law and threaten legal action, if necessary. If tutoring through the public schools does not work out (as in Maya's case), many cities have volunteer tutoring programs for children who cannot attend school. Tutoring can be done by a teenager (if the child is younger), college students in education programs, or retired teachers. The child who is still attending school needs to rest during gym and study hall. It helps to have a note from your doctor.

KEEP A REGULAR NONSTRESSFUL SCHEDULE. Stressors of any kind can worsen CFIDS in children, as they do in adults. To avoid as much physical stress as possible, make sure your child follows a fairly fixed schedule for eating, sleeping, and activities. Adjust his or her schedule accordingly during remissions, but remember that even if the child appears well, late bedtimes and overactivity will only cause a relapse. This is not a good time to burden children with too many expectations or insist on competitive activities, however normal they may be for others in their age group. Parents must walk that fine line between allowing normal activities, which are essential for a child's growth and happiness, and excesses, which court relapse. Learning to pace a child with CFIDS is one of the most difficult tasks a parent can master, but it is well worth it in the long run. Eventually the child learns to pace him- or herself. Let your child have fun, but keep an eye on his or her limits.

As you care for your child with CFIDS, don't forget to take care of yourself as well. Nothing is more heartbreaking than watching a child suffer. Seek out support groups, friends, and family members for moral support and take advantage of the resources available for children with long-term or disabling illnesses. Remember that, for your child, you are the most important person in the world. Take good care of yourself.

ORGANIZATIONS

CFIDS Youth Alliance (CYA)
PO Box 220398
Charlotte, NC 28222-0398
800-442-3437 (toll-free telephone)

National Information Center for Children and Youth With Disabilities
PO Box 1492
Washington, DC 20013

PEN-PALS

CFIDS Friendship Network
PO Box 7202
Gainesville, FL 32605

CFS Youth Outreach
c/o Sharon Walk
14 Shetland Road
Florham Park, NJ 07932-1813

Teen CFIDS Pen-Pal Connection
c/o Connie Howard
1810 Cliffwood Court
New Albany, IN 47150

WEBSITE

http://www.ypwcnet.org/ (provides extensive resources for children with CFIDS)

FURTHER READING

Journal of Chronic Fatigue Syndrome (Volume 2, Number 2, 1997) focuses on research and issues involving children with CFIDS.

Thorson, Kristin, ed. Fibromyalgia Syndrome and Chronic Fatigue Syndrome in Young People: A Guide for Parents. Tucson, Ariz.: Health Network, 1994.

Vanderzalm, Lynn. Finding Strength in Weakness. Grand Rapids, Mich.: Zondervan, 1995.

APPENDICES

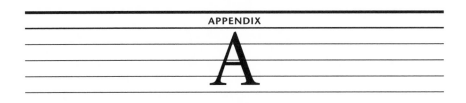

Resources

Selected CFIDS Books

Bell, David S. The Doctor's Guide to Chronic Fatigue Syndrome. New York: Addison-Wesley Publishing Co., 1994.

> Dr. Bell's guide, although ostensibly pitched to doctors, is not technical. The material is presented in a clear format, is easy to read, and is well organized. The strongest parts of the book are the overview and description sections. Dr. Bell's book is very useful for the new reader.

Berne, Katrina H. Running on Empty: Chronic Fatigue Immune Dysfunction Syndrome (CFIDS). Alameda, Calif.: Hunter House, 1992.

> This is one of the classics in the CFIDS literature. It contains information on testing, symptoms, resources, and a history of the illness, which together comprise the essential information every person with CFIDS must know. It has recently been updated.

Feiden, Karyn. Hope and Help for Chronic Fatigue Syndrome. New York: Simon & Schuster, 1990.

> This is one of the better practical guides for coping with CFIDS. It contains detailed and thoroughly researched information on the current theories concerning the cause of the illness, tests normally performed to help confirm a diagnosis, and standard treatment protocols. It concludes with an excellent resources section.

Goldstein, Jay A. Betrayal by the Brain. Binghamton, N.Y.: Haworth Medical Press, 1996. Courmel, Katie. A Companion Volume to Dr. Jay A. Goldstein's Betrayal by the Brain. Binghamton, N.Y.: Haworth Medical Press, 1996.

> This book by Dr. Goldstein gives insights into the limbic system dysfunction that characterizes CFIDS. Because it is geared to physicians, it is very technical. The companion guide by Katie Courmel provides the layperson with an easy-to-read interpretation of Dr. Goldstein's work ($14.95).

Hyde, Byron M, ed. The Clinical and Scientific Basis of Myalgic Encephalomyelitis/Chronic Fatigue Syndrome. Ottawa, Ontario: Nightingale Research Foundation, 1992.

> The Cambridge Easter Symposium on ME/CFS held in Cambridge, England, in April 1990 forms the bulk of this book. Despite the fact that the 75 papers included in this volume represent research that is several years old, the information contained in them, and in the review chapters, is not outdated. Chapter topics include historical reviews of

CFIDS epidemics, CFIDS in children, diagnosis, infectious origins of CFIDS (viral research), skeletal muscle and heart involvement, neurologic injury, neuropsychological changes, food sensitivities, immunology, blood cell changes, and treatment. For anyone who wishes to explore the more technical aspects of CFIDS, this book is a gold mine of information. As of this writing, it is available for the price of a membership in the Nightingale Research Foundation (see Appendix B).

Johnson, Hillary. Osler's Web, Inside the Labyrinth of the Chronic Fatigue Syndrome Epidemic. New York: Crown Publishers, 1996.

In this thoroughly researched book, Johnson tells the inside story of the recent medical and political events surrounding the CFIDS outbreaks of the 1980s.

Rosenbaum, Michael, and Susser, Murray. Solving the Puzzle of Chronic Fatigue Syndrome. Tacoma, Wash.: Life Sciences Press, 1992.

The authors offer a wide range of theories and ideas regarding CFIDS. Dr. Susser and Dr. Rosenbaum view CFIDS as a complex disorder, and in light of the fact that a single agent or pathogen has yet to be discovered, they suggest treating CFIDS as a mixed-infection syndrome. The authors test their patients for parasites, yeast, bacteria, and viruses and investigate possible underlying medical conditions that may mimic or worsen CFIDS (such as hypothyroidism, adrenal insufficiency, environmental illness, heavy metal poisoning, and allergies).

Thorson, Kristin, ed. Fibromyalgia Syndrome and Chronic Fatigue Syndrome in Young People: A Guide for Parents. Tucson, Ariz.: Health Network, 1994.

This book offers basic information on the care and management of children with CFIDS. It also provides appendices that detail the laws and services applicable to students in the United States. The guides in the back of the book are quite useful for teachers. To order, contact the Fibromyalgia Network, PO Box 31750, Tucson, AZ 85751-1750 (520-290-5508; fax: 520-290-5550) (58 pages; $10.00).

Vanderzalm, Lynn. Finding Strength in Weakness. Grand Rapids, Mich.: Zondervan, 1995.

Ms. Vanderzalm interviewed 70 people with CFIDS, and drew on her own experience as a mother of children with CFIDS (and ill herself) to write this book about the impact of CFIDS on a family. Her avowedly Christian perspective may put some people off. However, since it is one of the few books concerning this topic, the information it contains should be useful to all who read it. The Foreword is written by David Bell, M.D. To order, contact the CFIDS Association of America, PO Box 220398, Charlotte, NC 28222-0398 (286 pages; $11.00).

Wilkinson, Steve. Chronic Fatigue Syndrome: A Natural Healing Guide. New York: Sterling Publishing Co., 1990.

This is one of the more detailed books on alternative treatments for CFIDS. Wilkinson worked as an alternative health care practitioner in Great Britain and treated a number of patients for ME before he contracted the illness himself. The sections describing the benefits of acupuncture, aroma therapy, hypnosis, meditation, and dietary supplements, while brief, offer a good sampling of some of the alternative treatments considered useful for many CFIDS symptoms.

PERSONAL ACCOUNTS

Fisher, Gregg Charles. Chronic Fatigue Syndrome: A Victim's Guide to Understanding, Treating and Coping With This Debilitating Illness. New York: Warner Books, 1987.

This book is both a personal account of Gregg Fisher and his wife's illness and a CFIDS guide, including all that was known about the illness in 1987. He also has many helpful suggestions for dealing with the Social Security Administration, coping with the subjective fallout of having a major illness (emotional upset), and maintaining relationships with incredulous friends and acquaintances. The book has recently been revised and updated.

Kenny, Timothy. Living With Chronic Fatigue Syndrome: A Personal Story of the Struggle for Recovery. New York: Thunder's Mouth Press, 1994.

This book documents Tim Kenny's struggle with severe CFIDS. Kenny, a journalist, wanted to share his own battle with CFIDS to inspire others to keep up the fight. His essay on fatigue is particularly cogent (paperback, $12.95).

Journals and Periodicals

The CFIDS Chronicle

This quarterly journal of the Chronic Fatigue and Immune Dysfunction Association of America (see Appendix B) is perhaps the best, in terms of variety and depth of coverage, of all the publications offered by independent CFIDS organizations. Within its covers are the latest in fast-breaking research news, a complete listing of all related CFIDS materials (which can be conveniently ordered by phone from the Association), letters, book reviews, "Ask the Doctor," and myriad other highly useful resources. Back issues to 1989 are available. The March 1991 issue "Physician's Forum" is an excellent resource for currently available treatments from the four best-known CFIDS clinicians. To order, write the CFIDS Association of America, PO Box 220398, Charlotte, NC 28222-0398. (Subscription: $30.00 in U.S.; $40.00 in Canada; $55.00 overseas.)

Journal of Chronic Fatigue Syndrome

This is a highly technical quarterly medical journal edited by Dr. Nancy Klimas and Dr. Roberto Petarca. The basic mission of the journal is to blend basic scientific, clinical, and epidemiologic research in a peer-review format. Much of the research is also available in *The CFIDS Chronicle*. To order, write Hawthorn Press, 10 Alice Street, Binghamton, NY 13904-9981. (Subscription: $36.00.)

The CFIDS Inspiration

This newsletter, edited by Brenda Sheridan, helps people with CFIDS exchange personal ideas and information about coping with CFIDS. For a sample copy, send name, address and a $2.00 check to Lorri Coller-Nugent, The CFIDS Inspiration, 2419 S. 61st Street, Philadelphia, PA 19142-3215. (Subscription: $15.00 in U.S.; $17.00 international.)

CFS and FMS Teen Voices

This newsletter, published six times a year and edited by two adolescents with CFIDS, provides a phone support group and locates pen-pals. For more information, contact Jen Day, CFS and FMS Teen Voices, 205 Walnut Street, Red Oak, IA 51566 (712-623-2238—helpline). Website: jennyd@redoak.heartland.net (Subscription: $8.00.)

The National Link

This quarterly newsletter features creative writing, personal stories, and poetry dedicated to the experience of CFIDS/ME. To order, write PO Box 51952, Durham, NC 27727-1952. (Subscription: $15.00 in U.S.; $20.00 in Canada.)

Skywriters

This quarterly literary journal edited by Tara Allen contains submissions for people with CFIDS and related diseases (a self-addressed stamped envelope should be included with submissions). (Subscription: $20.00; make checks payable to Lyman Farris, Jr., 245 Spring Street SW, Concord, NC 28025.)

The Meeting Place

This newsletter of the ANZYME Society of New Zealand contains physicians' reports, letters from readers, and information about CFIDS. To order, write ANZYMES, Inc., PO Box 36307, Northcote, Auckland 1309, New Zealand. (Subscription: $35.00 U.S. for airmail; $28.00 U.S. for surface.)

The MEssenger

The monthly newsletter of the ME Association of Canada contains articles, treatment news, legal helpline information, medical information, letters from patients, conference reports, and book reviews. This newsletter is nontechnical and patient-centered. To order, write ME Canada, 400-246 Queen Street, Ottawa, Ontario, K1P 5E4 Canada. (Subscription: $40.00.)

1996 ME and FM Manual Newsletter

This 155-page informative guide was assembled by Doug Shore, vice president of the ME Society of British Columbia. To order, write PO Box 2591, Suman, WA 98295; or 235-32550 MacLure Road, Abotsford, BC V2T 4N3 Canada. (Subscription: $14.00 in U.S.; $19.00 in Canada.)

Videotapes

Living Hell: The Real World of Chronic Fatigue Syndrome (1 hour)

Produced in 1993 by Authentic Pictures and directed by Lennie Copeland, this video accurately and thoroughly represents CFIDS from the perspective of those who have the illness. It is emotionally charged, sometimes even shocking, which may limit its usefulness for physicians, caregivers, and those who are not personally worried about the more severe effects of CFIDS. ($32.00 from the CFIDS Association.)

CFIDS Diagnosis and Treatment: A Grand Rounds Medical Training Video (30 minutes)

Dr. Jonathan Rest instructs health care professionals on the diagnosis and treatment of CFIDS. ($30.00 from the CFIDS Association.)

CFS: Unraveling the Mystery (20 minutes)

Produced by CNN Newsource in October 1991, this four-part series gives a general but accurate description of CFIDS. It is useful for convincing skeptical friends and family members of the reality of CFIDS ($2.00 from the sale of each video goes to fund CFIDS research). ($12.00 from the CFIDS Association.)

Cheney Clinic Information Video

Produced by the Cheney Clinic, this presentation by Dr. Paul Cheney is meant to accompany a visit to his clinic, but provides an informative and clear account of some of the theories, mechanisms, and treatments frequently discussed in CFIDS books and journals. This is a good video to show your doctor. ($20.00 from the Cheney Clinic.)

Chronic Fatigue Syndrome: A Real Disease (90 minutes)

This clear and concise talk by Dr. Charles Lapp, a well-known CFIDS specialist, provides an excellent overview of the illness: its symptoms, possible causes, and effect on the immune system. Treatments are discussed and self-management strategies such as bed rest and vitamin therapy are emphasized. This tape is invaluable for support groups and friends and families of people who have CFIDS. It is of particular value for those patients with cognitive problems who may have difficulty reading more technical printed material. Most important, Dr. Lapp addresses some important questions: Is CFIDS contagious? Is CFIDS fatal? Can people with CFIDS recover? ($25.00 in U.S.; $30.00 in Canada; $35.00 overseas from the CFS Foundation of Greensboro, NC, 10 Partridge Court, Dept. NC, Greensboro, NC 27455.)

The CFS Foundation of Greensboro, NC also offers the following videotapes (each tape is $25.00 in U.S.; $30.00 in Canada; $35.00 overseas):

- *Recognition, Diagnosis & Treatment of CFS*. Dr. Charles W. Lapp (50 minutes)
- *CFS Update—Richmond, Virginia, Conference, November 1992*. Dr. Paul Cheney and Dr. Charles W. Lapp (2 hours)
- *U.S. and British Research Comparisons*. Dr. Byron M. Hyde (2 hours)
- *CFS in Children*. Dr. Michael Goldberg (75 minutes)

Articles, Information Packets, and Resource Guides

The CFIDS Association
PO Box 220398
Charlotte, NC 28222-0398
800-442-3437 (toll-free telephone)
704-362-2343 (local telephone)
704-365-9755 (fax)
704-365-2343 (resources)
http://cfids.org/cfids (Internet home page)
info@cfids.org (e-mail)

The Association provides a broad range of educational materials, including 17 key media and 13 classic medical articles. Contact the Association for a complete listing. ($1.00 to $4.00 per article, with discounts available for sets.)

CFIDS Pathfinder
PO Box 2644
Kensington, MD 20891-2644
301-530-8624 (telephone)

The Pathfinder is a comprehensive reference for CFIDS citations, including books, historical references, government press releases, government publications, congressional documents, research, periodicals, FOIA requests, computer bulletin boards, audiotapes, libraries, films, GPO bookstores, vertical files, pharmaceuticals, and where and how to finds CFIDS articles. It is compiled by a librarian with CFIDS and arranged in looseleaf notebook format to accommodate updates. (Pathfinder, $12.00, postage $1.05, or 60 cents for medical residents; Addenda, $6.00 each, postage $1.05, or 30 cents for medical residents.)

Division of Viral Diseases
Center for Infectious Diseases
Centers for Disease Control and Prevention
Atlanta, GA 30333
404-332-4555 (telephone)

> The CDC will send a copy of the booklet, *The Facts About Chronic Fatigue Syndrome,* and an article, "The Chronic Fatigue Syndrome: A Comprehensive Approach to Its Definition and Treatment," free on request. These two publications reflect the CDC's long-term position of denial of CFIDS and, as a consequence, provide little useful information for diagnosis or treatment. (According to the CDC, there is none.)

National Institutes of Health
National Institute of Allergy and Infectious Diseases (NIAID)
Office of Communications
9000 Rockville Pike
Building 31, Room 7A32
Bethesda, MD 20892
301-496-5717 (telephone)

> The NIAID's packet contains summaries of all their recent research concerning CFIDS, including articles on hormone deficiencies, immune abnormalities, patient resources, mononucleosis, Epstein-Barr virus, and fibromyalgia. A copy of the CDC booklet is also included. Both are free.

Computer Networks

For those who are bedridden or find themselves some distance from support groups, computer networking provides easy access to information, companionship, and news. Several commercial services provide access to the Internet.

America Online (800-827-6364) has a weekly live chat session on CFIDS and a library of files. Notes are posted in the Disabilities area.

CompuServe (800-848-8990) has a CFIDS discussion in the Health and Fitness Forum. Members can visit the section by entering "GO CFIDS." For more information, contact Ed Isenburg (505-898-4635); on CompuServe at 72303, 1236; or on the Internet at isenburg@rt66.com.

DRAGnet, a nonprofit group, provides inexpensive access to computer technology for people with disabilities. For more information, write DRAGnet, 119 N. 4th Street, Suite 405 Textile Bldg., Minneapolis, MN 55401 (voice TDD: 612-338-2535; fax: 612-338-2569). DRAGnet Information Service, which provides a wide array of disability information, can be reached by computer and modem at 612-753-1943 (ANSI emulation. 8-N-1).

GEnie (800-638-9636 in U.S.; 800-387-8330 in Canada) has a CFIDS category, library of files, and a monthly conference. Once on GEnie MOVE to page 970 (type M970) to get to the DisABILITIES RoundTable. From the main menu you can enter the Bulletin Board. The CFS Category is #18, or visit the CFS Library (#11 from the Library menu). For further help, contact CFS Category Leader Lucie Dorais at GE Mail address L. DO-RAIS.

Prodigy (800-776-3449) has a CFIDS discussion group. Go to Medical Support bulletin board, then to CFIDS for questions and up-to-date information.

Internet provides the following resources:
- *http:/www.cais.net/CFS—news/* is the best website for obtaining information about CFIDS.
- *CFS-News* is an electronic newsletter that provides the latest news on CFIDS. For subscription information, contact CFS-NEWS@LIST.NIH.GOV.
- *CFS Newswire* is a news article exchange network. Contact the CFS/ME Computer Networking Project at CFS-ME@SJUVM.STJOHNS.EDU.
- *Catharsis* is an electronic magazine that focuses on health and creativity. For information, contact the editor at CATHAR-M@SJUVM.STJOHNS.EDU.
- *CFS-L* is an international on-line discussion group for people with CFS. For information, contact the moderator at CFS-L-REQUEST@LIST.NIH.GOV.
- Website for Teens: http://www.ypwcnet.org/index.htm

For more information about electronic networking and computer resources, contact the CFS/ME Computer Networking Project at CFS-ME@SJUVM.STJOHNS.EDU. or send an inquiry with a legal-size self-addressed stamped envelope to PO Box 11347, Washington, DC 20008-0547 or 3332 McCarthy Road, PO Box 37045, Ottawa, Ontario K1V 0W0, Canada. From outside the United States or Canada, send to either address and include an International Reply Coupon to cover return postage (see *CFIDS Chronicle*, Spring 1995 for detailed information about computer networking).

Networking by Mail

Pen-pal services are available for those who prefer to write letters. Please specify your age when inquiring.

PWC Pen-Pal List
15865-B Gale Avenue
Box 818
City of Industry, CA 91745
  Send 25 cents and a self-addressed stamped envelope.

CFS Youth Outreach
c/o Sharon Walk
14 Shetland Road
Florham Park, NJ 07932-1813
  CYO also publishes a quarterly for children with CFS.

CFIDS Friendship Network
PO Box 7202
Gainesville, FL 32605
  Send $1.00 and a legal-size self-addressed stamped envelope.

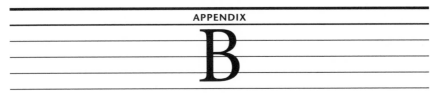

National and International Organizations

United States

The CFIDS Association of America
PO Box 220398
Charlotte, NC 28222-0398
800-442-3437 (toll-free telephone)
704-362-2343 (local telephone)
704-365-9755 (fax)
704-365-2343 (resources)
http://cfids.org/cfids (Internet home page)
info@cfids.org (e-mail)

> The CFIDS Association of America is the largest CFIDS organization in the United States. It publishes the quarterly, *The CFIDS Chronicle*, which contains treatment information, articles by leading CFIDS physicians, reports on national and international CFIDS conferences (including summaries of the presentations), updates on CFIDS research, as well as printing highly informative letters, editorials, and commentaries. The Association also distributes educational materials and will send a list of support groups and physicians in your area (send a self-addressed stamped envelope). The Association makes significant contributions to research efforts. Donations, which can be exclusively allocated to CFIDS research, are tax-deductible. Membership is $30.00.

CFIDS and Fibromyalgia Health Resource
1187 Coast Village Road, Suite 1-280
Santa Barbara, CA 93108-2794
800-366-6056 (toll-free telephone)
805-965-0042 (fax)

> The CFIDS and Fibromyalgia Health Resource offers high-quality supplements frequently recommended for people with CFIDS and publishes an informative newsletter, *Health Watch*, for members. Membership is free.

C.A.N.
PO Box 345
Larchmont, NY 10538
   or
720 Balboa Street
San Francisco, CA 94118
   C.A.N. (CFIDS Activation Network) represents two independent political advocacy networks.

National Chronic Fatigue Syndrome Association
3521 Broadway, Suite 222
   or
PO Box 18426
Kansas City, MO 64111
816-931-4777 (telephone)
   The National CFS Association publishes a quarterly, *Heart of America News,* and distributes several other publications at nominal cost. Membership is $25.00 for addresses from the United States and $35 for foreign addresses. The National CFS Association's board takes the position that there is no treatment for CFS or fibromyalgia.

RESCIND, Inc.
9812 Falls Road, Suite 114-270
Potomac, MD 20854
301-983-5644 (fax after 6:00 ET)
MAY12@American.edu (Internet address)
   RESCIND (Repeal Existing Stereotypes about Chronic Immunological and Neurological Diseases) was established to call attention to four similar conditions: CFIDS/ME, fibromyalgia, multiple chemical sensitivities, and Gulf War Syndrome. RESCIND is a nonprofit organization with no paid employees. Donations are gratefully accepted.

CHILDREN

National Information Center for Children and Youth With Disabilities
PO Box 1492
Washington, DC 20013
   The National Information Center for Children and Youth With Disabilities provides free information to assist parents, teachers, caregivers, and others in helping children become participating members of the community.

CFIDS Youth Alliance
PO Box 220398
Charlotte, NC 28222-0398
800-442-3437 (toll-free telephone)
   The CFIDS Youth Alliance (CYA), a daughter organization of the CFIDS Association of America, was founded by a 19-year-old girl whose main goals were to expand awareness about pediatric CFIDS and to represent the needs and concerns of people with CFIDS aged 24 years and younger. The CYA publishes a quarterly newsletter, *Youth Allied by CFIDS,* available to CFIDS Association members ($15.00 in U.S.; $20.00 in Canada; $25.00 overseas) and to nonmembers ($20.00 in U.S.; $25.00 in Canada; $30.00 overseas).

Pen-Pals

CFIDS Friendship Network
PO Box 7202
Gainesville, FL 32605
> The CFIDS Friendship Network will send a pen-pal questionnaire to help match you as closely as possible with a new friend (send a legal-size self-addressed stamped envelope with $1.00).

CFS Youth Outreach
c/o Sharon Walk
14 Shetland Road
Florham Park, NJ 07932-1813
> A pen-pal service for children only. CFS Youth Outreach also publishes a quarterly newsletter for children with CFS.

Teen CFIDS Pen-Pal Connection
c/o Connie Howard
1810 Cliffwood Court
New Albany, IN 47150
> Teenagers 10 to 19 years old who would like to write other teens with CFIDS can receive a brief questionnaire to be matched with a teen who shares similar hobbies and interests (send a self-addressed stamped envelope and 25 cents).

ORGANIZATIONS FOR HEALTH PROFESSIONALS

American Association for Chronic Fatigue Syndrome (AACFS)
Dr. Paul Levine, President
PO Box 895
Olney, MD 20832
> The objectives of the AACFS are to promote, stimulate, and coordinate the exchange of ideas related to CFS research, patient care, and treatment and to periodically review current CFS literature. Clinicians, research professionals, and health care workers engaged in CFIDS activities may apply for membership.

Medical Professionals/Persons With CFIDS (MPWC)
Lori Clovis
PO Box 144
Hinsdale, NY 14743
http://www.geocities.com/HotSprings/2744/ (website)
> MPWC, an organization for medical professionals, publishes the quarterly *MPWC News*. Subscription is $10.00 a year. For more information, send a legal-size self-addressed stamped envelope with a 64-cent stamp.

Gail E. Dahlen, R.N.
50 N. Cecil Avenue
Indianapolis, IN 46219
> This group was formed to help develop advocacy programs, exchange information, and provide mutual support for health care workers with CFIDS.

Thomas L. English, M.D.
PO Box 18267
Asheville, NC 28814

This group would like to hear from physicians with CFIDS. Tentative goals of the group are advocacy and physician education.

SUPPORT FOR CFS CAREGIVERS

Well Spouse Foundation
PO Box 801
New York, NY 10023
212-644-1241 (local telephone)
800-838-0879 (toll-free telephone)

REGIONAL ORGANIZATIONS

Note: Many state organizations provide information packets, referral services, hotlines, and up-to-date regional information.

Northeast

Massachusetts CFIDS Association
808 Main Street
Waltham, MA 02154

The Massachusetts CFIDS organization distributes several useful CFIDS publications for $5.00 each. All proceeds go to CFIDS research and education.
- *CFS: A Primer for Physicians and Allied Health Professionals* (excellent)
- *How to Apply for Social Security Disability Benefits If You Have CFS*
- *Training Manual for CFIDS Support Groups, CFIDS: Investigating the Mystery 1.1* (a computer program)

CFS Crisis Center
27 W. 20th Street, Suite 703
New York, NY 10011
212-691-4800 (telephone)

Greater New York CFS Coalition
880 Pine Avenue
West Islip, NY 11795
516-548-8237 (telephone)

South

Gulf Coast CFIDS Association
752 J Avenue Estancias
Venice, FL 34292-2316
813-484-0706 (telephone)

Midwest

Chicago CFS Association
818 Wenonah Avenue
Oak Park, IL 60304
708-524-9322 (telephone)

Wisconsin CFS Association
PO Box 442
Thiensville, WI 53092

West

Los Angeles CFIDS Association
PO Box 5414
Sherman Oaks, CA 91413
818-785-8301 (telephone)
818-458-9192 (recorded information)

Southern California CFIDS Association, Inc.
23732 Hillhurst Drive, #U-9
Laguna Niguel, CA 92677
714-249-6976 (telephone)

CFIDS New Mexico
PO Box 3642
Albuquerque, NM 87190-3642
505-899-0954 (telephone)
Publishes the *CFIDS Update* ($10.00).

Utah CFIDS Association, Inc.
PO Box 511257
Salt Lake City, UT 84151
801-461-3378 (telephone)

Canada

The M.E. Association of Canada
246 Queen Street, Suite 400
Ottawa, Ontario K1P 5E4, Canada
613-563-1565 (telephone)
613-567-0614 (fax)
http://www.mecan.ca/ (Internet home page)
info@mccan.ca (e-mail)

> The M.E. Association publishes a monthly newsletter, *The MEssenger,* distributed throughout Canada, England, and Australia. *The MEssenger* contains information about medical treatment, personal stories about people with CFIDS, articles (some in French), and book reviews. The Association provides physician and support group referrals on request and houses a walk-in library with literature on CFS/ME (also available worldwide free of charge on the Internet). Membership is $40.00.

The Nightingale Research Foundation
383 Danforth Avenue
Ottawa, Ontario K2A 0E1, Canada
613-728-9643 (telephone)
613-729-0825 (fax)
http://www.cyberus.ca/~bhyde/ (website)

> The Nightingale Research Foundation publishes a quarterly magazine on new medical information about CFIDS and a comprehensive, 750-page book on medical aspects of CFIDS (available at a considerable discount for people with CFIDS). It also conducts research and sponsors public education programs for the international CFIDS/ME community. Membership is $35.00.

National ME/FM Action Network
3836 Carling Avenue
Hwy 17B
Nepean, Ontario K2H 7V2, Canada

> The purpose of this patient support organization, formed in 1993, is to deal with patient issues, including insurance problems, government, children and the school system, media, lack of proper medical testing, physician and lawyer referrals. Dues are $20.00 a year.

United Kingdom

ME Association of Great Britain
Stanhope House
High Street
Stanford le Hope
Essex SS17 OHA
England
01375-642-466 (telephone)
01375-360-256 (fax)
http://www.compulink.co.uk/~deepings/welcome (Internet home page)

ME Association Northern Ireland
28 Bedford Street
Belfast BT2 7FE
Northern Ireland
01232-439-831 (telephone)

ME Association Scotland
52 St. Enoch Square
Glasgow G1 4AW
Scotland
01-41-204-3822 (telephone)

> The ME Association is Great Britain's largest national ME organization. It publishes a quarterly magazine, *Perspectives,* runs information and advice lines, distributes free leaflets, conducts seminars and training sessions, funds research, and provides advocacy and representation for employment and insurance problems. Dues are £15 a year (£25 outside the U.K.).

ME Action Campaign
PO Box 1126
London W3 ORY
England

Action for ME
PO Box 1302
Wells, Somerset BA5 2WE
England
> Dues are £12.5 a year.

New Zealand

A.N.Z.M.E. Society
PO Box 35-429
Browns Bay
Auckland 10
North Island

A.N.Z.Y.M.E., Inc.
PO Box 36307
Northcote
Auckland 1309
North Island
ejoconnl@ihug.co.n2 (e-mail)
> Publishes the quarterly magazine, *Meeting Place*. Dues are $35.00 a year.

Australia

ANZAMES
PO Box 645
Mona Vale, New South Wales 2103

ME Society of Western Australia
PO Box 75
Tuart Hill, Western Australia 6060
61-09-483-6667 (telephone)

ME/CFS Society of New South Wales
Royal South Sydney Community Health
  Centre
Joynton Avenue
Zetland, New South Wales 2017
61-02-382-8267 (information)
61-02-906-2906 (social worker)

ME/CFS Society of South Australia
PO Box 383, GPO
Adelaide, South Australia 500l
61-08-373-2110 (telephone)

ME/CFS Society of Victoria
23 Livingston Close
Burwood, Victoria
61-03-888-8991 (telephone)

ME Syndrome Society of Queensland
PO Box 938
Fortitude Valley, Queensland 4006
61-07-32-5217 (telephone)

Europe

ME Fonds
c/o Hanneke Los, Pres.
Kennedylaan 745
1079 MR Amsterdam
The Netherlands
31-020-644-5566 (telephone)
31-020-644-5440 (fax)
mef@xs4all.nl (e-mail)

ME Lobby
c/o Marc Fluks
de Bosch Kemperpad 136
l054 PM Amsterdam
The Netherlands
31-020-618-9095 (telephone)
melobby@dds.nl (e-mail)

ME Stichting
Robert Scottsstraat 4
1056 AX Amsterdam
The Netherlands

Ms. Alice Vertomme
Dorp 7
3221 Niew Rode
Belgium
32-16-570983 (telephone)

Danish ME/CFS Association
c/o A Midsem
Maglehoj 86
DK - 3520 Farum
Denmark

Norges M.E. Forening
Eikveien 96A
1345 Osteras
Norway
47-2-2 (telephone)

Selbsthilfegruppe CFS-Syndrome
c/o Birke Steinitz
An St. Swidbert 52, D-40489
Duesseldorf
Germany
49-211-404376 (telephone)

C.F.S. Associazione Italia
Segretaria: Via Moimacco 20
33100 Udin
Italy

Organizations for Related Conditions

American Academy of Allergy and
    Immunology
611 East Wells Street
Milwaukee, WI 53202
800-822-2762 (toll-free telephone)
    or
800 East Northwest Highway, Suite 1080
Palatine, IL 60067-6516
847-427-1200 (hotline)

American Chronic Pain Association
    Outreach
PO Box 850
Rocklin, CA 95677
916-632- 0922 (telephone)

American Sleep Disorders Association
1610 14th Street NW, Suite 300
Rochester, MN 55901

Arthritis Foundation
PO Box 19000
Atlanta, GA 30326
800-283-7800 (toll-free telephone)

Asthma Information Line
PO Box 1766
Rochester, NY 14603
800-727-5400 (toll-free telephone)

Candida Research Foundation
1638 B Street
Haward, CA 94511
510-582-2179 (telephone)

Chemical Injury Information Network
PO Box 301
White Sulphur Springs, MD 59645-0301
406-547-2255 (telephone)

Environmental Health Association
1800 S. Robertson Blvd., Suite 380
Los Angeles, CA 90035
301-837-2048 (telephone)

Environmental Health Network
PO Box 1155
Larkspur, CA 94977
415-541-5075 (telephone)

Fibromyalgia Network
5700 Stockdale Hwy, #100
Bakersfield, CA 93309
805-631-1950 (telephone)

Food Allergy Network
10400 Eaton Place, Suite 107
Fairfax, VA 22030-5647
800-929-4040 (telephone)

Human Ecology Action League
PO Box 49126
Atlanta, GA 30359
404-248-1898 (telephone)

Lupus Foundation of America
4 Research Place, Suite 180
Rockville, MD 20850-3226

National Center for Environmental Health
Strategies
1100 Rural Avenue
Voorhees, NJ 08043
609-429-5358 (telephone)

National Chronic Pain Association
7979 Old Georgetown Road, Suite 100
Bethesda, MD 20814-2429
301-652-4948 (telephone)

National Foundation of Chemical
Hypersensitivities and Allergies
PO Box 222
Ophelia, VA 22530
804-453-7538 (telephone)

National Gulf War Resource Center, Inc.
1224 M Street NW
Washington, DC 20005
202-628-2700, ext. 162 (telephone)
202-628-6997 (fax)
gulfvet@fwbell.net (e-mail)
www.gulfwar.org/resourcecenter/ (website)

National Organization for Rare Disorders
PO Box 8923
New Fairfield, CT 06812-8923
203-746-6518 (local telephone)
800-999-6673 (toll-free telephone)

National Organization for Seasonal
Affective Disorder
PO Box 40133
Washington, DC 20016

Rheumatoid Arthritis Foundation
615-646-1030 (telephone)

Sjögren's Syndrome Foundation, Inc.
333 N. Broadway, Suite 2000
Jericho, NY 11753
516-933-6365 (local telephone)
800-475-6473 (toll-free telephone)
516-933-6368 (fax)
http://www.sjogrens.com (website)

Society for Mitral Valve Prolapse Syndrome
PO Box 431
Itasca, IL 60143-0431

Other Useful Organizations

Government Entitlement Services
23930 Michigan Avenue
Dearborn, MI 48124
800-628-2887 (toll-free telephone)

Benefits Resource Network
Kennedy Krieger Institute
2911 East Biddle Street
Baltimore, MD 21213
410-767-7452 (telephone)

Clearinghouse on Disability Information
Office of Special Education and Rehabilitation Services
U.S. Department of Education
Room 3132, Switzer Building
Washington, DC 20202
202-205-8241 (telephone)

U.S. Social Security Administration
800-772-1213 (7:00 AM to 7:00 PM weekdays)

> The Social Security Administration pays disability benefits under two programs: the Social Security Disability Insurance Program and the Supplemental Security Income (SSI) Program. Medical requirements for both programs are the same. Eligibility for Social Security is based on prior work history and SSI benefits are based on financial need. Most people with CFIDS who apply for Social Security are denied once or twice and must go through an appeals process.

National Organization of Social Security Claimants Representatives
(a lawyer referral service)
800-431-2804 (telephone)

> Most people have greater success with experienced lawyers than with filing their own appeals. Lawyers who process Social Security appeals usually charge a percentage of back payments owed you by the government (if your appeal is successful).

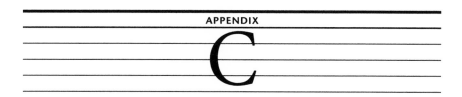

CFIDS Clinics, Clinicians, and Laboratories

The following is a list of clinics, clinicians, and researchers who have made contributions in the area of CFIDS treatment. It is by no means a complete list. A comprehensive directory is currently being marketed by Morgan-Rand Publishing in association with the CFIDS Association of America. It includes caregivers, physicians, clinics, hospitals, support groups, and advocacy groups for CFIDS in the United States. It is available through the CFIDS Assocation for $19.95 (for members) or can be purchased directly from Morgan-Rand Publishing for $34.90. For more information call 215-938-5511.

If you are seeking a clinician, either to diagnose or treat CFIDS, we strongly recommend you contact the appropriate national organization (see Appendix B) and ask for a listing of local support groups. Since most specialists require that you have a local primary health care physician to monitor treatments, it is well worth the effort to find a cooperative physician *before* you seek the services of a specialist. Your local support group leader should be able to provide a listing of recommended physicians in your area.

United States

Majid Ali, M.D.
Institute of Preventive Medicine
95 E. Main Street
Denville, NJ 07834
201-586-4111 (telephone)

David Bell, M.D.
77 South Main Street
Lyndonville, NY 14098
716-765-2060 (telephone)

Sheila Bastien, Ph.D.
2126 Los Angeles Avenue
Berkeley, CA 94707
510-526-7391 (telephone)

Center for Progressive Medicine
Steven Bock, M.D., and Kenneth Bock,
  M.D., Directors
Pinnacle Place, Suite 210
10 McKown Road
Albany, NY 12203
518-435-0082 (telephone)
  or
Rhinebeck Health Center
108 Montgomery Street
Rhinebeck, NY 12572
914-876-7082 (telephone)

Center for Specialized Immunology
400 Arthur Godfrey Road, Suite 504
Miami Beach, FL 33140
305-672-5009 (telephone)

Cheney Clinic
Paul Cheney, M.D., Ph.D.
10620 Park Road, Suite 234
Charlotte, NC 28210
704-542-7444 (telephone)

Chronic Fatigue Clinic
Dedra Buchwald, M.D., Director
Harborview Medical Center ZX-21
325 Ninth Avenue, 5 South, Room 36
Seattle, WA 98104
206-731-3111 (telephone)

Chronic Fatigue and Immune Disorder
  Center
Patricia Salvato, M.D., Medical Director
4140 Southwest Freeway
Houston, TX 77027
713-961-7100 (telephone)

Chronic Fatigue Syndrome Center
Benjamin Natelson, M.D., Director
90 Bergen Street, Suite 4100
Newark, NJ 07103-2499
201-982-2552 (telephone)

Chronic Fatigue Syndrome Institute
Jay Goldstein, M.D., Director
6200 East Canyon Rim Road, Suite 110D
Anaheim Hills, CA 92807
714-998-2780 (telephone)

Alexander Chester, M.D.
3301 New Mexico Avenue NW, #348
Washington, DC 20016
202-362-4467 (telephone)

Kristina Dahl, M.D.
133 East 73rd Street
New York, NY 10021
212-861-9000 (telephone)

Environmental Health Center
8345 Walnut Hill Lane, Suite 220
Dallas, TX 75231
214-368-4132 (telephone)
www.ehcd.com (website)

Fatigue Clinic of Michigan
Edward Conley, M.D., Director
G3494 Beecher Road
Flint, MI 48522
810-230-8677 (telephone)

Fibromyalgia Center
Paul Lasky, M.D., Director
747 Chestnut Ridge Road
Chestnut Ridge, NY 10977
914-578-1758 (telephone)

Jorge Flechas, M.D.
724 5th Avenue West
Hendersonville, NC 28739
704-693-3015 (telephone)

Fred Friedberg, Ph.D. (psychologist)
6 Yorktown Road
Setauket, NY 11733
516-751-4924 (telephone)
  or
111 Lambert Road
Sharon, CT 06069
860-364-1107 (telephone)

Leo Galland, M.D.
133 East 73rd Street
New York, NY 10021
212-861-9000 (telephone)

Michael Goldberg, M.D. (pediatric CFIDS)
5620 Wilbur Avenue, Suite 318
Tarzana, CA 91356
818-343-1010 (telephone)

Don Goldenberg, M.D. (fibromyalgia)
Newton-Wellesley Hospital
2000 Washington Street, Suite 304
Newton, MA 02162
617-243-5440 (telephone)

Linda Miller Iger, Ph.D.
Chronic Fatigue Syndrome Institute
6200 East Canyon Rim Road, Suite 110D
Anaheim Hills, CA 92807
714-998-2780 (telephone)

James Jones, M.D.
National Jewish Medical and Research
  Center
1400 Jackson Street
Denver, CO 80206
303-388-4461 (telephone)

Nancy Klimas, M.D.
Director, Diagnostic Immunology Clinic
   and Center for Specialized Immunology
400 Arthur Godfrey Road, Suite 504
Miami Beach, FL 33140
305-672-5009 (telephone)

Anthony Komaroff, M.D.
   (not accepting new patients)
Chief, Division of General Medicine
Harvard Medical School
Brigham and Women's Hospital
75 Francis Street
Boston, MA 02115
617-732-6077 (telephone)

Charles Lapp, M.D.
10724 Park Road
Bldg. 100, Suite 105
Charlotte, NC 28210
704-543-9692 (telephone)

Susan Levine, M.D.
200 West 86th Street
New York, NY 10021
212-472-4816 (telephone)
   or
889 Lexington Avenue
New York, NY 10021
212-472-4816 (telephone)

Mark Loveless, M.D.
Oregon Health Sciences University
Division of Infectious Diseases
3181 SW Jackson Park Road
Portland, OR 97201
503-494-8311 (telephone)

Daniel Peterson, M.D.
Sierra Internal Medicine
865 Tahoe Blvd., Suite 306
Incline Village, NV 89451
702-832-0989 (telephone)
   mailing address:
PO Box 7870
Incline Village, NV 89452

Sigita Plioplys, M.D., and Audrius Plioplys,
   M.D. (research)
CFS Center
Mercy Hospital
Chicago, IL 60616
312-445-0123 (telephone)

Richard Podell, M.D.
571 Central Avenue, Suite 106
New Providence, NJ 07974
908-464-3800 (telephone)

Michael Rosenbaum, M.D., and Murray
   Susser, M.D.
2730 Wilshire Blvd., Suite 110
Santa Monica, CA 90403
310-453-4424 (telephone)

I. Jon Russell, M.D., Ph.D. (fibromyalgia)
Director, Brady-Green Clinical Research
   Center
University of Texas Health Science Center
San Antonio, TX 78284
210-358-4000 (telephone)

Jay Seastrunk, M.D.
102 East Freeman Street
Duncanville, TX 75116
972-709-4834 (telephone)

Neil Singer, M.D. (internist)
Sedona Medical Center
3700 W. Highway 89-A
Sedona, AZ 86336
520-204-4900 (telephone)

Thomas Steinbach, M.D.
902 Frostwood, Suite 243
Houston, TX 77024
713-467-6471 (telephone)

Jacob Teitelbaum, M.D.
139 Old Solomons Island Road
Annapolis, MD 21401
410-224-2222 (telephone)

Ruth Walkotten, D.O.
427 W. Seminole Road
Muskegon, MI 49441
616-733-1989 (telephone)

Canada

Environmental Clinic
PO Box 1230
Fall River, Nova Scotia B2T 1K6
902-860-0057 (telephone)

Nightingale Research Foundation
Byron Hyde, M.D., and Anil Jain, M.D.
121 Iona Street
Ottawa, Ontario K2A OE3

Post-Polio Syndrome, CFS, Fibromylagia
  Clinic
Beverly Tompkins, M.D.
1228 Kensington Road, NW
Main Floor, Kensington Professional Center
Calgary, Alberta T2N 4P9
403-270-6896 (telephone)

United Kingdom

Ted Dinan
Professor, Department of Psychological
  Medicine
St. Bartholomew's Hospital (Medical
  College)
West Smithfield
London, England
0171-601-8138 (telephone)

Leslie Findley, M.D.
Devonshire Hospital
29-31 Devonshire Street
London, England
0171-486-7131 (telephone)

Laboratories

Great Smokies Diagnostic Laboratory
Martin Lee and Stephen Barrie Associates
63 Zillicoa Street
Asheville, NC 28801-1074
800-522-4762 (toll-free telephone in United States)
800-268-6200 (toll-free telephone in Canada)
  Intestinal permeability detection (leaky gut), parasites, Candida, and comprehensive
  stool analysis.

Immunocomp Laboratory, Inc.
James McCoy, M.D., Director
11919 Sunray Avenue, Suite C
Baton Rouge, LA 70816
504-293-3698 (telephone)
  Expert in lymphocyte-immune competence and identification of proper drug agents
  for disease treatment. Tests for exact dosage levels of drugs recommended by your
  physician for maximum effectiveness. Health insurance carriers reimburse 80% to
  100% of laboratory tests.

Immunosciences Lab, Inc.
8730 Wilshire Blvd., Suite 305
Beverly Hills, CA 90211
800-950-4686 (toll-free telephone)
310-657-1077 (local telephone)

> Tests for mycoplasma incognitas, Rnase-L inhibitor, immune system panel for CFIDS, viral panel for CFIDS (Epstein-Barr virus, human herpesvirus 6, cytomegalovirus), natural killer cells, interferon, Candida.

MetaMetrix Medical Laboratory
J. Alexander Bralley, Ph.D., Director
5000 Peachtree Industrial Blvd., Suite #110
Norcross, GA 30071
770-446-5483 (telephone)

> Nutritional testing, Organic Acids Test ($349.00), amino acids panels blood test ($310.00 for a 40-panel test; $263.00 for a 20-panel test), food antibodies test ($170.00 for 90 foods).

Ms. Sue Dorney
Department of Biological Sciences
The University of Newcastle
Callaghan, New South Wales 2308
Australia

> Test for the presence of CFSUM1 ($175.00 U.S.).

Mail-Order Suppliers

Nutritional Supplements

Bronson
1945 Craig Road, PO Box 46903
St. Louis, MO 63146-6903
800-235-3200 (toll-free telephone)
314-469-5741 (fax)
> Reasonably priced vitamins, amino acids, herbs, personal care products, digestive aids, minerals, and antioxidants obtained directly from the manufacturer.

CFIDS and Fibromyalgia Health Resource
1187 Coast Village Road, Suite 1-280
Santa Barbara, CA 93108-2794
800-366-6056 (toll-free telephone)
> High-quality vitamins, minerals, amino acids, CoQ10, and other food supplements used by people with CFIDS. A portion of the profits goes to support CFIDS research.

L&H Vitamins
37-10 Crescent Street
Long Island City, NY 11101
800-221-1152 (toll-free telephone)
> Name-brand vitamins, minerals, probiotics, enzymes, and food supplements at 20% to 40% discount; large selection, fast delivery.

NEEDS Catalogue
527 Charles Avenue, Suite 12-A
Syracuse, NY 13209
800-634-1380 (toll-free telephone)
315-488-6336 (fax)
> A huge selection of brand-name vitamins, supplements, herbs, Bach remedies, and glandular preparations at a discount.

Sun-Ray Supply
524 Shamrock Lane
Dawsonville, GA 30534
800-437-1765 (toll-free telephone)
706-265-4680 (fax)

> Sublingual CoQ10 troches, Reliv, UltraClear, oral spray vitamins, probioplex, pyc-nogenol, vitamins, minerals, herbs, water and air filters, and other natural products for people with CFIDS.

Trans-Pacific Health Products
3934 Central Avenue
St. Petersburg, FL 33711
800-336-9636 (toll-free telephone)

> Chinese herbs for sinus infections, allergies, yeast control, low blood sugar, PMS, arthritis, flu and colds, alertness, eyes, circulation, herpes, headaches, immune system, hair loss, liver function, and more.

Wellness Health & Pharmaceuticals
2800 South 18th Street
Birmingham, AL 35209
800-227-2627 (toll-free telephone)

> National brands, including Allergy Research Group, Kal, Montana Naturals, Nature's Way, Natrol, Schiff, Twinlab, Kyolic, Cardiovascular Research Ltd., and Rainbow Light, at a discount.

Willner Chemists
100 Park Avenue
New York, NY 10017
800-633-1106 (toll-free telephone)
212-685-2538 (local telephone)
212-685-0441 (local telephone)

> Wide selection of specialty supplements, personal care products, herbs, and naturo-pathic remedies.

Nontoxic Home and Health Products

AFM Enterprises, Inc.
1140 Stacy Court
Riverside, CA 92507
714-781-6860 (telephone)

> Nontoxic paints, stains, waxes, enamels, adhesives, caulking, carpet guards, mildew control, and other products especially formulated for people with chemical sensitivi-ties.

Allergy Resources, Inc.
557 Burbank Street, Suite K
Broomfield, CO 80020
800-873-3529 (800-USE-FLAX) (toll-free telephone)

> Air purifiers, food products, supplements, Lifespan vitamin protocols, natural cosmet-ics, cotton bedding, cleaning products, kitchen aids, water filters, and books for people with allergies and multiple chemical sensitivities.

Auro Organic Paints
Sinan Co. Natural Building Materials
PO Box 181
Suisun City, CA 94585
707-427-2325 (telephone)
> Manufactures paints, varnishes, waxes, glues, cleansers, and polishes made from beeswax, natural oils, chalk, plants, and other natural ingredients.

The Body Shop
106 Iron Mountain Road
Mine Hill, NJ 07803
201-984-2536 (local telephone)
800-541-2535 (toll-free telephone)
> Cosmetics, lotions, shampoos, soaps, body brushes, and other personal care products.

CFIDS and Fibromyalgia Health Resource
1187 Coast Village Road, Suite 1-280
Santa Barbara, CA 93108-2794
800-366-6056 (toll-free telephone)
> Nontoxic cleaners, soaps, shampoos, skin lotions, deodorants, and other chemical-free personal and home products.

Coast Filtration
142 Viking Avenue
Brea, CA 92621
714-990-4602 (telephone)
714-990-3951 (telephone)
> Reverse osmosis and carbon water filtration systems and ultraviolet lights. The staff is very helpful.

KB Cotton Pillows, Inc.
PO Box 57
De Soto, TX 75123
800-544-3752 (toll-free telephone)
> All natural cotton pillows (even the thread).

Living Source
Products for the Chemically Sensitive
PO Box 20155
Waco, TX 76702
817-776-4878 (local telephone)
800-662-8787 (voice mail)
817-776-9329 (fax)
> Large selection of personal care products, cotton mattresses, pillow covers, blankets, books, charts, pet care products, oxygen equipment, cotton masks, air and water filters, moisture absorbers, ozone purification systems, room heaters, juicers, water softeners, vacuums, cleaners, gardening products, and nontoxic building supplies. Many unusual and hard-to-get products.

Livos Plant Chemistry
2641 Cerrillos Road
Santa Fe, NM 87501
505-988-9111 (telephone)
> Manufactures paints, oil finishes, shellacs, stains, varnishes, adhesives, thinners, waxes, and polishes made from natural ingredients.

The Natural Bedroom
PO Box 2048
Sebastopol, CA 95472-2048
800-365-6563 (toll-free telephone)
707-823-0106 (fax)
> Natural and organic cotton products for the bedroom, including camisoles, night-shirts, bathrobes, towels, rugs, sheets, pillows, comforters, mattresses, and box springs.

NEEDS Catalogue
527 Charles Avenue, Suite 12-A
Syracuse, NY 13209
800-634-1380 (toll-free telephone)
315-488-6336 (fax)
> Large selection of cosmetics, household products, paints, air purifiers, water filters, and other products for people with chemical sensitivities. No order is too small.

Nigra Enterprises
5699 Kanan, #123
Agoura Hills, CA 91301
818-889-6877 (telephone)
> Water purification systems (carbon, reverse osmosis, home distillation), ultraviolet lights. Information given over the telephone.

Nontoxic Environments
PO Box 384
Newmarket, NH 03857
800-789-4348 (toll-free telephone)
> Nontoxic building supplies, air filters, water purifiers, cleaning products, books, videos, supplements, and more.

The Old Fashioned Milk Paint Company
436 Main Street
Groton, MA 01450-0222
508-448-6336 (telephone)
508-448-2754 (fax)
> Manufactures milk paint from milk protein, lime clay, and earth pigments; contains no lead, chemical preservatives, fungicides, or petrochemicals (available in 16 colors).

Priorities
70 Walnut Street
Wellesley, MA 02181
800-553-5398 (toll-free telephone)
> HEPA vacuums, water purifiers, lead, radon, and carbon dioxide testing kits, window air filters, and other products designed for people with allergies.

Real Goods
555 Leslie Street
Ukiah, CA 95482-5507
800-762-7325 (toll-free telephone)
> Nontoxic personal care products, face masks, laundry disks, dioxin-free paper products, solar and other environmentally conscious products.

Seventh Generation
360 Interlocken Blvd., Suite 300
Broomfield, CO 80021
800-456-1177 (toll-free telephone)
> Biodegradable soaps, natural shoe polishes, water filters, natural shampoos, and personal care products.

Audiotapes

Sounds True Catalogue
PO Box 8010
Boulder, CO 80306-8010
800-333-9185 (toll-free telephone)
303-665-3151 (local telephone)
> Self-help, psychology, meditation, inspirational, alternative health, and music with Deepak Chopra, Thich Nhat Hanh, Desmond Tutu, Ram Dass, Sogyal Rinpoche, and other spiritual luminaries. Over 300 audiotapes and videotapes.

Green Island Productions, Inc.
PO Box 368
Greenfield, MA 01301
800-438-0956 (toll-free telephone)
> Novels, poetry, history, interviews, science fiction, health. Hundreds of titles for sale or rent. Call for a free brochure.

E

CFIDS Treatment Survey

Your first name _____ State _____ Age _____ Sex _____

When did you first become ill? _____

Was onset sudden or gradual (over a few months or years)? _____

Has CFIDS been diagnosed? _____ By whom? _____

Please rate the severity of your illness (0 = bedridden; 10 = recovered):

| 0 | 1 | 2 | 3 | 4 | 5 | 6 | 7 | 8 | 9 | 10 |

What are your worst symptoms? _____

_____

_____

_____

_____

TREATMENTS

Please rate any treatments you have tried. Include dosage.

	Not sure	Harmful	No effect	Helpful	Very helpful
Pharmaceuticals					
Ampligen	_____	_____	_____	_____	_____
Antidepressants					
Sinequan	_____	_____	_____	_____	_____
Elavil	_____	_____	_____	_____	_____
Prozac	_____	_____	_____	_____	_____
Zoloft	_____	_____	_____	_____	_____
MAOIs: _____	_____	_____	_____	_____	_____
Wellbutrin	_____	_____	_____	_____	_____
Other: _____	_____	_____	_____	_____	_____

	Not sure	Harmful	No effect	Helpful	Very helpful
Pharmaceuticals—cont'd					
Antifungals	_____	_____	_____	_____	_____
Nystatin	_____	_____	_____	_____	_____
Diflucan	_____	_____	_____	_____	_____
Nizoral	_____	_____	_____	_____	_____
Sporanox	_____	_____	_____	_____	_____
Antihistamines					
Claritin	_____	_____	_____	_____	_____
Hismanal	_____	_____	_____	_____	_____
Benadryl	_____	_____	_____	_____	_____
Atarax	_____	_____	_____	_____	_____
Other:_____	_____	_____	_____	_____	_____
Antivirals					
Acyclovir	_____	_____	_____	_____	_____
Famvir	_____	_____	_____	_____	_____
Amantadine	_____	_____	_____	_____	_____
Benzodiazepines					
Klonopin	_____	_____	_____	_____	_____
Valium	_____	_____	_____	_____	_____
Xanax	_____	_____	_____	_____	_____
Other:_____	_____	_____	_____	_____	_____
Beta Blockers					
Atenolol	_____	_____	_____	_____	_____
Other:_____	_____	_____	_____	_____	_____
Calcium Channel Blockers					
Nicardipene	_____	_____	_____	_____	_____
Verapamil	_____	_____	_____	_____	_____
Other:_____	_____	_____	_____	_____	_____
CNS Stimulants					
Cylert	_____	_____	_____	_____	_____
Ritalin	_____	_____	_____	_____	_____
Other:_____	_____	_____	_____	_____	_____
Cytotec	_____	_____	_____	_____	_____
Diamox	_____	_____	_____	_____	_____
Flexeril	_____	_____	_____	_____	_____

	Not sure	Harmful	No effect	Helpful	Very helpful
Pharmaceuticals—cont'd					
Florinef	_____	_____	_____	_____	_____
Gamma Globulin	_____	_____	_____	_____	_____
Guaifenesin	_____	_____	_____	_____	_____
Hydrocortisone	_____	_____	_____	_____	_____
Kutapressin	_____	_____	_____	_____	_____
Naltrexone	_____	_____	_____	_____	_____
Nitroglycerin	_____	_____	_____	_____	_____
Oxytocin	_____	_____	_____	_____	_____
Pain Relievers					
NSAIDs:_____	_____	_____	_____	_____	_____
Acetominophen	_____	_____	_____	_____	_____
Narcotics	_____	_____	_____	_____	_____
Pentoxifylline	_____	_____	_____	_____	_____
Tagamet (cimetidine)	_____	_____	_____	_____	_____
Transfer factor	_____	_____	_____	_____	_____
Zantac (ranitidine)	_____	_____	_____	_____	_____
Other:_____	_____	_____	_____	_____	_____
Nutritional Supplements and Botanicals					
Alpha Ketoglutarate	_____	_____	_____	_____	_____
Amino Acids					
Carnitine	_____	_____	_____	_____	_____
Glutamine	_____	_____	_____	_____	_____
Glutathione	_____	_____	_____	_____	_____
Lysine	_____	_____	_____	_____	_____
Taurine	_____	_____	_____	_____	_____
Other: _____	_____	_____	_____	_____	_____
Bioflavonoids:_____	_____	_____	_____	_____	_____
Blue-Green Algae	_____	_____	_____	_____	_____
Butyric acid (Butyrex)	_____	_____	_____	_____	_____
CoQ10 (ubiquinone)	_____	_____	_____	_____	_____
DHEA	_____	_____	_____	_____	_____
Entero-Hepatic Resuscitation	_____	_____	_____	_____	_____

	Not sure	Harmful	No effect	Helpful	Very helpful
Nutritional Supplements and Botanicals—cont'd					
Essential Fatty Acids					
Evening primrose oil	____	____	____	____	____
Borage seed oil	____	____	____	____	____
Fish oils	____	____	____	____	____
Other:_____	____	____	____	____	____
Herbs					
Astragalus	____	____	____	____	____
Echinacea	____	____	____	____	____
Gingko	____	____	____	____	____
Ginseng	____	____	____	____	____
Licorice	____	____	____	____	____
Milk thistle	____	____	____	____	____
Valerian	____	____	____	____	____
Other:_____	____	____	____	____	____
LEM	____	____	____	____	____
Malic acid	____	____	____	____	____
Melatonin	____	____	____	____	____
Minerals					
Calcium	____	____	____	____	____
Magnesium	____	____	____	____	____
Zinc	____	____	____	____	____
Other:_____	____	____	____	____	____
NADH	____	____	____	____	____
Probioplex	____	____	____	____	____
Probiotics/acidophilus	____	____	____	____	____
Pycnogenol	____	____	____	____	____
Royal jelly	____	____	____	____	____
Sambucol	____	____	____	____	____
Vitamins					
Beta carotene	____	____	____	____	____
Vitamin B_{12}	____	____	____	____	____
Vitamin C	____	____	____	____	____
Vitamin E	____	____	____	____	____
Other:_____	____	____	____	____	____

	Not sure	Harmful	No effect	Helpful	Very helpful

Alternative and Complementary Medical and Supportive Therapies

	Not sure	Harmful	No effect	Helpful	Very helpful
Acupressure	____	____	____	____	____
Acupuncture	____	____	____	____	____
Aroma therapy	____	____	____	____	____
Bach remedies	____	____	____	____	____
Bed rest	____	____	____	____	____
Biofeedback	____	____	____	____	____
Chelation therapy	____	____	____	____	____
Chiropractic	____	____	____	____	____
Exercise	____	____	____	____	____
Homeopathy	____	____	____	____	____
Hydrotherapy	____	____	____	____	____
Hypnosis	____	____	____	____	____
Live cell therapy	____	____	____	____	____
Massage	____	____	____	____	____
Meditation	____	____	____	____	____
TENS	____	____	____	____	____
Visualization/imagery	____	____	____	____	____
Other: _____	____	____	____	____	____

Have you found any treatments or therapies particularly helpful? How? _____

_____

_____

_____

Have you found any treatments or therapies particularly harmful? How? _____

_____

_____

_____

Are there any treatments you would like to see added to this questionnaire? _____

_____

_____

_____

What would you prefer to name, or rename, this illness? _____

_____

Bibliography

GENERAL

Book of the Body: The Way Things Work. New York: Simon & Shuster, 1979.

Berne, Katrina H. Running on Empty: Chronic Fatigue Immune Dysfunction Syndrome (CFIDS). Alameda, Calif.: Hunter House, 1992.

Feiden, Karyn. Hope and Help for Chronic Fatigue Syndrome. New York: Simon & Schuster, 1990.

Hawk, Philip B, Oser, Bernard, and Summerson, William. Practical Physiological Chemistry. New York: McGraw-Hill, 1947.

Hyde, Byron M, ed. The Clinical and Scientific Basis of ME/CFS. Ottawa, Ontario: Nightingale Research Foundation, 1992.

Lehninger, Albert L. Biochemistry. New York: Worth Publishers, 1975.

Treatments

Balch, James F, and Balch, Phyllis A. Prescription for Nutritional Healing. Garden City Park, N.Y.: Avery Publishing Group, 1990.

Complete Drug Reference. New York: Consumer Reports Books, 1994.

The Doctor's Book of Home Remedies. Emmaus, Pa.: Rodale Press, 1990.

Kastner, Mark. Alternative Healing. La Mesa, Calif.: Halcyon Publishing, 1993.

Nurse's Handbook of Drug Therapy. Springhouse, Pa.: Springhouse Corporation, 1993.

Stanway, Andrew. Alternative Medicine: A Guide to Natural Therapies. London: Bloomsbury Books, 1979.

Winter, Ruth. A Consumer's Dictionary of Medicines: Prescription, Over-the-Counter and Herbal. New York: Crown Trade, 1993.

CHAPTER 1: THE MANY FACES OF CFIDS

Ali, Majid. The Canary and Chronic Fatigue. Denville, N.J.: Life Span Press, 1994.

Anderson, Dean. Recovery From CFIDS. CFIDS Chronicle, Winter 1996, pp 27-29.

Johnson, Hillary. Journey Into Fear: The Growing Nightmare of Epstein-Barr Virus. Rolling Stone, July 30 and August 13, 1987.

Johnson, Hillary. Osler's Web: Inside the Labyrinth of the Chronic Fatigue Syndrome Epidemic. New York: Crown Publishers, 1996.

Kenney, Kim. Treating CFIDS: Still More Art Than Science. CFIDS Chronicle, Winter 1994, pp 22-28.

Mangano, Joe. Could CFIDS Be a Radiation-Related Disorder? CFIDS Chronicle, Winter 1994, pp 36-38.

Rogers, Sherri. Tired or Toxic? Syracuse, N.Y.: Prestige Publishers, 1990.

Suhadolnick, Robert J, Peterson, Daniel L, et al. Biochemical Evidence for a Novel Low Molecular Weight 2-5A-Dependent RNase L in Chronic Fatigue Syndrome. Journal of Interferon and Cytokine Research 17(7):377-385, 1997.

CHAPTER 3: SPECIFIC SYMPTOMS AND TREATMENT TIPS

Airola, Paavo. Hypoglycemia: A Better Approach. Phoenix, Ariz.: Health Plus Publishers, 1977.

Balch, James F, and Balch, Phyllis A. Prescription for Nutritional Healing. Garden City Park, N.Y.: Avery Publishing Group, 1990.

Baranowski, Zane. Colloidal Silver: The Natural Antibiotic Alternative. New York: Healing Wisdom Publications, 1995.

Bell, David. The Disease of a Thousand Names. Lyndonville, N.Y.: Pollard Publications, 1991.

Bell, David. The Doctor's Guide to Chronic Fatigue Syndrome. New York: Addison-Wesley Publishing Co., 1994.

Benson, Herbert. The Relaxation Response. New York: Avon Books, 1976.

Blau, Sheldon Paul, and Schultz, Dodi. Lupus: The Body Against Itself. New York: Doubleday and Company, 1977.

Bloom, Floyd E, Lazerson, Arlyne, and Hofstader, Laura. Brain, Mind and Behavior. New York: W.H. Freeman and Co., 1985.

Bou-Holaigah, Issam, Rowe, Peter C, Kan, Jean, and Calkins, Hugh. The Relationship Between Neurally Mediated Hypotension and the Chronic Fatigue Syndrome. Journal of the American Medical Association 274(12):961-967, 1995.

Browning, David J. Eye Problems and CFIDS. CFIDS Chronicle, 1988 Compendium, pp 17-19.

Buchwald, Dedra. Comparison of Patients With Chronic Fatigue Syndrome, Fibromyalgia, and Multiple Chemical Sensitivities. Archives in Internal Medicine 154(18):2049-2053, 1994.

Carpman, Vicki. CFIDS Treatment: The Cheney Clinic's Strategic Approach. CFIDS Chronicle, Spring 1995, pp 38-45.

Chalker, Rebecca, and Whitmore, Kristene. Overcoming Bladder Disorders. New York: Harper & Row, 1990.

Chalmers, Andrew, Littlejohn, Geoffrey Owen, Salit, Irving E, and Wolfe, Frederick, eds. Fibromyalgia, Chronic Fatigue Syndrome, and Repetitive Strain Injury: Current Concepts in Diagnosis, Management, Disability, and Health Economics. Binghamton, N.Y.: Haworth Medical Press, 1995.

Cheney, Paul. Proposed Pathophysiologic Mechanism of CFIDS. CFIDS Chronicle, Spring 1994, pp 1-2.

Cheney, Paul. Midwest CFIDS Conference. CFIDS Chronicle, Summer 1996, pp 63-65.

Chester, Alexander. Chronic Fatigue of Nasal Origin: Possible Confusion With Chronic Fatigue Syndrome. In Hyde, Byron M, ed. The Clinical and Scientific Basis of ME/CFS. Ottawa, Ontario: Nightingale Research Foundation. 1992.

Courmel, Katie. A Companion Volume to Dr. Jay A. Goldstein's Betrayal by the Brain. Binghamton, N.Y.: Haworth Medical Press, 1996.

Crook, William. Chronic Fatigue Syndrome and the Yeast Connection. Jackson, Tenn.: Professional Books, 1992.

Cunha, Burke. Crimson Crescents: A Diagnostic Marker for CFS? CFIDS Chronicle, Summer 1993, p 47.

Demitrack, Mark A, Dale, Janet K, Straus, Stephen E, Laue, Louisa, Listwak, Sam J, Dreusi, Markus JP, Chrousos, George P, and Gold, Philip W. Evidence for Impaired Activation of the Hypothalamic-Pituitary-Adrenal Axis in Patients With Chronic Fatigue Syndrome. Journal of Clinical Endocrinology and Metabolism 73:1224-1234, 1991.

The Doctor's Book of Home Remedies. Emmaus, Pa.: Rodale Press, 1990.

Duchene, Lucy. CFS: Influence of Histamine, Hormones and Electrolytes. CFIDS Chronicle, Summer 1993, pp 31-35.

Fan, Thim Peng, and Blanton, Margaret Ellen. Clinical Features and Diagnosis of Fibromyalgia. Journal of Musculoskeletal Medicine April:24-42, 1992.

Fisher, Gregg Charles. Chronic Fatigue Syndrome: A Victim's Guide to Understanding, Treating, and Coping With This Debilitating Illness. New York: Warner Books, 1989.

Flechas, Jorge. Yeast and the CFIDS Patient. CFIDS Chronicle, Summer/Fall 1989, pp 40-42.

Gillespie, Larrian. You Don't Have to Live With Cystitis. New York: Avon Books, 1986.

Goldstein, Jay A. Dysfunctional Neuroimmune Network. CFIDS Chronicle, Fall 1991, pp 19-24.

Goldstein, Jay A. The Diagnosis of Chronic Fatigue Syndrome as a Limbic Encephalopathy. CFIDS Chronicle, Fall 1992, pp 20-34.

Goldstein, Jay A. Physician's Forum. CFIDS Chronicle, Fall 1993.

Goldstein, Jay A. Could Your Doctor Be Wrong? New York: Pharos Books, 1991.

Goldstein, Jay A. Betrayal by the Brain. Binghamton, N.Y.: Haworth Medical Press, 1996.

Guillory, Gerard. IBS: A Doctor's Plan for Chronic Digestive Troubles. Washington, D.C.: Hartley and Marks, 1991.

Hyde, Byron M, ed. The Clinical and Scientific Basis of ME/CFS. Ottawa, Ontario: Nightingale Research Foundation, 1992.

Hyde, Byron M, and Jain, Anil. Cardiac and Cardiovascular Aspects of ME/CFS, A Review. In Hyde, Byron M, ed. The Clinical and Scientific Basis of ME/CFS. Ottawa, Ontario: Nightingale Research Foundation, 1992.

Hyde, Byron M, and Jain, Anil. Clinical Observations of Central Nervous System Dysfunction in Post-Infectious, Acute Onset ME/CFS. In Hyde, Byron M, ed. The Clinical and Scientific Basis of ME/CFS. Ottawa, Ontario: Nightingale Research Foundation, 1992.

Israel, Leon. Premenstrual Tension. Journal of the American Medical Association 110:1721, 1938.

Ivker, Robert S. Sinus Survival: The Holistic Medical Treatment for Allergies, Asthma, Bronchitis, Colds, and Sinusitis. New York: Putnam Publishing Group, 1995.

Jacobsen, Soren, Danneskiold-Samsoe, Bente, and Lund, Birger, eds. Musculoskeletal Pain, Myofascial Pain Syndrome, and the Fibromyalgia Syndrome: Proceedings from the Second World Congress on Myofascial Pain and Fibromyalgia. Binghamton, N.Y.: Haworth Medical Press, 1993.

Janowitz, Henry D. Your Gut Feelings. New York: Oxford University Press, 1987.

Jessop, Carol. Moderated Questions and Answers. CFIDS Chronicle, Spring 1991, p 80.

Jovanovic, Lois, and Subak-Sharpe, Genell J. Hormones: The Woman's Answerbook. New York: Atheneum, 1987.

Krohn, Jacqueline. The Whole Way to Allergy Relief and Prevention: A Doctor's Complete Guide to Treatment and Self-Care. Washington, D.C.: Hartley and Marks, 1991.

Kuratsune, Hirohiko, and Plioplys, Audrius. Muscle and Mitochondia Studies CFIDS Chronicle, Winter 1995, pp 66.

Lauersen, Niels, and Stukane, Eileen. PMS and You: What It Is, How to Recognize It, and How to Overcome It. New York: Simon & Shuster, 1983.

LeRoy, Jim, Haney Davis, Trina, and Jason, Leonard A. Treatment Efficacy: A Survey of 305 MCS Patients. CFIDS Chronicle, Winter 1996, pp 52-53.

Lieberman, Allan. The Role of Rubella Virus in the Chronic Fatigue Syndrome. Clinical Ecology VII(3):51-54, 1990.

Loblay, Robert H, and Swain, Anne R. The Role of Food Intolerance In Chronic Fatigue Syndrome. In Hyde, Byron M, ed. The Clinical and Scientific Basis of ME/CFS. Ottawa, Ontario: Nightingale Research Foundation, 1992.

McCoy, James. Immunomodulatory Properties of DHEA as a Potential Treatment for CFIDS. CFIDS Chronicle, Fall 1993, pp 21-23.

Moldofsky, Harvey. Sleep, Neuroimmune and Neuroendocrine Functions in Fibromyalgia and Chronic Fatigue Syndrome. Advances in Neuroimmunology 5:39-56, 1995.

Nelson, Philip K. Fingerprint "Loss"—Is It a Sign of CFIDS? CFIDS Chronicle, Fall 1994, pp 49-50.

Norris, Ronald, with Sullivan, Colleen. PMS/Premenstrual Syndrome. New York: Rawson Associates, 1983.

Ornstein, Robert, and Thompson, Richard F. The Amazing Brain. Boston: Houghton Mifflin Co., 1984.

Orr, William C, Altshuler, Kenneth Z, and Stahl, Monte L. Managing Sleep Complaints. Chicago: Year Book Medical Publishers, 1982.

Patarca, Roberto, Klimas, Nancy, Garcia, Maria, et al. Dysregulated Expression of Soluble Immune Mediator Receptors in a Subset of Patients With Chronic Fatigue Syndrome. Journal of Chronic Fatigue Syndrome 1(1):81-96, 1995.

Pellegrino, Mark J. The Fibromyalgia Survivor. Columbus, Ohio: Anadem Publishing, 1995.

Pisetsky, David S. The Duke University Medical Center Book of Arthritis. New York: Fawcett Columbine, 1991.

Poland, Russell. Research Conference. CFIDS Chronicle, Summer 1993, pp 56, 62.

Randolph, Theron. Human Ecology and Susceptibility to the Chemical Environment. Springfield, Ill.: Charles C Thomas, 1962.

Rapoport, Alan, and Sheftell, Fred. Headache Relief. New York: Simon & Shuster, 1990.

Restak, Richard. The Brain. New York: Bantam, 1984.

Restak, Richard. The Receptors. New York: Bantam, 1994.

Restak, Richard. Brainscapes. New York: Hyperion, 1995.

Rosenbaum, Michael, and Susser, Murray. Solving the Puzzle of Chronic Fatigue Syndrome. Tacoma, Wash.: Life Sciences Press, 1992.

Rous, Stephen. The Prostate Book: Sound Advice on Symptoms and Treatment. New York: W.W. Norton & Co., 1988.

Rowe, Peter C, Bou-Holaigah, Issam, Kan, Jean S, and Calkins, Hugh. Is Neurally Mediated Hypotension an Unrecognized Cause of Chronic Fatigue? Lancet 345:623-624, 1995.

Russell, I Jon. Fibrositis/Fibromyalgia Syndrome. In Hyde, Byron M, ed. The Clinical and Scientific Basis of ME/CFS. Ottawa, Ontario: Nightingale Research Foundation, 1992.

Sheppard, Leslie, and Hawkridge, Audry. Tinnitus: Learning to Live With It. Bath, England: Ashgrove Press, 1989.

Starlanyl, Devin, and Copeland, Mary Ellen. Fibromyalgia and Chronic Myofascial Pain Syndrome. Oakland, Calif.: New Harbinger Publications, 1996.

Stern, Kathy. Oral Health Symptoms of Chronic Fatigue Syndrome. CFIDS Chronicle, Fall 1994, pp 42-43.

Sulman, Felix G. Short- and Long-Term Changes in Climate. Boca Raton, Fla.: CRC Press, 1982.

Thompson, W Grant. Gut Reactions: Understanding the Symptoms of the Digestive Tract. New York: Plenum Press, 1989.

Thomsen, Thomas. Shingles. New York: Cross River Press, 1990.

Whitaker, Samuel. Research Conference. CFIDS Chronicle, Summer 1993, pp 56, 62.

Wood, Lawrence. Your Thyroid: A Home Reference. Boston: Houghton Mifflin Co., 1982.

Wood, Lawrence C, Cooper, David S, and Ridgway, E Chester. Your Thyroid: A Home Reference. New York: Ballantine Books, 1982.

Wurtman, Judith J. The Serotonin Solution. New York: Fawcett Columbine, 1996.

Wyckoff, Betsy. Overcoming Migraine. Barrytown, N.Y.: Station Hill Press, 1991.

CHAPTER 4: PHARMACEUTICALS AND PRESCRIPTION DRUGS

Ablashi, DV, Bernman ZN, Lawyer C, Kramorsky B, Ferguson DM, Komaroff AL. Antiviral Activity In Vitro of Kutapressin Against Human Herpesvirus 6. In Vivo 8(4):581-586, 1994.

Ablashi, DV, Bernman, Z, et al. Kutapressin Inhibits In Vitro Infection of Human Herpesvirus Type 6. Clinical Infectious Diseases 18(Suppl 1):S113, 1994.

Ablashi, DV, Bernman, Z, et al. Poly(I)-Poly(C12U) Inhibits In Vitro Replication of Human Herpesvirus 6. Clinical Infectious Diseases 18(Suppl 1):S113, 1994.

Bell, David. The Doctor's Guide to Chronic Fatigue Syndrome. New York: Addison-Wesley Publishing Co., 1994.

Bou-Holaigah, Issam, Rowe, Peter C, Kan, Jean, and Calkins, Hugh. The Relationship Between Neurally Mediated Hypotension and the Chronic Fatigue Syndrome. Journal of the American Medical Association 274(12):961-967, 1995.

Brooks, Barbara, and Smith, Nancy. CFIDS, An Owner's Manual. Silver Spring, Md.: BBNS Publishers, 1990.

Carpman, Vicki. CFIDS Treatment: The Cheney Clinic's Strategic Approach. CFIDS Chronicle, Spring 1995, pp 38-45.

Carpman, Vicki. Cough Syrup for Pain? CFIDS Chronicle, Fall 1996, pp 46-47.

Cheney, Paul. Physician's Forum. CFIDS Chronicle, 1991, pp 2-6.

Conley, Edward J. Treatment of HHV-6 Reactivation in CFIDS. CFIDS Chronicle, Fall 1993, pp 15-17.

Crook, William G. Chronic Fatigue Syndrome and the Yeast Connection. Jackson, Tenn.: Professional Books, 1992.

Crook, William G. The Yeast Connection: A Medical Breakthrough. Jackson, Tenn.: Professional Books, 1986.

Demitrack, Mark A, Dale, Janet K, Straus, Stephen E, Laue, Louisa, Listwak, Sam J, Dreusi, Markus JP, Chrousos, George P, and Gold, Philip W. Evidence for Impaired Activation of the Hypothalamic-Pituitary-Adrenal Axis in Patients With Chronic Fatigue Syndrome. Journal of Clinical Endocrinology and Metabolism 73:1224-1234, 1991.

DeVinci, C, Levine, PH, Pizza, G, et al. Lessons From a Pilot Study of Transfer Factor in Chronic Fatigue Syndrome. Biotherapy 9:87-90, 1996.

Filsinger, Joan D. Coughing up CFIDS; A Patient's Experience With Guaifenesin. The Mass CFIDS Update, Summer 1996, p 10.

Fisher, Gregg. Chronic Fatigue Syndrome; A Comprehensive Guide to Symptoms, Treatments, and Solving the Practical Problems of CFS. New York: Warner Books, 1997.

Flechas, Jorge. A Theoretical Paper on CFS and Oxytocin. CFIDS Chronicle, Spring 1995, pp 49-52.

Friedberg, Fred. Coping With Chronic Fatigue Syndrome: Nine Things You Can Do. Oakland, Calif.: New Harbinger Publications, 1990.

Goldstein, Jay A. Betrayal by the Brain. Binghamton, N.Y.: Haworth Medical Press, 1996.

Goldstein, Jay A. Chronic Fatigue Syndrome: The Limbic Hypothesis. Binghamton, N.Y.: Haworth Medical Press, 1993.

Goldstein, Jay A. The Evolving Hypothesis: The Role of the Suppressor T Cell in CFIDS. CFIDS Chronicle, 1988 Compendium, pp 7-10.

Goldstein, Jay A. The Evolving Hypothesis IX: Toward a New Decade. CFIDS Chronicle, Spring/Summer 1990, pp 48-53.

Goldstein, Jay A. The Neuropharmacology of Chronic Fatigue Syndrome. CFIDS Chronicle, Fall 1993, pp 24-27.

Goldstein, Jay A. New Treatments for CFS. CFIDS Chronicle, Summer 1994, pp 2-6.

Goldstein, Jay A. Nitroglycerin: A Potential Mediator for Hypoperfusion in CFS. CFIDS Chronicle, Summer 1993, pp 36-39.

Goldstein Jay A. Physician's Forum. CFIDS Chronicle, Spring 1991, p 10.

Jackson, Dennis. Gamma Globulin—Therapy for CFIDS? CFIDS Chronicle, Summer/Fall 1989, pp 51-53.

Jessop, Carol. Moderated Questions and Answers. CFIDS Chronicle, Spring 1991, p 80.

Keim, Katherine. Improve Your Sleep; Feel Better. CFIDS Chronicle, Winter 1994, pp 20-21.

Keller, Robert. Immune Dysfunction in CFIDS: Why You Feel the Way You Do. CFIDS Chronicle, Fall 1994, pp 34-42.

Kenney, Kim. Ampligen: Past, Present and Future. CFIDS Chronicle, March 1991, pp 18-20.

Kenney, Kim. Treating CFIDS: Still More Art Than Science. CFIDS Chronicle, Winter 1994, pp 22-28.

Klimas, Nancy. Research Conference. CFIDS Chronicle, Spring 1991, p 50.

Kramer, Peter D. Listening to Prozac. New York: Penguin Group, 1993.

Lapp, Charles. The Practical Treatment of CFIDS: One Doctor's Approach. CFIDS Chronicle, Summer/Fall 1989, pp 16-21.

Lapp, Charles. Physician's Forum. CFIDS Chronicle, Spring 1991, p 15.

Levin, Alan S, and Zellerbach, Merla. The Type 1/Type 2 Allergy Relief Program. Los Angeles, Calif.: Jeremy P. Tarcher, 1983.

Levine, Susan. Allergy, Immune Fuction and Endocrinological Disorders in CFIDS. CFIDS Chronicle, January/February 1989, p 32.

Lloyd, Andrew, Hickie, Ian, Wakefield, Denis, Boughton, Clem, and Dwyer, John. Intravenous Immunoglobulin Therapy in Patients With Chronic Fatigue Syndrome. In Hyde, Byron M, ed. The Clinical and Scientific Basis of ME/CFS. Ottawa, Ontario: Nightingale Research Foundation, 1992.

Lloyd, Andrew, Hickie, Ian, et al. Immunological Therapy With Transfer Factor in Patients With Chronic Fatigue Syndrome—A Double-Blind, Placebo-Controlled Trial. American Journal of Medicine 89:561-568, 1990.

Low, P, Gilden, J, Frieman, R, et al. Efficacy of Midodrine vs. Placebo in Neurogenic Orthostatic Hypotension: A Randomized Double-Blind Multicenter Study. Journal of the American Medical Association 277:1046-1051, 1977.

McCoy, James L. Immunomodulatory Properties of DHEA as a Potential Treatment for CFIDS. CFIDS Chronicle, Fall 1993, pp 21-23.

Mena, Ismael. Research Conference. CFIDS Chronicle, Spring/Summer 1990, pp 7-8.

Orens, Perry A. U.S. Scientists Study Transfer Factor. CFIDS Chronicle, Fall 1993, p 14.

Peterson, Daniel L, Strayer, David R, et al. Clinical Improvements Obtained With Ampligen in Patients With Severe Chronic Fatigue Syndrome and Associated Encephalopathy. In Hyde, Byron M, ed. The Clinical and Scientific Basis of ME/CFS. Ottawa, Ontario: Nightingale Research Foundation, Ottawa, 1992.

Peterson, Phillip. Research Conference. CFIDS Chronicle, Spring/Summer 1990, p 12.

Peterson, Phillip, Shepard J, et al. A Controlled Trial of Intravenous Immunoglobulin G in Chronic Fatigue Syndrome. American Journal of Medicine 89:554-560, 1990.

Rosenbaum, Michael, and Susser, Murray. Solving the Puzzle of Chronic Fatigue Syndrome. Tacoma, Wash.: Life Sciences Press, 1992.

Rosenfeld, E, Salimi, B, O'Gorman, MR, Lawyer, C, Katz, BZ. Potential In Vitro Activity of Kutapressin Against Epstein-Barr Virus. In Vivo 10(3):313-318, 1996.

Rowe, Katherine. Double-Blind Randomized Controlled Trial to Assess the Efficacy of Intravenous Gamma Globulin for the Management of Chronic Fatigue Syndrome in Adolescents. Journal of Psychiatric Research 31:133-147, 1997.

Simpson, OL. Nondiscocyte Erythrocytes in Myalgic Encephalomyelitis. New Zealand Medical Journal 2(864):126-127, 1989.

Snorrason, Ernir, Geirsson, Arni, and Stefansson, Kari. Trial of a Selective Acetylcholinesterase Inhibitor, Galanthamine Hydrobromide, in the Treatment of Chronic Fatigue Syndrome. Journal of Chronic Fatigue Syndrome 2:2-3, 1996.

St. Armand, R Paul. One Disease—Two Names. CFIDS/FM Health Resource, Fall 1996, pp 4-5.

Steinbach, Thomas, and Hermann, William. The Treatment of CFIDS With Kutapressin. CFIDS Chronicle, Spring/Summer 1990, pp 25-30.

Steinbach, Thomas, and Hermann, William. The Use of Kutapressin in CFIDS. CFIDS Chronicle, Spring 1991, pp 50-54.

Straus, Steven, Dale, JK, Tobi, M, et al. Acyclovir Treatment of the Chronic Fatigue Syndrome. New England Journal of Medicine 26:1692-1698, 1988.

Strayer, David R, Carter, William A, et al. A Controlled Clinical Trial With a Specifically Configured RNA Drug, Poly(I)-Poly(C12U), in Chronic Fatigue Syndrome. Clinical Infectious Diseases 18(Suppl 1):S88-S95, 1994.

Suhadolnick, Robert J, Peterson Daniel L, et al. Biochemical Evidence for a Novel Low Molecular Weight 2-5A-Dependent RNase L in Chronic Fatigue Syndrome. Journal of Interferon and Cytokine Research 17(7):377-385, 1997.

Theoharides, Theoharis C, and Sant, Grannum R. Bladder Mast Cell Activation in Interstitial Cystitis. Seminars in Urology IX(2):74-87, 1991.

Vercoulen, JH, Swanink, CM, Zitman FG, et al. Randomized Double-Blind, Placebo-Controlled Study of Fluoxetine in Chronic Fatigue Syndrome. Lancet 347:858-861, 1996.

Viza, Dimitri, and Pizza, Giancarlo. Can Specific Transfer Factor Be an Effective Treatment for CFS? CFIDS Chronicle, Fall 1993, pp 11-13.

Wakefield, Denis. The Use of Gamma Globulin in CFS. CFIDS Chronicle, Spring 1991, pp 41-50.

Wein, Alan, and Hanno, Phillip. American Urological Association Update Series, Lesson 10. Volume VI, 1985, p 5.

CHAPTER 5: NUTRITIONAL SUPPLEMENTS AND BOTANICALS

Ali, Majid. The Canary and Chronic Fatigue. Denville, N.J.: Life Span Press, 1994.

Balch, James F, and Balch, Phyllis A. Prescription for Nutritional Healing. Garden City Park, N.Y.: Avery Publishing Group, 1990.

Baschetti, Riccardo. Letter. New Zealand Journal of Medicine 108:156:157, 1995.

Behan, Peter O, Behan, WMH, and Horrobi, D. Effect of High Doses of Essential Fatty Acids on the Post Viral Fatigue Syndrome. Acta Neurologica Scandinavica 82:209-216, 1990.

Bock, Steven, and Boyette, Michael. Stay Young the Melatonin Way. New York: Dutton Press, 1995.

Bralley, J Alexander, and Lord, Richard S. Treatment of Chronic Fatigue Syndrome with Specific Amino Acid Supplementation. Journal of Applied Nutrition 46(3):74-78, 1994.

Carpman, Vicki. CFIDS Treatment: The Cheney Clinic's Strategic Approach. CFIDS Chronicle, Spring 1995, pp 38-45.

Casson, Peter, Andersen, Richard, Herrod, Henry, Stentz, Frankie, Straughn, Arthur, Abraham, Guy, and Buster, John. Oral Dehydroepiandrosterone in Physiologic Doses Modulates Immune Function in Postmenopausal Women. St. Louis: Mosby–Year Book, 1993.

Castleman, Michael. The Healing Herbs. Emmaus, Pa.: Rodale Press, 1991.

Cheney, Paul. Ask the Doctor. CFIDS Chronicle, Spring 1995, p 53.

Cheney, Paul R, and Lapp, Charles W. Entero-Hepatic Resuscitation in Patients With Chronic Fatigue Syndrome: A Pyramid of Nutritional Therapy. CFIDS Chronicle, Fall 1993, pp 1-3.

Cox, IM, Campbell, MJ, and Dowson, D. Red Blood Cell Magnesium and Chronic Fatigue Syndrome. Lancet 337:757, 1991.

Cunha, Burke A. Beta-Carotene Stimulation of Natural Killer Cell Activity in Adult Patients With Chronic Fatigue Syndrome. CFIDS Chronicle, Fall 1993, p 18.

Farber, Paul. The Silver Micro Bullet. Houston, Tex.: Professional Physicians Publishing and Health Services, 1977.

Friedberg, Fred. Coping With Chronic Fatigue Syndrome: Nine Things You Can Do. Oakland, Calif.: New Harbinger Publications, 1995.

Graham, Judy. Evening Primrose Oil. Rochester, Vt.: Healing Arts Press, 1989.

Housecalls. Health, September 1997, p 144.

Kuratsune, Hiroko, Yamaguti, Kouzi, et al. Acylcarnitine Deficiency in Chronic Fatigue Syndrome. Clinical Infectious Diseases 18(Suppl 1):S562-567, 1994.

Lapp, Charles. Physician's Forum. CFIDS Chronicle, March 1991, pp 13-16.

Lapp, Charles W, and Cheney, Paul R. The Rationale for Using High-Dose Cobalamin (Vitamin B_{12}). CFIDS Chronicle, Fall 1993, pp 19-20.

Letter to the Editor. CFIDS Chronicle, Summer 1996, p 4.

Leung, Albert Y. Chinese Herbal Remedies. New York: Universe Books, 1984.

Mass CFIDS Update, Fall 1995.

McCoy, James L. Immunomodulatory Properties of DHEA as a Potential Treatment for CFIDS. CFIDS Chronicle, Fall 1993, pp 21-23.

Melatonin Still Unproven as Sleep Aid. The MEssenger, May 1997, p 5.

Moore, Michael. Medicinal Plants of the Mountain West. Santa Fe, N.M.: Museum of New Mexico Press, 1979.

Plioplys, Audrius V, Plioplys, Sigita. Amantadine and L-Carnitine Treatment of Chronic Fatigue Syndrome. Neuropsychobiology 35(1):16-23, 1997.

Rigden, Scott. Entero-Hepatic Resuscitation Program. CFIDS Chronicle, Spring 1995, pp 46-48.

Rudin, Donald O, and Felix, Clara, with Schrader, Constance. The Omega-3 Phenomenon. New York: Avon Books, 1987.

Russell, IJ, Michalek, JE, Flechas, JD, Abraham, GE. Treatment of Fibromyalgia Syndrome With Super Malic: A Randomized, Double-Blind, Placebo-Controlled, Crossover Pilot Study. Journal of Rheumatology 22:953-958, 1995.

Schmidt, Patti. Dr. Paul Cheney Discusses Nutritional Supplements. CFIDS Chronicle, Fall 1994, p 31.

Spurgin, Maryann. The Role of Red Blood Cell Morphology in the Pathogenesis of ME/CFIDS. CFIDS Chronicle, Summer 1995, pp 55-58.

Theodasakis, Jason, Adderly, Brenda, and Fox, Barry. The Arthritis Cure. New York: St. Martin's Press, 1997.

Wilkinson, Steve. Chronic Fatigue Syndrome: A Natural Healing Guide. New York: Sterling Publishing Co., 1990.

Winther, Michael. Essential Fatty Acid Therapy for Myalgic Encephalomyelitis. In Hyde, Byron M, ed. The Clinical and Scientific Basis of ME/CFS. Ottawa, Ontario: Nightingale Research Foundation, 1992.

CHAPTER 6: ALTERNATIVE AND COMPLEMENTARY MEDICAL AND SUPPORTIVE THERAPIES

Anderson, Dean. Recovery From CFIDS. CFIDS Chronicle, Winter 1996, pp 27-29.

Ashendorf, Douglas. The Ability of Low Level Laser Therapy (LLLT) to Mitigate Fibromyalgia Pain. CFIDS Chronicle, Fall 1993, pp 28-29.

Bailey, Covert. Smart Exercise. Boston: Houghton Mifflin Co., 1994.

Blate, Michael. The Natural Healer's Acupressure Handbook. Falkynor Books, 1983.

Borysenko, Joan. Minding the Body, Mending the Mind. New York: Addison-Wesley Publishing Co., 1987.

Carpman, Vicki L. Natelson's Niche. CFIDS Chronicle, Winter 1996, pp 42-44.

Collinge, William. Recovering From Chronic Fatigue Syndrome. New York: The Body Press/Perigee Books, 1993.

Garloch, Karen. Chronic Fatigue Syndrome Treatment Patented. CFIDS Chronicle, Spring 1994, p 7.

Lapp, Charles. Dublin Conference. CFIDS Chronicle, Summer 1994, p 35.

Preston, Myra. A New Test. CFIDS Chronicle, Winter 1996, pp 50-51.

Tansey, Michael A. EEG Neurofeedback and Chronic Fatigue Syndrome: New Findings With Respect to Diagnosis and Treatment. CFIDS Chronicle, Fall 1993, pp 30-32.

Walker, Morton. The Chelation Way: The Complete Book of Chelation Therapy. Garden City Park, N.Y.: Avery Publishing Group, 1990.

Weiner, Michael. The Complete Book of Homeopathy. Garden City Park, N.Y.: Avery Publishing Group, 1989.

Wilkinson, Steve. Chronic Fatigue Syndrome: A Natural Healing Guide. New York: Sterling Publishing Co., 1990.

Worwood, Valerie Ann. The Complete Book of Essential Oils and Aromatherapy. San Rafael, Calif.: New World Library, 1991.

CHAPTER 7: STRESS REDUCTION AND ELIMINATION

Anderson, Dean. Recovery From CFIDS. CFIDS Chronicle, Winter 1996, pp 27-29.

Cheney, Paul. Physician's Forum. CFIDS Chronicle, March 1991, p 3.

Chrousos, George P, and Gold, Philip W. The Concepts of Stress and Stress System Disorders. Journal of the American Medical Association 267:1244-1252, 1992.

Cousins, Norman. Anatomy of an Illness. New York: Bantam Books, 1981.

Demitrack, Mark A, Dale, Janet K, Straus, Stephen E, Laue, Louisa, Listwak, Sam J, Kreusi, Markus JP, Chrousos, George P, and Gold, Philip W. Evidence for Impaired Activation of the Hypothalamic-Pituitary-Adrenal Axis in Patients With Chronic Fatigue Syndrome. Journal of Clinical Endocrinology and Metabolism 73:1224-1234, 1991.

Friedberg, Fred. Coping With Chronic Fatigue Syndrome: Nine Things You Can Do. Oakland, Calif.: New Harbinger Publications, 1995.

Goliszek, Andrew G. Breaking the Stress Habit. Carolina Press, 1987.

Hyde, Byron M. The Clinical and Scientific Basis of ME/CFS. Ottawa, Ontario: Nightingale Research Foundation, 1992.

Kenny, Timothy. Living With Chronic Fatigue Syndrome: A Personal Story of the Struggle for Recovery. New York: Thunder's Mouth Press, 1994.

Sapolsky, Robert. Why Zebras Don't Get Ulcers: A Guide to Stress, Stress-Related Diseases, and Coping. New York: W.H. Freeman and Co., 1994.

CHAPTER 8: CLEANING UP: ELIMINATING TOXINS IN THE HOME

Bruning, Nancy. Breast Implants: Everything You Need to Know. Alameda, Calif.: Hunter House, 1992.

Carpman, Vicki. Chemical Warfare: CFIDS, Multiple Chemical Sensitivity and Silicone Implant Disorder. CFIDS Chronicle, Fall 1993, pp 33-41.

Dadd, Debra Lynn. Nontoxic and Natural. Los Angeles: Jeremy P. Tarcher, 1984.

Dadd, Debra Lynn. The Nontoxic Home. Los Angeles: Jeremy P. Tarcher, 1986.

Elkington, John, Hailes, Julia, and Makower, Joel. The Green Consumer. New York: Penguin Books, 1990.

Hunter, Linda Mason. The Healthy Home: An Attic to Basement Guide to Toxin-Free Living. Emmaus, Pa.: Rodale Press, 1989.

LeRoy, Jim, Haney Davis, Trina, and Jason, Leonard A. Treatment Efficacy: A Survey of 305 MCS Patients. CFIDS Chronicle, Winter 1996, pp 52-53.

Mangano, Joseph. Could CFIDS Be a Radiation-Related Disorder? CFIDS Chronicle, Winter 1994, pp 36-38.

Millar, Myrna, and Millar, Heather. The Toxic Labyrinth. Vancouver, B.C.: NICO Professional Services, 1995.

Ware, George W. The Pesticide Book. San Francisco: W.H. Freeman and Co., 1978.

Wittenburg, Janice Strubbe. The Rebellious Body: Reclaim Your Life From Environmental Illness or Chronic Fatigue Syndrome. New York: Insight Books, 1997.

CHAPTER 9: FOOD AND DIET

Brostoff, Jonathan, and Gamlin, Linda. The Complete Guide to Food Allergy and Intolerance. New York: Crown Publishers, 1989.

Dumke, Nicolette M. Allergy Cooking With Ease. Lancaster, Pa.: Starburst Publishers, 1992.

Hale, Mary, and Miller, Chris. The Chronic Fatigue Syndrome Cookbook. New York: Birch Lane Press, 1994.

Loblay, Robert H, and Swain, Anne R. The Role of Food Intolerance in Chronic Fatigue Syndrome. In Hyde, Byron M, ed. The Clinical and Scientific Basis of ME/CFS. Ottawa, Ontario: Nightingale Research Foundation, 1992.

Winter, Ruth. A Consumer's Dictionary of Food Additives. New York: Crown Publishers, 1989.

CHAPTER 10: SPECIAL NEEDS OF CHILDREN WITH CFIDS

Bell, David. Chronic Fatigue Syndrome in Children. Journal of Chronic Fatigue Syndrome 1(1):9-33, 1995.

Bell, David. Special Bulletin. CFIDS Chronicle, November 1993.

Carpman, Vicki. Educating the Educators: The Special Needs of Children With CFIDS. CFIDS Chronicle, Spring 1995, pp 13-15.

Lang, Karen. Calen's Story: A Child's Journey Through CFIDS. CFIDS Chronicle, Winter 1994, pp 1-6.

ME and the Young Sufferer. The MEssenger, April 1995.

Thorson, Kristin, ed. Fibromyalgia Syndrome and Chronic Fatigue Syndrome in Young People: A Guide for Parents. Tucson, Ariz.: Health Network, 1994.

Vanderzalm, Lynn. Finding Strength in Weakness. Grand Rapids, Mich.: Zondervan, 1995.

Vanderzalm, Lynn. The Challenges of Parenting a Child With CFIDS. CFIDS Chronicle, Winter 1996, pp 15-16.

Index

A

Absence seizures, 115
Acceptance, role of, in recovery, 284
Acebutolol; *see* Sectral
Acetaminophen, 88, 94, 107, 193, 328; *see also* Tylenol
Acetaminophen poisoning, 206
Acetazolamide; *see* Diamox
Acetylcholine, 38, 61-62, 63, 96, 210, 241
  pesticides and, 304-305
  royal jelly and, 241
  sleep disorders and, 127, 129
Acetylsalicylic acid, 192
Acid foods, sensitivity to, 320
Acid-free C powder, 250
Acidophilus bacteria, 47, 48, 65, 119, 239-240
Acne, 123
Acne vulgaris, 186
Acquired immunodeficiency syndrome (AIDS)
  Ampligen and, 152
  Diflucan and, 163
ACTH; *see* Adrenocorticotropic hormone
Activated-carbon filter, 309
Activated charcoal, 65, 72
Acupressure, 65, 254-255
Acupuncture, 81, 90, 148, 254, 255-257
  for children with CFIDS, 328
  fibromyalgia and, 99
  joint problems and, 95
  pain relief and, 107
Acupuncture analgesia, 256
Acyclovir (Zovirax), 83, 122, 167-168
  chickenpox and, 113
  shingles and, 118
Acylcarnitine, 98, 204-205, 317
ADD; *see* Attention deficit disorder
Addison's disease, 76, 291, 292
Additives, food, 317-318

Adenosine triphosphate (ATP), 78, 79, 183, 237
  alpha ketoglutarate and, 202
  CoQ10 and, 213
  exercise and, 266, 268
  malic acid and, 230
Adrenal exhaustion, 141
Adrenal glands, 76-77, 290
Adrenal hormones, 91-92, 96, 141, 292
Adrenal stimulants, 77
Adrenaline, 49-50, 76, 155, 209, 290, 297
Adrenocorticotropic hormone (ACTH), 292
Advil (ibuprofen), 88, 94, 191, 192, 193, 220
Aerobic cell metabolism, 69, 98
Aerobic exercise, 266-268
Afrin, sinusitis and, 121
Aged cheese, sensitivity to, 319
Agitated exhaustion, 80-81
Agnosia, facial, 55
AIDS; *see* Acquired immunodeficiency syndrome
Air contaminants, chemical sensitivities and, 43
Air duct systems, mold and, 308
Air quality, household toxins and, 308-309
Air travel, sinusitis and, 121
Airborne allergens, 38-40
Air-conditioning systems, weather sensitivity and, 142
ALA; *see* Alpha-linoleic acid
Alcohol
  CFIDS diet and, 315-316
  echinacea and, 225
  hydrogen peroxide and, 90
  sinusitis and, 120
  wood, aspartame and, 316
Alcohol addiction, naltrexone and, 188
Alcohol intolerance, 315
Alcohol-based mouthwashes, 316
Algae, blue-green, 81, 210-211, 315

Outdoor chemical air contaminants, chemical
  sensitivities and, 43
Oxytocin, 96, 190-191

P

Pain, 106-108
  hearing problems and, 90
  joint, 93-95
  treatment tips for, 107-108
Pain relievers, 191-195
Pain threshold, 107
Pallor, skin problems and, 122
Palpitations, 49
Pamelor (nortriptyline), 157
Panic disorder
  benzodiazepines and, 170
  seizures and, 114
Pantothenic acid, 77, 241, 248
Paradoxical reactions, benzodiazepines and, 170
Parasympathetic nervous system, 61-62
Paresis, 100-101
Paresthesias, 124, 327
Parnate (tranylcypromine), 160
Paroxetine; *see* Paxil
Partial seizures, simple, 115
Passion flower, 129, 296
Patchouli essential oil, 142
Pau d'arco, 47
Paxil (paroxetine), 59, 159
Peeling skin, 122-123
Pemoline; *see* Cylert
Penicillin, 122, 225
Pen-Pal organizations, CFIDS, 345
Pentoxifylline (Trental), 56, 195
Pepper, black, sensitivity to, 319
Peppermint, 68, 120, 257, 258, 259
Peppers, sensitivity to, 319
Peptic ulcers, pentoxifylline and, 195
Periodicals about CFIDS, 337-338
Periodontitis, 103
Peripheral vision, loss of, 137
Permeable intestine, 66-67
Personal care products
  chemical sensitivities and, 44
  sensitivity to, 306-308
Pesticides, 42-43
  toxicity of, 304-306
PET; *see* Positron emission tomography
Petit mal seizures, 115
Petroleum derivatives, sensitivity to, 43, 299, 317
Petroleum distillates, in household cleaning
  products, 301
Pettigraine essential oil, 142

PGE_1; *see* Prostaglandin E_1
Pharmaceuticals and prescription drugs, 151-
  199
  acetaminophen, 193-194
  acyclovir, 167-168
  Amantadine, 169
  Ampligen, 152-154
  antidepressant drugs, 154-161
  antifungal agents, 161-164
  antihistamines, 164-167
  Antivert, 167
  antiviral agents, 167-169
  aspirin, 192-193
  Atarax, 166
  Benedryl, 165-166
  benzodiazepines, 169-172
  beta blockers, 172-173
  calcium channel blockers, 173-175
  central nervous system stimulants, 175-176
  chemical sensitivities and, 43-44
  Chlor-Trimeton, 166
  Claritin, 165
  Cylert, 175-176
  Cytotec, 176-177
  Desyrel, 160-161
  Dexedrine, 175-176
  Diamox, 177-178
  Diflucan, 163-164
  Effexor, 161
  Elavil, 157
  Famvir, 169
  Flexeril, 178-179
  Florinef, 179-180
  gamma globulin, 180-183
  guaifenesin, 183-185
  Hismanal, 165
  hydrocortisone, 185-186
  Ionamin, 175-176
  Klonopin, 170
  Kutapressin, 186-188
  monoamine oxidase inhibitors, 159-160
  naltrexone, 188-189
  narcotics, 194
  Nardil, 160
  nicardipene, 173-175
  nifedipine, 173-175
  nimodipine, 173-175
  nitroglycerin, 189-190
  Nizoral, 164
  Norpramin, 157
  NSAIDs, 193
  nystatin, 161-163
  oxytocin, 190-191

ORDERING INFORMATION

Additional copies of *Chronic Fatigue Syndrome: A Treatment Guide* or any of QMP's consumer health books listed below may be purchased from most booksellers, via e-mail, from our home page on the Internet at http://www.qmp.com, by fax, or by mailing the following order form. Substantial discounts on orders of 10 or more books are also available. For information, call QMP's Special Sales Division toll-free at 800-348-7808.

Book Title	Unit Price	# Copies	Total
Berger/Bostwick: *A Woman's Decision, 2/e* (ISBN 1-942219-04-X)	$18.50	_____	_____
Berger/Bostwick: *What Women Need To Know About Breast Self-Examination* (ISBN 1-942219-99-6)	$ 1.95	_____	_____
Berger/Bostwick: *What Women Want To Know About Breast Implants* (ISBN 1-942219-61-9)	$ 6.00	_____	_____
Jenks/Spiniello: *The Patient's Little Instruction Book* (ISBN 1-57626-022-4)	$10.00	_____	_____
Pokluda: *Understanding Managed Health Care* (ISBN 1-57626-021-6)	$ 6.50	_____	_____
Salowe: *Prostate Cancer* (ISBN 1-57626-023-2)	$15.00	_____	_____
Sarnoff/Swirsky: *Beauty and the Beam* (ISBN 1-57626-059-3)	$23.50	_____	_____
Verrillo/Gellman: *Chronic Fatigue Syndrome* (ISBN 1-57626-053-4)	$23.00	_____	_____
Wiseman: *Pediatric Home Companion* (ISBN 1-57626-036-4)	$15.00	_____	_____

POSTAGE & HANDLING:
Add $3.00 for first book;
$2.00 for each additional book

Postage & Handling _____

Amount Enclosed _____

METHOD OF PAYMENT: ❏ Check enclosed
Charge my credit card: ❏ MC ❏ VISA ❏ AMEX
#_____ Exp. date_____
Signature_____

SHIP ORDER TO:
Name _____
Address _____
City/State/Zip _____
Telephone _____
Fax _____ e-mail _____

Mail this form with payment to:

QUALITY MEDICAL PUBLISHING, INC.
11970 Borman Drive • Suite 222 • St. Louis, MO 63146

or   phone: 800-348-7808 • fax: 314-878-9937 • e-mail: qmp@qmp.com

VG0534